PERFORMATIVE PRAXIS

Jean Baxen

PERFORMATIVE PRAXIS

Teacher Identity and Teaching in the Context of HIV/AIDS

PETER LANG
Bern · Berlin · Bruxelles · Frankfurt am Main · New York · Oxford · Wien

Bibliographic information published by Die Deutsche Nationalbibliothek
Die Deutsche Nationalbibliothek lists this publication in the Deutsche Nationalbibliografie; detailed bibliographic data is available on the Internet at ‹http://dnb.d-nb.de›.

British Library Cataloguing-in-Publication Data:
A catalogue record for this book is available from *The British Library,* Great Britain

Library of Congress Cataloging-in-Publication Data

Baxen, Jean, 1957-
Performative praxis : teacher identity and teaching in the context of HIV/AIDS / Jean Baxen.
p. cm.
Includes bibliographical references and index.
ISBN 978-3-03911-612-6 (alk. paper)
1. HIV infections--Prevention--Study and teaching--South Africa--Western Cape.
2. HIV infections--Prevention--Study and teaching--South Africa--Mpumalanga.
3. AIDS (Disease)--Prevention--Study and teaching--South Africa--Western Cape.
4. AIDS (Disease)--Prevention--Study and teaching--South Africa--Mpumalanga.
5. Teachers--South Africa--Western Cape--Attitudes.
6. Teachers--South Africa--Mpumalanga--Attitudes. 7. Performative (Philosophy)
I. Title.
RA643.86.S62W473 2010
362.196'97920096827--dc22

2009048386

Cover illustration: from iStockphoto.com © Beau Meyer
Cover design: Thomas Jaberg, Peter Lang AG

ISBN 978-3-03911-612-6

Hochfeldstrasse 32, CH-3012 Bern, Switzerland
info@peterlang.com, www.peterlang.com, www.peterlang.net

Printed in Germany

To Dad: Strong and Phenomenal

Acknowledgements

Knowingly or not, any work of this magnitude that takes years to complete has many people working in the background to support and edge on the 'producer.' Many have contributed to make this work possible and help it come to fruition.

Two projects gave impetus to this work. First, special thanks go to DFID/British Council for initial financial support through a link established between the University of Cape Town and Sussex University, U.K. Second, this work contributed to and was part of the project "Schooling, Cultural Values and HIV/AIDS". The ground work and data collection process, therefore, was made possible through generous financial support and joint funding from the National Research Foundation and Norway Research Council.

Special thanks to the participants who unreservedly welcomed and allowed me into their lives. They trusted me with their deeply private worlds and generously shared their stories. May this work serve to enhance understandings of their lived realities and may we, together through this story, make the world a better place.

Appreciation goes to Professor Crain Soudien, Director in the School of Education at the University of Cape Town; my supervisor, mentor, and kind friend. Thank you for your generosity of spirit, your gentleness and for having the vision that sustained me when I did not believe I could complete this work.

Heartfelt thanks and gratitude goes to my family: You all know how special you are. Thanks for your support.

To my dear son, Aegean: you had to endure many days, weeks, and months without me. Thank you for your patience.

Professor Anders Breidlid from Oslo University College, Norway, co-principal investigator in the project, 'Schooling, Cultural Values and HIV/AIDS' provided support, read, and commented on a draft of this work, thank you.

Kent State University hosted and supported me in the early stages of this work. I am particularly grateful to Ken Cushner and members of College of Education at White Hall, especially those at the Centre for

International Studies. Linda Robertson was instrumental in making my stay very fruitful.

My gratitude goes to Faith McClure for editing and commenting on a draft of this work.

Thanks to Marilyn Smith, Dianne Steele, Nuroo Ismail and Seta Jackson from Knowledge Commons at the Chancellor Oppenheimer Library, University of Cape Town for technical support.

It would be dangerous to begin naming the many dear friends who contributed indirectly to the completion of this work. You know who you are. Thank you for the many hours of laughter and joy.

Contents

Introduction 13

Part I
Context and contours of the research

Introduction 27

1 The study 29

Part II
A theoretical framework for understanding teachers and their work: towards a 'performative' subject

Introduction 47

2 Dominant sociological debates in understanding social action . . 51

3 Subject formation and Bourdieu's theory of practice 55

4 Subjectivity and Giddens's theory of structuration 69

5 Subject positioning and Butler's theory of performativity 79

Part III
Limitations in dominant epistemological orientations and research on teachers, teaching and HIV/AIDS

Introduction 91

6 The limitations of dominant epistemological orientations and interpretations of teachers and teachers' work 93

7 The limitations of dominant epistemological orientations and discourses in influencing the understandings of, responses to, and interpretations of HIV/AIDS 117

8 Limitations of dominant discourses and epistemological and methodological orientations in researching HIV/AIDS ... 131

Part IV
Dominant factors shaping teachers' lives

Introduction 149

9 Social and material conditions shaping teachers' lives 153

10 Dominant factors shaping teachers' subjective experiences .. 191

11 Subject positioning and teaching: understanding the performative teacher 269

Part V
Unintended consequences of 'performing' teaching

Introduction 301

12 Teacher performativity and classroom discourse 303

Appendices 313

List of References 321

Index 331

List of Tables

Table 1: Western Cape: Teacher and School Profile 34

Table 2: Mpumalanga: Teacher and School Profile 34

Table 3: Community, Region, Economic and Social Cluster and Selected Number of Schools 162

Table 4: Geographic Population Groups: Western Cape 167

Table 5: Geographic Population Groups: Mpumalanga 168

Table 6: Language Profile of Communities in the Western Cape 169

Table 7: Western Cape: Teachers' Profile 195

Table 8: Mpumalanga: Teachers' Profile 196

List of Diagrams

Diagram 1: Layers of Influence on Teachers' Social Identity and Discourses on HIV/AIDS: Understanding the Context 151

Diagram 2: Factors and Four Levels of Influence Shaping Teachers' Subjective Experiences 193

Diagram 3: Early Influences and Subject Positions 231

Diagram 4: Teachers, Perceptions of Teaching and Subject Positions 241

Diagram 5: Iterativity of Factors and Four Levels of Influence Shaping Teachers' Subjective Experiences and Patterns of Performativity 267

Introduction

HIV/AIDS prevalence amid heterosexual populations in Sub-Saharan Africa is amongst the highest in the world. As one of the countries in this region, South Africa experienced an increase in its infected population from about 3.5 million in 1999 (World Bank, 2000) to almost double the number in a very short space of time (about 6.5 million in 2002 according to the ASSA model by Dorrington, Bradshaw and Budlender (2002). Figures from UNAIDS (2006) show the number of those living with HIV in South Africa to be at about 5.5 million (available at http:/data.unaids.org/pub/EPISlides/2007/071118_epi_revisions_factsheet_en.pd). Projections of the pandemic's potential devastation on the economic and social well-being of the country are well documented (see Coombe, 2000; Dorrington, Bradshaw & Budlender, 2002; Barnett & Whiteside, 2002).

The accuracy of these projections is not of consequence here. Suffice it to say that their significance is twofold: they indicate both on the magnitude of the problem and the consequences for government, in terms of planning at the systemic level and taking proactive steps to combat the disease and provide support for those infected and affected. In the wake of these projections, many strategies and programmes have been developed and implemented to educate the South African population against infection and to combat rates of infection. These have included, among others, the development of policies (national,[1] provincial and local); mass media campaigns (television,[2] billboards,[3] newspapers); peer education, workplace training and support; and free access to condoms (Baxen, 2005). In some regions, such as in the Western Cape, a website has been developed that provides information for educators, learners, and parents. In sum education has been identified as crucial in the fight against HIV/AIDS, not only in South Africa but also around the world (Coombe, 2000; Gallant & Maticka-Tyndale, 2003; Kelly, 2000).

1 National Health Care on HIV/AIDS.
2 For example, *Soul City* and Scamtu.
3 For example, *LoveLife*.

Indeed education is arguably "the single most powerful weapon against HIV transmission" (Kelly, 2000: 9). In particular, within formal schooling, guidance and Lifeskills programmes seem the most likely and accessible environments in which messages about safe and safer sex might be conveyed. The expectation is that such information will equip learners to make informed sexual choices, and that this will lead to a reduction in the infection rate. Gallant and Maticka-Tyndale (2003) elaborate on some commonly held perspectives for such an emphasis in formal school settings. First, schools are recognized as the largest single site where youth can be reached and, therefore, 'naturally' the most 'obvious' spaces for the dissemination and mediation of preventive messages. Second, in the Sub-Saharan region, 67% of children of school-going age remain in school at least until Grade 5. It is logical, therefore, for governments to spend resources on prevention strategies, such as education, rather than on the health care system to help those already infected. Third, studies indicate that youth in Sub-Saharan Africa become sexual active while still of school-going age. It would make sense, therefore, to provide them with safe sex messages to enable them to make informed choices, thereby minimising the potential risk of infection. Indeed, programme evaluation reviews, such as those by Kaaya, Mukoma, Flisher and Klepp (2002) point to evidence that prevention programmes initiated in primary schools, before sexual debut, are successful in lowering sexually transmitted infections. Lastly, schools are familiar spaces: their structure, *modus operandi* and general patterns of practice are known, and this renders them natural sites for knowledge mediation and transmission (Baxen, 2005).

South Africa has identified this role for schools. Evident within South Africa's National and Provincial Departments of Education policy documents is an emphasis on providing learners with accurate information about HIV/AIDS (modes of contraction and transmission, and prevention), as well as on ensuring that they are taught about sexuality. Content is clearly articulated for each grade of the Life Orientation[4] learning programme, one of eight learning programmes that comprise the Revised National Curriculum of 2002. Education departments have also embarked on training lifeskills teachers in the proposed content.

4 The curriculum for the General Education and Training Band (Grades 1–9 compulsory schooling period) comprises eight learning areas. Lifeskills is an area of the curriculum within the Life Orientation learning programme.

Although the argument about the situatedness and positioning of schools as obvious spaces for safe and safer sex message transmission is compelling, fundamental questions remain about what actually happens in schools and classrooms. What is actually taught? What do children actually learn about sexuality and HIV/AIDS in schools? How is knowledge about HIV/AIDS and sexuality mediated in classrooms? Who are the mediators and what determines the content and how it is taught? Do teachers feel confident or competent in addressing these issues? What, in their own experience and understanding of the disease, do teachers bring into the classroom? How are teachers positioned and how do they position themselves in teaching about what is taken for granted in everyday social practice as 'the deeply private'? The fundamental question that I pose in this book is: What actually happens in lifeskills classrooms when teachers teach sexuality and HIV/AIDS?

The study that serves as a basis for this book sought to address some of these questions by paying attention to two interrelated issues. The first relates to the content and form of HIV/AIDS and sexuality discourses in schools. The study raised questions concerning the epistemological origins and the frames of references underpinning constructions of HIV/AIDS and sexuality classroom discourse. Put differently, the question it responded to was: What informs constructions of HIV/AIDS and sexuality classroom discourse as articulated by the teacher in lifeskills lessons? The study also posed questions about how teachers mediate sexuality and HIV/AIDS. It asked how teachers position themselves and how they understand, produce, and reproduce discourses of HIV/AIDS and sexuality at the chalk-face. Through examining factors shaping their experience, understanding, and mediation of HIV/AIDS and sexuality, the study explored the nexus between the production of teacher identities and classroom discourse.

Teachers are rarely the focus of research pertaining to HIV/AIDS. Most studies are either concerned with the delivery of teacher development programmes and evaluating their effectiveness, or they research teachers as implementers of curricula. There is research that points to the catastrophic effects of the pandemic on teachers' work experience, either through an increase in their workload (due to sick personnel) or a variation in the nature of their work (supportive and caring demands made by sick or orphaned children, causing changed role expectations) (Simbayi, Skinner, Letlape & Zuma, 2005). But there is little research that questions what actually happens in classrooms. This is at odds with the general assumptions that have been made about the efficacy of education, assumptions that led to the types of questions posed in this work. Few questions are directed at *who* mediates sexuality and HIV/AIDS knowledge and how, in this mediation process, teachers are positioned or indeed, position themselves. Still fewer questions are focussed on *how* and *what* occurs during the mediation process. Little is known of the conditions that shape the processes and outcomes of mediation in HIV/AIDS and sexuality classrooms. In fact, little is known about what happens in lifeskills classrooms where teachers mediate knowledge about HIV/AIDS and sexuality.

The paucity of literature in this area led me to examine how Life Orientation (Lifeskills)[5] teachers in the General Education and Training Band understand, experience, and teach sexuality and HIV/AIDS in the context of a complex HIV/AIDS hermeneutic space, one highly contested and riven by multiple and competing interpretations. This book, therefore, reports on a study that examined how the discursive space of the Lifeskills classroom works as a site of production for particular teacher identities. The assumption the study made is that while teachers are, educationally at least, strategically positioned to mediate knowledge that might lead to change in sexual behaviour, this knowledge, and the meanings they transact, as well as the process of mediation they set in motion, cannot be understood outside the broader context of social action in which individual and collective meaning is constructed, reconstructed and re-articulated. The argument is that as agents, teachers make choices irrespective of the formal curriculum; they act to produce and reproduce while at the same time being produced within complex discursive spaces of social action. Knowledge and mediation processes are themselves not neutral but charged and contradictory, and they also function to produce and reproduce competing identities. What teachers consciously and unconsciously choose to foreground in the teaching encounter (what and how they teach), therefore, is mediated in and through particular subject positions that are constructed within complex networks of social relations. "Social relations" in this instance refers to relations among social

5 Life Orientation is one of eight learning areas taught in the General Education and Training Band. Lifeskills forms part of the larger Life Orientation learning area. It is within the Lifeskills programme that sexuality and HIV/AIDS education is taught.

agents themselves and the nexus between social agents and institutions, rules and regulatory practices that shape and are influenced by social actors (Hall & Du Gay, 1996). Importantly in this work, social relations presuppose an audience even when the audience includes the individual in dialogue with the 'self' (McLaren, 2005). This work, therefore, is about productions of the 'self' in a complex HIV/AIDS hermeneutic space.

Through the use of in-depth, semi-structured interviews with teachers and participant classroom observations in some purposively selected primary and secondary schools in the Western Cape and Mpumalanga, the study traced what happens in the act of teaching when teachers mediate sexuality and HIV/AIDS. The study began by asking questions about who the teachers are and what it is about themselves that they bring into the classroom. This in turn provoked questions about what happens in classrooms when teachers invoke the body in its physical and sexual form, a body usually absent in the public arena of the classroom. The underlying premise of the study was that factors shaping understanding, as well as individual and collective experiences, serve as mediatory resources teachers draw on to produce and reproduce knowledge and teacherly enactments in the classroom. Such an argument challenges constructions of, on the one hand, teachers as mere *deliverers* of an uncontested, sanitised and agreed upon body of content and, on the other hand, schools as stable or neutral environments where safe sex messages are effortlessly delivered by a complying teacher to a relatively passive audience. Thus the study focused on examining factors that shape teachers' understanding, experience, and teaching of sexuality and HIV/AIDS in some schools in the Western Cape and Mpumalanga. Three core questions formed the basis for this exploration.

- Amongst this cohort, what social and cultural practices shape Lifeskills teachers' understanding, experiences, beliefs, attitudes, and responses to sexuality and HIV/AIDS? Put simply, what factors accompany teachers into Lifeskills classrooms when they teach sexuality and HIV/AIDS?
- How do some Lifeskills teachers in the General Education and Training Band[6] teach sexuality and HIV/AIDS in the socio-political context of HIV/AIDS in South Africa? In other words, how are teachers posi-

6 This refers to the compulsory years of schooling in South Africa and comprises Grades 1–9.

tioned and how do they position themselves when teaching sexuality and HIV/AIDS?

- How does teaching sexuality and HIV/AIDS shape, produce, and reproduce a particular teacher identity? What are the patterns of teacher behaviour, and what teacherly performances are invoked when teachers teach sexuality and HIV/AIDS? How are these produced or reproduced and how do such invocations work to produce and reproduce 'the teacher'? What are the slippages and ruptures in teacher performance in teaching sexuality and HIV/AIDS?

Interest in understanding who teachers are and what it is in (and about) themselves that plays into what and how they teach, led me to pose questions about identity and its constitutive form in social order and social action. Such a focus directed me to a number of interrelated aspects that needed attention: subject formation, subjectivity, subject positioning and in this instance, their articulation with content and classroom practice. Since I was interested in understanding teacher subject positioning and teaching, I developed a theoretical framework that explained the nexus between the two.

To do this I drew first on social theory. In particular, I used Bourdieu's theory of practice, Giddens's theory of structuration, and some components from Goffman's presentation of the self in the everyday, to develop a conceptual framework that gives an account of subject formation and subjectivity. This framework offered some insight into how social and cultural practices shape lived experience and how the former is said to structure social action. While these theorists offer different theoretical perspectives on the phenomenon, they all make a valuable contribution to this work by offering explanatory tools to examine (a) the constituted nature of social action; (b) how subjects are constituted and constitute themselves in social action; and (c) teachers' subjective experiences. They also help to explain how teachers not only come to hold particular attitudes, beliefs, and values about themselves as individuals, but also how these become the frames of references they use to make meaning of themselves and their work in relation to the pandemic. However, this framework had limited application since I was unable to apply it to understand what actually happens in the classroom when teachers teach sexuality and HIV/AIDS. In particular, I was unable to explain some aspects of the empirical data that seemed to throw doubt on the deterministic claims regarding social action made by these theorists. In part, the problem was that applying such a framework allowed only limited possibilities for teachers to act differently, outside the experience amassed in their lifetime. The difficulty, as I saw it, related to constructions of power: how it is explained by these theorists and how it is brought into play in subject formation. Their explanations do not offer an understanding of subject formation beyond describing an already determined subject who is constrained by, rather than dependent on, power for 'survival.'

The inadequacy of conceptions of power in this explanatory framework led me to explore components of psychoanalysis and feminist theory that shed light on the role of power in subject formation, subjectivity and subject positioning. Such a focus enabled me to analyse the articulation between teacher positioning and classroom practice. In theorising the use of power in understanding subjection, domination, resistance, resignification and identification, the theories I used for the second part of the conceptual framework made it possible to shift from describing and explaining the conditions under which teachers come to understand who they are, to analysing the subject positions they take up in the classroom. The analytical framework thus relies primarily but not exclusively on Butler's theory of performativity. In deploying this theory, I refer to Foucault's notion of power and discourse, and Lacan's and Althusser's emphasis on the role of language in subject formation. Through highlighting the limitations in their explanations of subjection, I insert Butler's theory of performativity as the framework that offers possibilities for a different reading of subject positioning, resistance, identification and resignification.

It was through applying Butler's theory of performativity that I was able to respond to another key aspect of the main question, namely, how teachers are positioned and how they position themselves in the classroom when they teach sexuality and HIV/AIDS. This work advances Bourdieu's notion of *habitus* and Giddens's theory of structuration beyond conceptions of a predetermined subject. It illuminates how subjectivity is constituted *in and through* relations of power. Power here is understood as not only constraining or enabling but as the actual condition the subject relies on for its very existence (Butler, 1997). Such a perspective made it possible for me to explain the dialectic relationship between subject positioning and social practice, thereby enabling me to explicate the complex interrelationship between teacher subject positioning and teaching. This work challenges commonly held conceptions that (a) teachers merely deliver an uncontested or incontestable body of knowledge in an unproblematic fashion to achieve externally determined outcomes, (b) they are well placed to mediate knowledge on sexuality and HIV/AIDS, and (c) schools are the best repositories for sexuality and HIV/AIDS messages.

Overview of the book

This book comprises five parts.

Part I is a detailed description of the study. It offers insight into the particular research process followed and accounts for the choices I made in gathering and managing the empirical evidence. It also outlines the epistemological decisions made in this process.

Part II, which includes Chapters 2–5, describes the theoretical framework of the study. I introduce this part with a synopsis of the path I followed in developing an explanatory and analytical framework. I describe the assumptions made about teachers and their work and argue that any exploration of teachers and their work cannot be done outside a framework that accounts for who teachers are. Such an argument led me to situate this work within a sociological framework and pose questions about the constitutive nature of identity and its articulation in social practice. In particular, I posed questions about subject formation, subjectivity and subject positioning and how these are understood to be constituted in social practice. It is here that I outline the theories I rely on to develop a conceptual and analytical framework. I offer an explanation of why I use a range of perspectives on identity by describing each theory, its usefulness as well as its limitations. I end this section by formulating a theoretical and analytical framework that made it possible to examine (a) in the empirical evidence, the multiplicity of identity positions and their articulation in social practice; (b) the limitations of dominant epistemological discourses in selected literature on teachers and their work; (c) identity resources teachers draw on in constructions of sexuality and HIV/AIDS discourses; and (the main question addressed in the study) (d) levels of influence or factors shaping teachers' understanding, experience and teaching of sexuality and HIV/AIDS.

Part III contextualises the study within teacher and HIV/AIDS research. It comprises three chapters, each with a different focus. Common to all, though, is an orientation towards the literature that critically examines the epistemological and methodological limitations in research on teachers in general and their work in relation to sexuality and HIV/AIDS in particular. Chapter 6 reviews selected literature on teachers and teaching. It provides a rationale for the particular epistemological orientation on teachers' work followed in this study. Rather than offer a general review of teacher literature, I trace how dominant epistemological and methodological orientations influence constructions of the teacher subject. I argue that these orientations offer limited understandings of the complex interplay between structure and agency and, as such, limit understanding of the interconnectedness of teacher subject positioning and classroom discourse. I end this section by offering recent feminist and critical theory as alternative epistemologies to the above. I argue that within recent feminist orientations, subject positioning is not only proposed as constituted through and within relations of power, but as the condition on which subjects rely to constitute their identity. This orientation provides this study with an epistemological framework to examine teachers and their work, especially in teaching sexuality and HIV/AIDS which, as will become clearer in Chapter 11, requires a particular teacher subject positioning that is often not invoked in the public space of the classroom.

In preparation for the argument pursued later in the book, Chapter 7 introduces some dominant discourses that act as structures shaping constructions and interpretations of HIV/AIDS and sexuality. These include discourses on sexuality, disease and the politics of HIV/AIDS in South Africa. I trace how these discourses act as foregrounding as well as interpretive lenses for the meanings people attribute to the pandemic. First, a short historical overview of the dominant discourses shaping ways of knowing and understanding sexuality and disease is provided. Then I comment on the way epistemological frameworks used to describe and understand sexuality and disease shape interpretations of the phenomenon in general, and the HIV/AIDS research agenda in particular. This section is preparation for the argument in Chapter 8, where I illustrate how the dominant discourses under discussion influence orientations in research on HIV/AIDS. The relevance of this discussion lies in its importance as a contextual backdrop for understanding constructions and interpretations of HIV/AIDS and sexuality and concomitant classroom discourses. Importantly though, locating HIV/AIDS within the meta-narratives of sexuality and disease offers a way of exploring classroom discourse and teacher identity, since such discourses act as interpretive and reproductive scripts within, through, and from which teachers produce and reproduce individual and collective identities.

Chapter 8 continues with descriptions of how epistemological and methodological frameworks used to understand sexuality and disease are imposed on researching HIV/AIDS, thus setting limits to the nature of the research conducted, the type of questions posed and the meanings people attach to the pandemic. This is done by outlining the epistemological assumptions and methodological frameworks underpinning constructions of HIV/AIDS, which shows how, framed by the dominant discourses on sexuality and disease, these become the dominant research frameworks shaping research on HIV/AIDS, globally, on the African continent and in South Africa. I also show how these play out in research in education, particularly in examining teachers and their work. This lays the groundwork from my argument that such discourses shape what is taught about sexuality and HIV/AIDS, and how it is taught. I end this section by arguing that bringing together the discourses of sexuality, disease, and HIV/AIDS not only highlights ways in which the classroom text is constructed, but puts the very process of construction, production, and reproduction under the spotlight. As a site of production, this discursive space draws attention to those who speak, the positions from which they speak, as well as what is produced and reproduced in their speech. Such a space, I argue, is not neutral but embedded within unequal relations of power and is thus open to negotiation, contestation, and disruption.

Part IV focuses on the empirical data and is presented in three chapters. Chapters 9 and 10 are contextual and serve to situate the cohort of teachers in the study within a specific space and time. These two chapters offer perspectives on the specificity of context as a critical indicator in the understanding ofsocial identity, subject formation, and social positioning. They anchor what follows in the final chapter of this section, namely, descriptions of the patterns of behaviour that teachers enact in Lifeskills classrooms. The first two sections also offer a textual landscape from and through which not only to situate this group of teachers, but also to understand context as discursively constituted by structures and discourses that are only visible through performative behaviours within that site of practice. This is exemplified in in the present context by what happens in classrooms when teachers mediate sexuality and HIV/AIDS.

Observational data are presented in Chapter 11. Rather than select episodes from the behaviour of a range of teachers, I give detailed accounts of eight teachers in four categories. Each of the four categories identifies particular behaviours that exemplify the performative.

Part V of the book summarizes insights yielded by the study. I do not offer a conclusion because, like the theory on which this work depends, I see the work as neither complete nor conclusive. I do, however, outline the policy, teacher training and curriculum implications of the study and in so doing raise more questions than provide easy solutions. This section emphasizes the need for the application of epistemological and methodological orientations that offer a more nuanced reading of the HIV/AIDS landscape in South Africa.

Part I
Context and contours of the research

Introduction

This section outlines the methodological decisions made in crafting a research plan to examine factors shaping teachers' understanding and experience of teaching sexuality and HIV/AIDS. A study of this nature requires an approach that takes into account how people come to know and understand themselves; an approach that pays particular attention to constructions of social reality in the setting in which it occurs. In seeking to understand the meanings and interpretations people give to experiences, such an approach must not only allow for the inclusion of people's voices, but also be sensitive to the discursive spaces in which meaning is constructed and mediated. In short a methodological orientation was required that could enable me to illustrate how subjects come to know and the levels of influence that shape this.

1 The study

Methodological orientation

The main question to which this study responded was that of the factors shaping teachers' understanding, experience and teaching in a hermeneutic space of HIV/AIDS. Since I was interested in examining how a particular cohort of teachers made meaning of themselves and their work, I adopted a qualitative mode of inquiry which enabled me to pay attention to, not only how teachers viewed their social world, but also to how they were positioned and positioned themselves within their particular social worlds.

A case study approach was followed. According to Denzin & Lincoln (1994: 204) a case is "a phenomenon of some sort occurring in a bounded context-the unit of analysis, in effect." Usually, in a case study approach there is a focus and loosely defined physical and/or social boundaries within which the research is carried out. Foci and /or boundaries can be identified by large or small social units, e.g. individuals, groups, institutions, organisations. (Denzin & Lincoln, 1998). In this instance, teachers were the unit of analysis and as such constituted the 'case'. A life history approach was applied to gain access to a central source of information namely, teachers' life stories.

Life history is defined by Goodson as "a narrative, influenced by the cultural conventions of telling, by the audience, and by the social context" (1992: 236). Life histories and biographies have been used to gain an understanding of "individual – collective praxis and socio-historical change in the organisation of individual life data and more specifically in the interplay between teachers' individual identities and the socio-historical context in which they work" (Stephens, 2002: 16). According to Stephens, life history research focuses on two interrelated worlds, namely that of the individual with his or her particular life history, and that of the "past, present and future contextual world though which the individual travels" (2002: 16).

Goodson, though, makes a distinction between life stories and life history by suggesting that the former is the story as related by the person "who lived and experienced the life" while the latter is "influenced by cultural conventions of telling, by the audience, and by the social context" and is "life as told" by the life story teller and researcher, a collaborative process that seeks to produce an "intercontextual account, the life history" (1992: 236). In providing a rationale for studying teachers' lives (and by implication using a life history approach), Butt, Raymond, McCue and Yamagishi (1992: 57) argue that:

> The notion of the teacher's voice is important in that it carries the tone, the language, the quality, the feelings that are conveyed by the way the teacher speaks or writes. In a political sense the notion of the teacher's voice addresses the right to speak and be represented. It can represent both the unique individual and the collective voice; one that is characteristic of teachers as compared to other groups.

Goodson (1992) suggests a number of reasons why it is becoming increasingly necessary to focus on teachers' lives, one of these being that it emphasises the need to "understand and give voice to an occupational group that have been historically marginalized" (Goodson, 1992: 15). Furthermore, this type of study offers insights into the "deeply personal aspects of identity" (Goodson, 1992: 15). The rationale for an investigation into teachers' lives rested upon an understanding that *who* teachers are (their identity) and the context in which they live and work shapes their beliefs and hence their actions in the classroom.

Sites

The sampling strategy was purposive. This technique was appropriate because decisions had already been made that only teachers who taught Lifeskills in the General Education and Training Band would be considered for participation. Further, the age appropriateness of the content prohibited the inclusion of all grades. In order to include the perspectives of a diverse group of teachers across the social organisational categories of class, race, ethnicity and gender, the racial and social classifications imposed on the South African landscape and used in categorizing schools prior to the democratic government of 1994, had to be employed in the choice of schools. It was important that the sample included primary and secondary schools since teachers rather than schools or grades were the unit of analysis.

Schools

I applied a purposive sampling technique to select schools since I wanted to analyse the understanding, experience and teaching of a range of teachers. In selecting schools, I took account of their geographic location, demographic profile as well as their socio-historical locatedness during the Apartheid era.

The following procedures were used in selecting schools. First, I selected two regions, Mpumalanga and the Western Cape. The former ranked as one of four provinces in the country with high rates of HIV-infection, while the Western Cape had the lowest rate of infection. Another consideration was convenience. I reside in the Western Cape and it was thus easy to access schools in the region. Mpumalanga was included because permission had already been granted by the Education Department for the researcher, as principal investigator, to conduct research in the region as part of a project funded by DFID/British Council.[7] As this study contributed to and was located within a larger project on 'Schooling, Cultural Values and HIV/AIDS in South Africa',[8] the schools in the Western Cape pre-selected for this project were the ones in which the following selection process took place.

All the schools in the Western Cape metropolis were grouped according to their grade levels (primary or secondary). Thereafter, each group was separated into the categories used prior to the democratic elections of 1994, i.e. ex-House of Representatives (coloured), ex-House of Assembly (white), ex-Department of Education and Training (black) and ex-House of Delegates (Indian). The latter ex-Department (ex-House

7 The project investigated the policy and practice effects of HIV/AIDS on female teachers in two provinces in South Africa (Western Cape and Mpumalanga). I was the principal investigator in this project.

8 I was the principal investigator in this study funded jointly by the National Research foundation and Norway Research Council.

of Delegates) was omitted since there were only four schools under its jurisdiction in this region and they would have been too easily identifiable.

Simple random sampling was then applied. Each school was assigned a number that was placed in a box denoting the ex-department. The secondary school sample comprised one school from each of the three selected ex-Departments. However, two schools were selected from the ex-House of Representatives because they comprise the largest number of schools in the region. Thus, in total, four secondary schools were included in the study.

One school was selected from each of the three ex-departments in the primary school sample. Once the research was underway, the primary school from the ex-House of Assembly dropped out and was replaced with an additional ex-Department of Education and Training School. This resulted in three primary schools being included in the study. Therefore, the final number of primary and secondary schools in the Western Cape was seven.

All the schools in Mpumalanga were from the ex-Department of Education and Training. Simple random sampling was also applied to select four primary and four secondary schools. The total sample of schools, therefore, was fifteen, with seven from the Western Cape and eight from Mpumalanga.

Letters requesting permission to conduct research in the schools were written to the respective provincial Education Departments. Once permission was received, letters were sent to the regional offices notifying them of the research as well as the selected schools. After the regional office acknowledged receipt and approved access to schools, letters were sent to principals requesting an introductory meeting. At this meeting I explained the purpose and outcome of the research, sometimes to the entire staff and at other times to Lifeskills teachers only.

Teachers

Participation by teachers was voluntary. The focus was on those teaching Lifeskills in the General Education and Training Band of compulsory schooling. In considering the grades to focus on, three criteria were applied: age; appropriateness of the curriculum content I wanted to observe; and availability of teachers. Grade 9 was selected in the secondary school since, in most instances, teachers in these schools taught classes across the whole range of grades. Grade 6 was selected in the Intermediate Phase of the primary school. The Grade 7 teachers at the respective schools were reluctant since this was the final year of primary school and they did not want to have the additional pressure of participating in a project of this nature. In most instances, in the participating schools, more than one teacher taught Lifeskills. When more than one teacher volunteered from a school, s/he was simply included. The final sample of teachers was therefore more than the number of participating schools.

The Western Cape sample comprised seven secondary and three primary school teachers and the Mpumalanga sample four primary and four secondary teachers. While the same number of teachers was selected in each of the two provinces, the final sample consisted of only eighteen teachers because, upon arrival at two participating schools in Mpumalanga, it was discovered that two of the teachers who volunteered to participate no longer taught Lifeskills. Their names are italicised in the table below. While they were not selected for classroom observations, they were interviewed and were thus included in Chapter 10.

I tried to maintain the same number of primary and secondary school respondents as well as an equal number of males and females, but this was not possible. Reasons for this become clear in the analysis in Chapter 10. This factor did not adversely influence the results, however because non school level and the gender were the focus of the research. This notwithstanding, I deemed it important to include the perspectives and experiences of a broad spectrum of teachers across the school system. As a result, the final sample consisted of thirteen secondary school teachers and seven primary teachers. Tables 1 and 2, below, outline the school and teacher sample in each of the respective regions.

Table 1: Western Cape: Teacher and School Profile

Teacher	*Gender*	*Race*	*School*	*School Level*
Kobie	Male	White	Bloukoop	Secondary
Vera	Female	White	Bloukoop	Secondary
Pauline	Female	Coloured	Parktown	Secondary
Gwen	Female	Coloured	Parktown	Secondary
Paul	Male	Coloured	Redhill	Secondary
Carol	Female	Coloured	Redhill	Secondary
Shahida	Female	Coloured	Macadamia	Primary
Zodwa	Female	Black	Mzondi	Secondary
Xola	Male	Black	Vuyani	Primary
Gugu	Female	Black	Zondi	Primary

Table 2: Mpumalanga: Teacher and School Profile

Teacher	*Gender*	*Race*	*School*	*School level*
Mzi	Male	Black	Vuyisile	Secondary
Sipho	Male	Black	Hamba	Secondary
Lizzie	Female	Black	Hamba	Secondary
Thandi	Female	Black	Khonzani	Secondary
Volene	Female	Black	Buyisa	Secondary
Patricia	Female	Black	Buyisa	Secondary
Jenni	Female	Black	Yiso	Primary
Ester	Female	Black	Siyabonga	Primary
Dorothy	Female	Black	Mbazani	Primary
Jabulani	Female	Black	Hambani	Primary

Research path

I used interviews, participant observation and documentary analysis to collect information. Using multiple methods was important in that it ensured some form of verification and reliability in the data. According to Denzin, a researcher "deploys 'different methods' – such as interviewing, exploration of census data, and document checking – to 'validate' findings" (1998: 358). Such methods have traditionally been accepted as having the same set of assumptions, including the assumption that "there is a 'fixed point' or 'object' that can be triangulated" (Denzin & Lincoln, 1998: 358). The postmodernist perspective rejects this and prefers the notion of 'crystallization' to 'data validation'. Accordingly, my purpose in triangulating was not to find a 'fixed point', but to examine the phenomenon using a range of 'lenses' (Denzin & Lincoln, 1998).

A series of semi-structured interviews lasting about an hour each were conducted with the selected group of teachers. Each interviewed was taped, with permission from the teachers. Because the nature of the data collection process was inductive, teachers were interviewed more than once, with each interview having a different focus. The first set were narrative or life history type interviews (Sarantakos, 1994: 185), conducted to gain insight into teachers' lives as a way of understanding the influences shaping their identities.

The second series of interviews focused more closely on teachers' classroom practice. In all cases teachers taught two Lifeskills lessons, and in almost all cases, teachers were interviewed directly after the lesson. Where this was not possible, teachers were interviewed later the same day. In a few exceptional cases, however, the researcher had to return to the school to conduct the post-observation interview. No schedule was used for these interviews as questions were based on the specific lessons observed. However, to maintain a level of consistency, interviews focused mainly on the aim, proposed outcome and the choices teachers had made in the lesson, regarding particular responses to learners, strategies employed and content selected. All the interviews were audio-recorded after permission had been granted by individual teachers. These were transcribed and used in conjunction with field-notes kept throughout the data collection process.

Participant observation strategies were also used, both to collect data pertaining to the school culture of each participating school, and to collect data on teaching. Information on the former was critical to understanding the context in which the participating teachers work and was, therefore, integral to the study.

During the initial visit to each school, field-notes were, made on the daily life of the school: its ethos, codes of conduct, and discipline strategies. I observed in staffrooms and had informal conversations with many teachers as a way of ascertaining general information about the respective schools. I also observed the interaction and relationships among teachers within and beyond the staffroom, and between teachers and learners on the playground as well as in the selected Lifeskills classes.

The second observation period at each school focused on specific Lifeskills lessons that teachers had prepared beforehand. In all cases, teachers taught a lesson on sexuality or HIV/AIDS. Each teacher presented me with a lesson plan as well as copies of the tasks and resource material used in the lesson. I sat at the back of the room taking comprehensive notes during the first series of lessons. On the second occasion, each teacher was video-recorded after they had given their consent. The focus was primarily, but not exclusively, on the teacher. I observed the manner in which knowledge was mediated, the teaching strategies used, how teachers gave 'voice' to the messages they foregrounded, what they responded to and what they omitted or ignored in their interaction with the learners. Since I was interested in teacher behaviour, I often listened to learners' responses but did not always record these. Thus I noted the gist of discussions, while recording the 'teacher talk' in its entirety.

In addition to observing Lifeskills lessons, I spent a day with each teacher observing them teach other subjects. This was to gain insight into the strategies these teachers employed in teaching subjects that did not necessarily invoke a physical, sexed body in the way teaching about sexuality and HIV/AIDS had the potential to do. Each day was video-recorded and replayed.

Using participant observation strategies was challenging because I was faced with the dilemma of being both an insider and an outsider. By this I mean that I was "simultaneously a member of the group [I was] studying and a researcher doing the study" (Babbie, *et al.*, 2001: 292). This notwithstanding, using such a strategy enabled me to experience the natural context in which the phenomenon to be studied occurs (Babbie, *et al.*, 2001).

I found it increasingly difficult to interview and record field-notes as the interviews progressed. Rather, I chose to listen and write down key words during the interview. Immediately thereafter, I made comprehensive notes of the things that struck me as important, the mood in the interview, the gestures teachers used and a general impression of the interview. The same was done during the observations. These notes proved useful during the analysis in recalling moments, events and gestures that the audio equipment missed and may otherwise have been lost. The inductive nature of the research meant that I was able to go back to teachers when aspects of what had been observed were not clear.

I simultaneously took notes and reflected on the data as well as on the research process as I went along. During this period, I was continually aware of my own positionality and the subject positions I invoked as I interviewed, observed and finally wrote this work. I was aware, too, of how I framed the questions, responses and probes, and how I made choices concerning what and what not to privilege both in the interviews and in the field-notes.

Finally, I relied on various reports and data sets to gain statistical information about HIV-prevalence rates in the respective provinces, regions and districts (see Chapter 9). This information was used descriptively for the purpose of supporting rather than proving or making assertions about the descriptions outlined in this chapter.

As a way of contextualizing the schools and respondents, Census Reports, the *South African Yearbook* and the *Labour Law Survey* were used to develop the provincial, regional and community social and material profiles presented in Chapter 9.

My intention initially was to gain access to the mission and vision statements and policies of schools as a way of developing a profile of the schools. However, as the research process unfolded, it became unnecessary since I was able to obtain opposite information about the school from respondents themselves. In addition, the decision was reached that while school influences were important in shaping what teachers did in the classroom, the primary focus was on what teachers drew from their own lives. Thus, detailed information about the school was deliberately backgrounded. Nonetheless, I drew on teachers' subjective experiences to produce profiles of the schools in Chapter 10.

Managing the information

The interviews were transcribed soon after completion of the first series of twenty. Each interview was replayed while I read the transcriptions to ensure accuracy. The first round of analysis involved gaining familiarity with the respondents' life stories. In using the field-notes, I was able to develop nuanced profiles of each respondent. I wrote notes on the side of each transcript incorporating descriptions of 'the moment of instantiation' as had been recorded in my journal. I identified emerging patterns in the transcripts. At this preliminary stage, I also kept a separate file with respondents' names and additional questions that had arisen from reading the transcripts. I was aware that it would be possible to pose additional questions for clarification the next time I saw the respondents, either for observations or during the second series of interviews.

After the preliminary preparation phase described above, the next phase in the analysis was the development of individual teacher narratives. This was a cumbersome and lengthy but useful process in that it enabled me to develop rich descriptions of each respondent. However, as I state in the introduction to Chapter 10, these proved too bulky to include in the final analysis. The process was useful in that it submerged me in the data, making me well acquainted with the respondents and their life stories.

The outcome of the initial process of analysis led me to explore different ways of presenting the data. Once I reached the decision that I would develop themes and categories around emerging patterns, I used NVIVO, a programme frequently used to analyse qualitative data. It provided tools to identify units of analysis. While I used the theoretical structure I describe in Part 2 to frame and analyse the data, I applied a Foucauldian analysis of discourse as a way of extrapolating the units for analysis. To Foucault, discourse analysis is not structural analysis where statements are assumed to emanate from an "unspoken structure that secretly animates every statement" (Andersen, 2003: 10).

Rather, discourse analysis is about the examination of the statement in its moment of instantiation, in its '*positivity*' (Andersen, 2003). Statements have meaning in the moment of their utterance or in the moment of invocation and, therefore, have to be taken for what they are in the moment of utterance. To him a statement is a '*function of existence*' that "enables groups of signs to exist" (Andersen, 2003: 11).

Four identifiable features comprise what Foucault would qualify as a statement: object, subject, conceptual network and strategy (Anderson, 2003). Foucault believes that a statement is only a statement if it produces objects that are external to the signifier. Objects are discursively constituted and are discernable in the statement itself. Second, a statement can only be regarded as such if agents take up subject positions and a discursive space is created through which subjects invoke a position. Third, it can only be regarded as a statement if its "elements of signification" (Andersen, 2003: 11) are multipliable and can be duplicated. In other words, a statement can only be identified as such if there is a recognisable association with other statements that precede and follow it. In this instance, connectivity is critical if a statement is to be defined as such. Thus, statements are only identifiable as statements when there is some association between what was said before and what comes after. Lastly, a statement can only be identified as a statement if it is embedded, as Giddens (1984) suggests, in a situated content bound by time and space. To be defined as a statement, it cannot be disembedded or decontexualised. Statements have meaning only in as much as they are supported in a material and social universe. Applying the principles of Foucault's discourse analysis, and bearing in mind the features constituting a statement, I utilized NVIVO to identify nodes (or categories) that served as units of analysis. Through the use this programme, I was able to generate integrated node reports (placing all the common nodes across transcripts together) that were later used to develop themes.

The same process was undertaken with the analysis of the observational data. The audio recordings were extracted from the video recordings and transcribed. As in the case of the interviews, each video tape was reviewed while I read the transcriptions for accuracy. As with the interview data, field-notes were used to develop richer descriptions of the observations by adding the anecdotal evidence the researcher had recorded. Thereafter, the data was transposed into rich text format for use in the NVIVO programme. Unlike the process described above, where the focus was on developing themes that described factors shaping teachers' lives outside the classroom, the focus in developing nodes using observational data was to identify two interrelated themes: namely, what teachers taught and what behaviour they exhibited.

In the analysis described in Part IV, data were not separated in the way this section suggests. Relevant aspects of data generated from the various tools were integrated to develop the final product, a process that animates the performative in this work and highlights the subject positions invoked in its production.

I was aware that in dealing with human subjects, attention had to be given to certain ethical considerations. Three key elements were considered in this regard: informed consent, the right to privacy and protection from harm.

Consent to conduct this research was granted by the two provincial Departments of Education, the schools and the teachers concerned. Teachers and schools were assured that privacy and confidentiality would be upheld and that the information would only be used for the purposes of this research. To ensure privacy and anonymity, pseudonyms were used in all the sections in Part IV to denote schools and teachers. The participants were also assured that the information would not be used in ways that could bring harm to them the learners, the school or their families. Ethical issues regarding interviews have emerged as a debate within social research. The question is whether the techniques used, irrespective of whether or not respondents grant consent, can be regarded as manipulative. As Denzin & Lincoln state, "the techniques and tactics of interviewing are really ways of manipulating respondents while treating them as objects or numbers rather than individual human beings" (1998: 71). While the study went a long way to address this concern (through triangulating methods of data collection, conducting cyclical interviews, and developing a rapport with respondents), I acknowledge that respondents themselves may have given me what they thought I wanted to hear and observe.

Teachers often reported that they were comfortable teaching the topic despite its sensitivity. This, in part, was due to their knowledge of the purpose of the research and that they purported to 'know' me. Transparency in the intention of the research and respect for the teachers' privacy made access to information easy. They were assured that it was appropriate for them to retract any information they had offered me.

The code of ethics laid down by the University of Cape Town formed the basis for the *modus operandi* in this research.

Researcher positionality

Much has been written about the ethical difficulties attendant on having access to peoples' private spaces in very intimate ways.

While I applied ethical principles within my own research work over the last ten years, the process of conducting research about a topic as sensitive as this raised issues that few people have written about. Some social scientists suggest rules of conduct for the researcher, while others discuss self-disclosure as a technique to verify data and account for one's positionality as researcher. Few describe the multiple roles in which the researcher as well as the respondent become involved, and the difficulties these evoke.

I entered the field with certain assumptions about my role as a researcher and ill-prepared for what unfolded as I collected data and continually reflected on my role in the research process. What follows is a brief description of myself, the researcher, and the context in which the research took place.

I am a black (termed 'coloured' by the previous Apartheid government) female South African, born in White River, a rural town in Mpumalanga. I matriculated in Johannesburg and completed my Primary Teacher's Diploma in Durban. I taught in Durban for one year after which I relocated to Cape Town where I have resided for the last 27 years. I have had many career changes. I still maintain strong associations with Mpumalanga even though I have not lived there since my teen years.

The discussion that follows illuminates some of the issues that emerged and raised my awareness of the complexity, not only of the site where the research was conducted, but also of the whole process of research. I use the experience of conducting research in Mpumalanga only as an example that draws attention to the issues.

I speak isiSwati, the main language spoken in Mpumalanga. This placed me in a privileged position in more than one way. First, I could offer respondents the option of speaking either in English or isiSwati, with many opting to speak in both languages during the interviews. Second, speaking isiSwati gave me access to information that was best described in the vernacular. Any attempt to translate information was difficult because the interpretation was either inappropriate or downplayed an account of something profound. Third, my ability to speak the language combined with my roots as one from the region, positioned me as an insider. Respondents 'accepted' me as 'one of their own' and as one who 'understood' their contexts and the meanings implicit in their descriptions and accounts. The upshot of this was that teachers volunteered deeply private information that many said they had not divulged before (e.g., disclosure of their HIV status). Finally, being identified as black, insider and woman contributed to, and in part accounted for, the nature of the process: the enunciations, declarations and representations teachers offered as markers of their identities.

In reflecting on this experience I was conscious of the multiplicity and complexity of my own subject position and the roles I played or was expected to fulfil as a researcher. I also took into account the consequences of the research process and how my role in collecting life stories set up unintended and consequently, unfulfilled expectations. These included expectations of my being a counsellor, advisor, role model, and mentor. While it is beyond the scope of this work to provide a detailed account of these, suffice it to say that, managing the research process while being aware of teachers' expectations was a real challenge.

The research process also had consequences for the researched. Many teachers reported feeling special and privileged to be selected for participation.[9] The interview process, some reported, clarified aspects of their identity and gave them perspective. It illuminated their role in making their own life scripts and the choices they had or had not exercised. For others the process was more dramatic in that it was the catalyst for decisions they subsequently made about their lives.

In post-observation interviews, I posed questions about how teachers' experienced my presence in the classroom. Many in this region perceived the relationship (between the researcher and researched) as unproblematic. This they attributed to my perceived 'insider' status and the knowledge they held about the aim of the research. In some instances teachers perceived me as a critical friend. The effect of this was that teachers settled into their roles as mediators with little visible signs of discomfort. My sitting at the rear of the classroom may have added to this sense of comfort. Generally, I was not introduced except in some

9 The same may be said for many schools even though the impact of the research on schools is not unknown.

primary school classes. Learners were usually curious and would come to me enquiring about my presence during the intervals.

In the post-observation interviews, teachers commented on how being under scrutiny made them reflect on their teaching. They suggested that this research process was a reminder of how important it was to continually reflect on one's practice.

The unintended consequence of this process was that none who participated was left unchanged. The sentiments teachers expressed about the benefits of participation put me at ease – temporarily, that is, because as the main thesis in this work suggests, that this was not the whole story.

Part II
A theoretical framework for understanding teachers and their work: Towards a 'performative' subject

Introduction

Attempting to understand factors shaping how teachers in two regions of South Africa understand, experience and teach sexuality and HIV/AIDS required first asking broader questions about how teachers actually come to know who they are and how this knowing is instantiated in social practice. Questions about how this knowing influences their experiences and teaching about sexuality and HIV/AIDS became particularly pertinent. The study worked from the premise that what teachers do in the classroom is not neutral; that what they do with the subject content goes beyond merely delivering it to fulfil externally determined outcomes. The assumption was that teachers teach from particular subject positions influenced by how they understand themselves as individuals, as teachers and as members of different groups (family, school, professional, community, religious, etc.) within society. Importantly, too, this work was premised on the notion that the curriculum and teacher's work are complexly intertwined and that each operates reflexively to produce the other. Any question, therefore, about how and what teachers teach invoked broader questions about the constituted nature of 'the teacher.' Trying to explain teachers and their work required some explanation of the constituted nature of identity; in particular, subject formation, subjectivity and subject positioning. As I proceeded, what became apparent was the need to explain (a) how teachers come to know and understand themselves, (b) how this knowing is shaped by layers of influence (social and cultural) that is sometimes but not always hierarchically constituted, and (c) the extent to which these influences are instantiated (reproductively or transformatively) in social action (teaching). Since I was interested in how teachers' experience (their identity and the conditions they draw on) shapes their classroom practice, it seemed important to explore *two fundamental* questions that have permeated the discussion so far. First, how is the subject constituted, or rather, how does the subject construct the 'self' and what are the conditions under which the subject is 'formed'? Second, how is the self expressed or denied in social practice? In other words, what is it that subjects "harbour and preserve in the beings that [they] are" (Butler, 1997: 2) when a position is invoked? These questions, I understood, would help me explore the components constituting the main question, namely, factors influencing understanding, experience and teaching sexuality and HIV/AIDS.

A fundamental principle on which this work builds is that identity is constructed in a complex interrelationship between structure and agency. Construction, in this sense, is defined by Butler as constituted within relations of power and as the "effect of productive constraint" (1993: x), a conception that becomes clearer in the latter part of this section.

This work is thus as much about identity as it is about sexuality and HIV/AIDS. Therefore, to begin, I draw on social theory for an account of subject formation and subjectivity and provide a brief description of the two dominant epistemological orientations in social theory. I do this to highlight ways in which epistemological origins influence constructions of social action, the formation of society as well as the interrelationship between structure and agency in subject formation. Importantly, though, this brief description serves to locate the selected theorists epistemologically and offers a rationale for the theoretical orientation informing the ensuing sections.

Following on from this, the next section gives descriptions of selected theories that are drawn upon to develop the first part of the framework in Part II. Here, I use a combination of Bourdieu's theory of practice, Giddens's theory of structuration, and Goffman's notion of co-presence and framing to explain subject formation and subjectivity. I begin with a description of Bourdieu's theory of practice. This theorization of social life offers a useful explanation of subject formation and describes how we are socialised into the attitudes and practices we hold through what Bourdieu (1990) calls 'cultural fields'. For understanding factors shaping teachers' lives, I briefly explain three fundamental concepts that form the basis of this theory, namely capital, field and *habitus.* I give brief descriptions of each concept and explain how, through his theory of practice, Bourdieu offers an explanation of the structures that act as dominant frames of references shaping social action. These concepts serve as useful tools for exploring what comes later on in the book, namely, descriptions of the material and social conditions within which and the position from which this cohort makes meaning of their lives. This framework also gives insight into how early experiences recounted by the teachers serve to shape the attitudes, beliefs and values they hold about themselves and about sexuality and HIV/AIDS, and how these act to frame the positions from which they speak. I end this section with the argument that this explanation of subject formation and social life underplays the role of power and its 'availability' to agents. For Bourdieu, agents are constrained by the *habitus* and as such reproductions of power are those that work to maintain or reproduce rather than transform and redistribute power in a field of practice. Subjects are portrayed as passive and already determined through the *habitus* they inhabit. When applied to this work, Bourdieu's theory positions teachers as people who have little control over their actions in the classroom or over the curriculum material and learning outcomes. This is partly because those who have power in the field determine what is valued and partly because teachers, by and large, act in compliance to maintain rather than transform their position in the field. So, while useful in explaining the conditions under which teachers come to hold their beliefs, attitudes and values, Bourdieu's theory is unable to offer insight into how teachers not only produce identity in relations of power, but also how they *rely* on power in productions of 'self.'

The limitations in Bourdieu's theory led me to Giddens's (1984) theory of structuration. His theory offers a more nuanced explanation of subjectivity through a conception of the relationship between structure and agency as dialectic rather than dualistic, as Bourdieu suggests.[10] Rather than assume, as Bourdieu does, that people operate in a pre-structured world, structures in Giddens's view serve as resources people draw on in order to map out their plans of action. To him structures enable as well as constrain people's actions. Unlike Bourdieu, Giddens proposes that structures do not function outside the individual. Rather, agents embody structures that operate as "memory traces" that they instantiate or call up through their practices (Giddens, 1984: 25). He argues that structures comprise certain features that are long lasting and not bound by, but extend beyond, time and space. Such an expansion, however, is only achievable because of the likelihood that agents, in developing their own theories of social systems, reify systems thus making them seem durable and unalterable. In this section, I also briefly describe how Giddens relies on Goffman's

10 While Bourdieu's proposes a shift in arguments on structure and agency, he introduces a different dialectical set of relations, between those who do and those who do not possess power. So while on the one hand he moves away from some dichotomies, he reinserts a different set of dualistic relations and often renders the subject passive, unable to exercise agency apart from maintaining and reproducing the same sets of power relations.

concepts of co-presence and framing to expand his ideas on subjectivity. His explanation was useful for this work in that it offered tools to unearth and describe the resources teachers draw on to construct a 'self'. So while Bourdieu offered tools to describe and reveal the conditions and broader context in which the self is constructed, Giddens offered tools to explain how this construction occurs through a dialectic relationship between structures and agency. The explanations of both these theorists, however, do not go far enough in explaining difference or in offering insight into the way in which subjects – in this case, teachers – 'take up' different subject positions outside the normative script. The role and use of power is underplayed in subject formation and there is no explanation beyond its constitutive role in dominating and regulating social action. These theorists do not give an account of the ambivalent relationship between the social and the psyche and offer little insight into ways in which subjects are not only dominated by, but also rely on power for their very existence (Butler, 1997).

Limitations in the theories adumbrated above led me to draw on aspects of psychoanalysis and feminist theory to explain subject positioning. The framework I use to end Part II relies primarily but not exclusively on Butler's theory of performativity. In explaining this theory, I draw indirectly on Foucault's notion of power and discourse, and Lacan's and Althusser's emphasis on the role of language in subject formation. These theorists argue that one cannot explain subject formation without explaining how power works internally (relied on by the subject) and externally (as a form of domination). This differs from the theories discussed above, in which constructions of power are construed only as a process or means of domination. It is this framework that helped me tease out how teachers, rather than unthinkingly reproducing learning outcomes, make choices, act and position themselves in ways that sometimes comply but at other times work against or subvert the very discourse they invoke in the first place. Butler's theory of performativity helped me explain the topological complexity of teachers' positions as well as how teachers are not only produced in relations of power, but also how they use power to produce particular subject positions in teaching sexuality and HIV/AIDS. As already stated in the introduction, such explanations of teacher positioning challenge the notions that schools are the best spaces for mediating sexuality and HIV/AIDS, and that teachers are strategically positioned to mediate. In fact, it brings the process of mediation under scrutiny.

2 Dominant sociological debates in understanding social action

Fundamentally, social science is concerned with how we claim to understand social action and activity. Early explanations of how society works tended to describe it in terms of the "fixed arrangements of the parts of the social system that constrain the actions of actors in that system" (Cheal, 2005: 137). As will become clearer later in the discussion, more recent explanations have evolved to include an explanation of structures as fluid, unstable and open to change. Cheal (2005) identifies five broad concepts that he claims constitute the major debates in social theory. These include debates over the unit of analysis; modes of explanation, key factors to be used in explanations of social evolution; the relationship between sociology and ideology, and finally the debate over structure and agency (2005: ix). While these factors are interrelated, the key issue for the purpose of this discussion is the tension between structure and agency and its relevance in understanding social action.

I limit the discussion here since my unit of analysis is the teacher and the interactions that occur in the Lifeskills classroom when sexuality and HIV/AIDS are taught. Even though teachers are the focus, I start from the premise that they are situated in contexts in and through which they make meaning of their lives, as individuals and as teachers, but also to which they contribute. Therefore, the basis of the work this book reports on is the notion that the interconnection between structures (in this case teachers' [hi]stories and lived experience, discourses of sexuality, disease, HIV/AIDS, teaching, schooling) and their individual lives and experiences (as role model, partner, wife/husband, mother/father, son/daughter, colleague, and so forth) is complex, and open to negotiation, competition, contradiction, production, reproduction, and transformation.

Humans are distinguished from other living things by their ability to reason, act, and know what they are doing (Giddens, 1987). Giddens states that humans are, "concept-bearing agents, whose concepts in some part constitute what it is they are up to, not contingently, but as an inherent element of what it is they are up to" (1987: 2–3). In other words, as human beings we can articulate reasons for our actions in ways that enable us to make meaning of our daily lives. Moreover, and for the most part, we are able to explain our actions. In some way, Giddens (1987) argues, our actions hold some 'truth' for us, some reason for doing what we do or else those actions would not be conceived or established or continued in the first place. Fundamentally, how we come to know, to reason and act, is the question that divides groups of social scientists. In other words, it is reason, and the epistemological basis of reason that comprise a key area of disagreement among social scientists (Dodd, 1999). For some, one can reach a level of 'truth' by systematically applying reason and forming deducible conclusions. For others, reason means "rigorous and methodical doubt" (Dodd, 1999: 5). Another group considers reason to be culturally determined and, as such, culture specific (Dodd, 1999; Giddens, 1987). In other words, one cannot assume that taken-for-granted practices in one context are transferable or understood to mean the same thing in another context. Nevertheless, in a familiar context and for the most part, we are able to describe and offer a rationale for our actions in a way that is understandable to those who share some understanding of the practices in which the action is displayed. Put differently, we can find a way of explaining the conventions that govern our lives. Giddens points out that much of what we come to know about the practices that shape our lives, is not only contextual; it is "practical and *ad hoc* in nature" (1987: 7). However, he suggests that we are often not able fully to describe or verbalise reasons for our actions. The reasons we put forward for particular actions, he suggests, are not always the complete story. To him, the conversations about our actions and the reasons we put forward do not comprise complete disclosure (either of our actions or the reasons for our actions), but rather reveal only certain aspects of what we do in our daily lives. There is what he calls "a highly non-discursive side to our activities" (1987: 7), which is of interest in this work.

Often, two broad classificatory frameworks, modernist and post-modernist, are used to describe differences in social theory perspectives. Briefly and generally, modernists tend to hold objectivist perspectives and post-modernists, subjectivist views (Dodd, 1999). Dodd makes the point that these two concepts are not so much theories as they are projects relating to standards that regulate social action or social order. He defines such a normative project as "a system of thought and belief which is concerned in some way with improving society" (1999: 2). To him, there is an explicitness about the way rules and regulations prescribe how society reproduces itself even though the conventions governing values and beliefs are not explicit or fixed (Dodd, 1999).

Dodd (1999) suggests that in the modernist project, reason is used as the epistemological foundation for understanding social theory and, as such, is not dependent on or determined by culture or context. Postmodernists, on the other hand, assume that one cannot understand reason outside of culture and context. Within such a view, reason is understood as caught up in the dynamic of power and, as such, is a "distortion of attempts by theorists to make sense of the world" (Dodd, 1999: 5). These positions and interpretations of reason form the fundamental points of difference amongst early social scientists (see Delanty, 1999; Dodd, 1999; and Giddens, 1982 for discussion of the origins, arguments, and critiques of social theory).

Distinctions in social theory can also be understood as differences in perspectives between functionalists and structuralists on the one hand and hermeneutic and interpretive social scientists on the other (Cassell, 1993). Functionalists and structuralists are similar in that they conceive of the social system in a naturalistic, positivistic, objectivist and holistic manner. Structures act to order and regulate individuals that make up the system to simply perform pre-scripted roles.

Functionalists appeal to biology and naturalist constructions to explain social order and action. To them these are organizing frameworks for understanding structure and the operation of the social system.

Structuralists, on the other hand, are averse to functionalist notions of evolution and biological determinism. To them, "the homology between natural and social science is primarily a cognitive one in so far as each is supposed to express similar features of the overall constitution of mind" (Cassell, 1993: 88).

Hermeneutic theorists postulate that society cannot be explained outside human experience. As Cassell states, "subjectivity is the preconstituted centre of the experience of culture and history and as such provides the basic foundation of the social and human science" (1993: 89). He suggests that what lies outside of subjective experience is a material world that is governed by "impersonal relations of cause and effect" (Cassell, 1993: 89). Whereas in structuralist and functionalist perspectives primacy is given to the role of structures and their constraining effects on human action, interpretive and hermeneutic constructions of social action advance theories that propose human action as having priority over structures (Cassell, 1993).

Significant shifts in thinking have occurred within discourses on social theory in the last few decades (see Giddens, 1982). The main shift, as Giddens sees it, is a notable emphasis on the "active reflexive character of human conduct" (1982: xvi). In other words, most theorists tend now to work from the premise that human action is not dictated by external structures that the individual does not understand or control. Recent perspectives incorporate an understanding of the complexity of the relations between social institutions or practices and human action, while also acknowledging the fundamental role of language in explaining aspects of our daily life (Giddens, 1982).

What is clear from the above is that many social theorists have turned to more inclusive frameworks in their attempt to explain the complexity of human social activity. This notwithstanding, many still find it a challenge to put aside the objectivist and subjectivist binaries. Often theorists begin from a position where they refute the usefulness or highlight the difficulty of using these categories, but end up rehabilitating these very categories in their attempt to develop a different theory or perspective. The theorists I rely on in this work do exactly that; they explain why the binaries are unhelpful but at the same time invoke them to produce, displace, and reintroduce their positions. Each of the social theorists I use, therefore, offers more complex perspectives on social activity through explaining subject formation and subjectivity. For the purposes of this work, they put forward arguments that not only shed light on how teachers come to understand who they are, but also on ways in which dominant structures influence their understanding, experience and subsequent action.

3 Subject formation and Bourdieu's theory of practice

Bourdieu (1990) finds debates on structure and agency unhelpful since they do not adequately address the complexity inherent in social relations. He argues that debates polarise notions of social practice, creating an oppositional stance between subjectivism and objectivism. Instead, he suggests that social life is best understood when one considers the interrelationship between the "objective material, social and cultural structures and the constituting practices and experiences of individuals and groups" (Postone, LiPuma & Calhoun, 1993: 3).

Bourdieu's theory of practice is essentially concerned with how to understand and explain the interaction between "people's practices and the contexts in which those practices occur" (Webb, Schirato & Danaher, 2002: 21). To Bourdieu, subjects act as agents in the construction, modification, and transformation of society, social practices, and institutions. It is in their activity that they construct, reproduce, modify and transform social action. In essence, one cannot understand "social activity outside the action of the subjects" (Krais, 1991: viii). Bourdieu proposes that people are constituted within and by the practices in which they participate. Importantly though, they act to produce and transform the practices that serve to produce their actions in the first place. These practices include discourses, institutions, rules, regulations, and values. Further, these attitudes and values are not simply understood, produced, and reproduced, but are also where those participating act to produce the practice. Calhoun, *et al.* put it this way: "the various practical projects of different people, the struggles in which they engage, and the relations of power which push and pull them nonetheless reproduce the field of relations of which they are a part" (1993: 72).

Bourdieu refers to structures or contexts as 'cultural fields', which include, but are not restricted to discourses, rules, rituals, conventions, values, institutions, and regulations (Webb, *et al.*, 2002). These structures are constituted as hierarchized, meaning that within any constituted discursive space, certain discourses and activities are produced and legitimated as more authoritative than others. But importantly, too, he argues that 'cultural field' is also composed out of and a result of conflict that arises when groups or individuals challenge that which is understood as constituting capital in the field. To Bourdieu, the cultural field, constituted within power relations, is a dynamic discursive space that is not only made up of rules and institutions but also of the interrelationships between institutions, rules and practices (Webb, *et al.*, 2002). It is in the cultural field, Bourdieu (1990, 1977) suggests, that attitudes and practices are produced and transformed, since subjects actively participate to produce them just as they are produced by them. As Postone, *et al.* suggest, social life is "a mutually constituting interaction of embodied knowledge of those structures and enduring orientations to action which, in turn, are constitutive of social structures" (1993: 4). This means that these courses of action are simultaneously 'structured structures', and 'structuring structures' (Calhoun, *et al.*, 1993: 4). Put differently, structures influence human action in as much as they structure and are structured by, in and through social practice. Practice in this sense is understood as resulting from a process of 'improvisation' that is shaped by cultural factors, personal life paths/cycles, and the capacity to "play the game of social interaction" (Postone, *et al.*, 1993: 4). Bourdieu (1990) accepts that cultural fields have a role to play in the production, dissemination and authorisation of different versions of social reality. He insists that such fields are motivated and informed primarily by self-interest and internal competition. How competition plays out is discussed later in this section.

Societies, Bourdieu argues, are constituted by a range of independent *fields*. A field is "a structure of relationships between positions" (in Cheal, 2005: 155). Postone, *et al.* suggest that Bourdieu's concept of *field* is "to provide the frame for 'relational' analysis,' by which he means an account of the multi-dimensional space of positions and the position taking of agents" (1993: 5). Positions result from an interaction between a "person's *habitus* and his/her place in a field of positions as defined by the distribution of the appropriate form of capital" (Postone, *et al.*, 1993: 5). According to Bourdieu (1992) these positions are constituted objectively but have material effects on agents within any specific field. They are constituted within and through power relations and that within any field, one finds a distribution of capital along lines of power and superiority, the latter of which results from the amount of capital an agent has at his/her disposal (Bourdieu & Wacquant, 1992). Bourdieu compares the distribution of power and superiority and how these are constituted relationally in a field to understanding 'the game'. To him people play the game in relation to the amount of capital available to them and in relation to each other. In other words, those who have capital have the power to authenticate and validate what constitutes capital in a specific field. Sometimes but not always, what is valued as 'authentic' capital in one field does not translate as 'authentic' in another field. However, there are times when overlaps may occur. This also means that in order to participate or play the game, there has to be some co-operation between those who have and those who do not have capital. Not all those operating in the field are allowed or given access to play the game. A characteristic feature of *field*, then, is the distinction between those who are allowed to play the game and those who are denied access to the rules of the game. This relationship is constituted in competition and is, therefore, not so simple.

Each *field* is located within an "institutional field of power, and even more broadly, in a field of class relations" (Postone, *et al.*, 1993: 6). Capital (economic or symbolic) accumulated in one field is sometimes transposable to another. Fields are, therefore, not wholly autonomous. The amount (quantitatively and qualitatively) of capital one accumulates through life defines and/or determines one's social standing as well as one's life chances. As such, capital works to produce class stratification. The upshot is that within society, agents will endeavour competitively to gain capital of whatever form within fields. Each discursive field is by its very nature conflictual and within it are struggles and contestations of power. Competition, therefore, is an inherent feature of the field, since those operating in a specific field either vie for capital or to define what capital is valued. Those who obtain 'valued capital' make the rules and thereby gain access to play the game. Competition may also exist within and between fields because fields sometimes have to compete to be defined as a field (Postone, *et al.*, 1993: 5). Class and capital are defining features within and between fields.

Agents employ strategies either to stay in the game, conserve or gain capital, or transform the field by changing the rules of the game. Those who have a monopoly will usually work to conserve power and withhold the rules from those who do not have much capital. Bourdieu (1992) argues that rules can be changed only when values associated with the type of capital are changed. Sometimes, those who are not as invested work to undermine the capital of the dominant group, employing strategies that are often subversive. The suggestion here is that different groups compete in self-interest irrespective of the social class or status. Each competes for capital (symbolic and economic) and does so in ways that are not obvious or explicit.

Capital, Bourdieu (1977, 1990) suggests, refers to a form of worth associated with culturally legitimated and authenticated practices, tastes, dispositions, patterns of utilization, characteristics and competencies deemed valuable or 'worthy' within a field (Bourdieu, 1984; Webb, *et al.*, 2002). According to Bourdieu (1991), capital offers access to power in a field during specified periods of time. As Cheal suggests, capital refers to "a possession that gives individuals the ability to do certain things, such as exercising domination over other(s)" (2005: 156). Capital, as such, is constituted in relations of power: those who possess capital in the field have the power to legitimate, authenticate, and distinguish practices of worth. Possessing capital means that one has "control over one's own future and that of others, making power an integral ingredient" (Postone, *et al.*, 1993: 4).

Bourdieu (1986) suggests that capital functions to structure society through the differentiated and unequal distribution of social, cultural, and economic capital. Briefly, social capital is "the sum of resources, actual or virtual, that accrue to an individual or a group by virtue of possessing a durable network of more or less institutionalized relations of mutual acquaintance and recognition" (Bourdieu & Wacquant, 1992: 119). Social capital is 'accumulated' or made available through interactions and associations with other people who possess social, cultural, and economic capital. It is, however, not only the number of people with whom one interacts, but also the quality of people that offer social capital. In other words, the more one associates with those who possess economic or cultural capital, the greater one's own social capital (Bourdieu, 1986). Social capital, therefore, is constituted by group membership or social network. Networks or relationships are constituted, sustained, and practiced in and through material and symbolic exchanges. The mutual obligations (to be seen as contributing to maintaining relationships) and benefits (resulting from this association) provide the reason for sustaining the relationship because they invoke subjective feelings of gratitude, respect and friendship (Cheal, 2005). This mutual interrelationship requires work, active participation, and contribution by members in the network.

Exchanges in a social network require access to resources (economic, time, etc.). The more resources at one's disposal, the more viable one's social capital. Therefore, those with economic capital stand a better chance of gaining social capital, especially if this resource is coupled with social competencies and knowledge of 'social relations' (Cheal, 2005: 158).

One has economic capital when one has access to financial resources that are easily convertible into money. Those who own shares in the financial market and have property that they can convert into money, have access to economic power. Those with economic power are generally, but not always, high on the hierarchical social ladder because, in the final analysis, economic capital is one of the key indicators in class differentiation (Bourdieu, 1986). While Bourdieu accepts this as important in understanding how capital works, he also rejects any Marxist, objectivist interpretation that uses economic capital in simplistic ways as the primary classificatory tool or mode for explaining class and social inequalities. He states that a Marxist perspective on the association between economic capital and social class does not provide an explanation that considers the "specific contributions that representations of legitimacy make to the exercise and perpetuation of power" (in Swartz & Zolberg, 2004: 39).

Cultural capital is "the knowledge and tastes that are transmitted within families and schools, and that mark those who possess them as socially superior to those who do not" (Cheal, 2005: 158). For Bourdieu, cultural capital is a marker of social class, an aspect that is important for understanding social stratification. In *Distinction* (1984), Bourdieu offers an elaborated explanation of how knowledge and tastes are acquired and mediated through socialisation and education. Families maintain class membership through making available to their offspring the means to continuing education and through a development of taste in art (aesthetics). To him, an interest in art is one manifestation of cultural gains and is closely associated with educational and social capital. Cultural capital is appropriated only by understanding the meanings associated with, for example, the art form, or mathematical equations, literary texts, etc. and in order to do so, one must already "possess the necessary schemes of appreciation and understanding" (Swartz & Zolberg, 2004: 41). Acquiring dispositions and tastes is a lengthy process that requires investment of time (e.g. the educational processes of schooling and university). Cultural capital is also not static but dynamic and results from interactions mediated by power relations in the cultural field. As Swartz and Zolberg (2004: 43) state:

> Because cultural capital exists in an incorporated state, as a system of internalised dispositions, the payoff is contingent on the existence of gate-keeping mechanisms that regulate access to desirable dispositions by somehow taking account of cultivated dispositions – by attending, for example, to the intangibles of style and manner.

Bourdieu refers to symbolic capital as the "power of constructing reality" (1991: 166). He argues that Marxist objectivist notions do not consider the importance of symbolic capital and how it is constituted, maintained, and reliant on relations of power. Symbolic capital is the "capacity to construct beliefs about the world and make them seem real" (Cheal: 2005: 159). In other words, symbolic capital in a sense embodies the other three capitals even though it is not reliant on any for its maintenance. The currency of this form of capital is symbols and their representation and signification. In some instances, symbolic capital can take the form of reputation, prestige or fame and at other times it can be the trust and respect associated with certain symbols. Swartz and Zolberg (2004: 39) state that:

> Symbolic capital and economic capital are distinct though (under certain conditions and at certain rates) mutually convertible forms of power, obeying distinct logics of accumulation and exercise; and that the logic (of symbolic or economic) self-interest underlying certain practices (including contemporary society, most practices in the cultural domain) is misperceived as a logic of disinterest, and that this misperception is what legitimates these practices and thereby contributes to the reproduction of the social order in which they are embedded.

Bourdieu (2000) also explains how struggle for capital (power) operates in a field by introducing two constructs: reproduction and transformation. Those in the field will, for the most part, modify their expectations of what capital might be available to them. They make deductions based on what he calls "subjective hope and objective chances" regarding whether or not the action is worth the risk. The effect is that agents will adjust expectations according to how they are positioned in the field and how likely they think they are to change that position. If they deduce that the 'profit' might be low, the chances that they will participate in playing the game are low. They base their expectations and the likelihood of change on their social and family background, status and class, and the like. Often, therefore, those with the least capital are less ambitious and less likely to participate in competing for capital in the field. They would often seem more acquiescent, even fatalistic, about their position. Bourdieu (2000: 217) describes it this way:

> The realistic, even resigned or fatalistic, dispositions which lead members of the dominated classes to put up with objective conditions that would be judged intolerable or revolting by agents otherwise disposed can have the appearances of purposiveness only if it is forgotten that, by a paradoxical counterfinality of adaptation to reality, they help to reproduce the conditions of oppression.

Sometimes, though, agents with the least capital compete in the field. In some cases, they experience a level of success or win, thereby increasing their value and affecting a change in their status. Under more drastic circumstances, such transformations might lead to a change of authenticated or legitimated capital in a specific field, thereby leading to a change in what is valued in that field. Bourdieu is, however, fatalistic in his outlook about whether or not such transformations are possible. He suggests that the likelihood of such transformations occurring is low because children are already implicated or predisposed by their '*habitus*'. The '*habitus*' is described as the way individuals "on the one hand become themselves – develop attitudes and dispositions – and, on the other hand, ways in which those individuals engage in practices" (Webb, *et al.*, 2002: xii)". The *habitus* of the agent (for example, family background) disqualifies them from entry into the game. Bourdieu argues that social games are not fair and that "without being, strictly speaking, rigged, the competition resembles a handicap race that has lasted for generations ..." (2000: 215). In essence, Bourdieu suggests that fields reproduce themselves and that the forms of symbolic capital regulate how and how not (or whether or not) capital is distributed and redistributed. The way in which fields maintain the type of symbolic power and the capital that is valued in the field is through four strategies or modes of operation: misrecognition, improvisation, *illusio* and universalisation (Webb, *et al.*, 2002).

Bourdieu believes that symbolic power is in evidence when agents "voluntarily give up power, because they believe that the particular person has the power to do things" (Cheal, 2005: 161). Symbolic power is maintained, in the first instance, not in the form of domination or self-interest but in the form of perceived benefit for others: for the universal or general good. For the most part, self-interest is objectified. Symbolic power here exists "because the person who submits to it believes that it exists" (Bourdieu, 1991: 192). Because people believe that those who have symbolic capital have power, they give over their own power voluntarily.

But, Bourdieu, in agreement with Nietzsche (1966), posits that people always act out of self-interest under all circumstances. He suggests that there is no such thing as a 'disinterested act' and that people have a 'will to power' (Nietzsche, 1966). They masquerade their specific acts as universal when in effect all activities are informed by the notion of self-interest. All activities, Bourdieu (1991) suggests, are embedded in and governed by the rules of the specific field in which the activity takes place, as well as by the agent's place in that field.

Bourdieu (1990) explains that self-interest works to mask what is actually happening on two levels. For the one holding symbolic power, self-interest is masked as a person operating in the interest of the field. However, for those holding the least power, it is viewed as the way the world is anyway and, as such, power is voluntarily given over. Any action, he suggests, is only conceivable in self-denial. One way in which these mutually dependable forms of practice operate and are separated, (and, therefore, sustainable) is through the use of a style of language (abstracted and referential) that seems to have little connection with the social world. Bourdieu, like Nietzsche and Wittgenstein (in Webb, 2002), understands language "not as a mirror reflecting a pre-given reality but as a *practice* that 'makes the world' or at least determines how we understand it" (Webb, *et al.*, 2002: 13).

Being able to play the game, therefore, requires knowing the rules and the associated style and use of language characteristic of the specific field. But it also requires an understanding of the meanings attached to the language. All forms of language have a historicity while at the same time, are "empty content" (Webb, *et al.*, 2002: 14). Those who assume authority within and across fields compete to inscribe their respective meanings of language, and its concomitant symbolic capital. In this regard Bourdieu writes, "the obstacles to comprehension, perhaps especially when social things are in question, have less, as Wittgenstein observed, to do with the understanding than with the will" (2000: 8)

Another manifestation of symbolic power is through what Bourdieu (1990) calls symbolic violence. Misrecognition is fundamental to understanding symbolic violence. Violence here is understood as the enforcement of power in ways that cannot be explained in rational or justifiable terms. But this enforcement is not forceful; rather it operates through complicity. For Bourdieu, symbolic violence is that which is done to the agent with his or her complicity, essentially because he/she misrecognises the conditions of his/her existence. Agents are complicit in the act, because as Bourdieu suggests, they are caught up in it. They implicitly recognise the existence of hierarchy in the field but rationalise it as the way the world is, as 'natural' and given (Webb, *et al.*, 2002; Cheal, 2005). Bourdieu (2000: 142–43) puts it this way:

> The agent engaged in practice knows the world but with a knowledge which, as Merleau-Ponty showed, is not set up in the relation of externality of a knowing consciousness. He knows it, in a sense, too well, without objectifying distance, takes it for granted, precisely because he is caught up with it; bound up with it; he inhabits it like a garment [*un habit*] or a familiar habitat. He feels at home in the world because the world is also in him, in the form of *habitus*, a virtue made of necessity which implies a form of love of necessity.

Understanding it as 'the way it is' means that people do not question the hierarchical nature of relations but reproduce it because they are encased in the *habitus*. He uses the term '*illusio*' to explain this. '*Illusio*' refers to the way in which agents almost blindly adhere to the rules of the game, the capital, and its symbolic value because the rules are carried in their '*habitus*'. The rules of the game, according to Bourdieu, are always in one's head.

Explaining the third construct of Bourdieu's theory of practice, '*habitus*', is important in order to understand the agent's capacity for what Bourdieu calls 'structured improvisation'. I have already alluded to this above, but briefly, *habitus* is

> [...] a system of general generative schemes that are both durable (inscribed in the social construction of the self) and transposable (from one field to another), function on an unconscious plane, and take place within a structured space of possibilities (defined by the intersection of material conditions and fields of operation). (Calhoun, *et al.,* 1993: 4)

Put simply, *habitus* is a set of dispositions embodied by an agent as a result of the social, economic, and cultural resources available, particularly early on in a person's life. These act as internal radar and predispose the agent to act or respond in a certain way. As Cheal puts it, "[t]he dispositions generate perceptions, attitudes and practices which are predictable without being consciously articulated or governed by any rule" (2005: 160). As conditions change under new circumstances, the *habitus* is affected by them in ways that either reinforce or modify it (Bourdieu & Wacquant, 1992). People are socialised through the day-to-day practices in their everyday lives. *Habitus,* therefore, is acquired in practice. Practices differ across space and time and thus people within the same field can certainly acquire different *habitus* through various social trajectories that are embedded in a context. In other words, practices have a historicity and are thus structured. The *habitus* acts as the lens or frame of reference through which new experiences are filtered. Bourdieu suggests that early experience is dominant and is in some way deterministic in shaping later behaviour, attitudes, and values. To him, these early experiences solidify an agent into a position that is difficult to change (Cheal, 2005).

Bourdieu's theory of practice is useful in that it offers tools to explain social practice as constituted in a complex interaction between structure and agent. He offers a useful critique of the objectivist/subjectivist dichotomy by demonstrating, particularly through the concept of *habitus,* how the agent inhabits structure, and how the agent is produced and at the same time acts to produce and reproduce structures. Bourdieu explains social practice as the interconnection between "class *habitus* and current capital as realized within the specific logic of a given field" (Calhoun, *et al.*, 1993: 6). He also provides a persuasive argument concerning the ways in which power produces and is produced in fields of practice. Accordingly, an agent's capital is an outcome of the *habitus* in as much as the distinctive nature of a field is an "objectified history that embodies the *habitus* of agents who have operated in the field" (Bourdieu, 1993: 6). The self-reflective nature of the *habitus* is underscored, in that each time it is invoked in practice, it displays itself as both embodied and as objectified history (Calhoun, *et al.*, 1993).

Understanding the interrelationship between field, *habitus* and capital enables us to develop, according to Calhoun, *et al.* (1993), a reflexive approach to social life, and goes a long way in helping us understand the production of social structure and its associated dispositions and attitudes; an understanding located within concepts of emancipation. To Bourdieu, the examination of human life is unproductive if it does not provide the chance for agents to understand the significance of their own actions within and between fields. As Calhoun, *et al.* indicate, "[his] approach seeks to illuminate the social and cultural reproduction of inequality by analysing processes of misrecognition: that is, by investigating how *habitus* of the dominated groups can veil the conditions of their subordination" (1993: 6).

Bourdieu's theory of practice was helpful in a number of ways for this work. First, it provided a framework for managing and reporting the data in a systematic way (see Chapters 9 and 10). Bourdieu's insistence on the importance of context in shaping early experiences became one of the key indicators shaping these chapters. In Chapter 9, I provide a description of the material and social conditions in which this cohort of teachers makes meaning of their day-to-day experiences. This chapter applies Bourdieu's theoretical tools to describe and explain the nature and quality of the capital that teachers draw on. It also serves to situate the content of the following chapter of the analysis (10), namely a description of the dominant early influences on subject formation and subjectivity. I not only describe the early influences, but also indicate ways in which this cohort of teachers is positioned and indeed, how they position themselves in the respective fields of practice in which they operate.

Application of Bourdieu's theory, therefore, made it possible for me to identify and describe dominant structures, as well as explain how they are constituted. In addition, I was able to trace how rules in one field of practice get transposed or modified and operationalised in another field. Importantly too, I was able to describe how teachers modify their behaviour in one field as a result of the rules applicable in another field of practice. In essence, Bourdieu's theory of practice enabled me to explain how these teachers come to be who they are as well as to describe the conditions that shape their attitudes, beliefs, and experiences. However, as the next section explicates, Bourdieu's theory cannot tell the whole story since it offers no insight into how teachers exercise agency to make choices outside a predetermined script.

Limitations in Bourdieu's theory of practice

Bourdieu's theory of practice takes as its point of departure the assumption that people act and are acted upon, mostly in 'unconscious', 'amnesiac', or 'mindful forgetfulness' ways. For the most part, people act out of self-interest to position and determine their role, status, and power in the social field. They also, through misrecognition, and through an embodied *habitus*, reproduce positions and relations of dominance and subordination. As indicated above, such a theorisation is useful for developing the argument that early experiences shape identity. It is also useful in tracing how agents might act in complicit ways to reproduce hierarchical relations of power. However, it is simply not the case that agents are always complicit. They often act to reproduce different sets of power relations. Yet for Bourdieu, action more often than not produces and reproduces in order to maintain rather than transform relations of power and redistribute capital (i.e. change the rules of the game). The resilience of *habitus* in his explanation is problematic in a number of ways. *Habitus* is understood as predisposing an agent and thereby serving as a constraint limiting the chances for transformation. Bourdieu also introduces a different dialectical set of relations, between those who have and those who do not possess power. Power is divisive since the struggles in the field revolve around control and capital gain.

Bourdieu defines power as primarily external to the individual; as residing in structures that, as Butler says, "press on the subject from the outside" (1997: 2). In his conception, power, closely associated with capital, is that which emanates from positioning by the '*habitus*' and acts to subordinate, constrain, and maintain capital status. His concept of power foregrounds a subject who has very little maneuverability outside the predetermined script because structures are imposed from the outside. While he describes an embodied subject, to him forms of embodiment are only relevant in as much as they reproduce and maintain existing forms of power. To him power informs and maintains the status quo. In other words, he does not account for how power *forms* (my emphasis) the subject; how the subject depends on it for its existence (Butler, 1977). He, therefore, pays little attention to concepts of power that describe how subjects are formed in and through relations of power rather than only through power dynamics. Such an omission reinforces a deterministic orientation and leaves little room for agency.

Second, the inherent features in his explanation of *habitus* assume that societies are largely stable entities that reproduce themselves through the practices or actions of those operating within them. Change occurs only as a function of reproduction as opposed to transformation. Societies are slow to change because practices that serve as mechanisms of production and reproduction are constant.

Bourdieu's construction of *habitus* is also problematic for feminists who are offended by the absence of a nuanced account of gender in his work. His theory tends to naturalize gender, and he underplays the extent to which dominant discourses depend upon masculinised constructions of social reality.

Relatedly, constructions of the body are under-theorised in his work. As de Silva (2005: 91) puts it, Bourdieu "places emphasis on the body as the site from which the naturalisation processes of masculine domination proceed." In his theory the sexed body, standing outside culture and history, is used to frame distinctions between the masculine and the feminine. Sex thus provides the site for the construction of gender, explicitly understood as "sexually characterised *habitus*" (Bourdieu, 2001: 3). He makes nature, and particularly an understanding of the biologically sexed body, central in his attempt to reveal and explain the constancy of the *habitus* of a sexually ordered social order. He does not account for societies where sex differences are not characteristically the defining feature and in so doing assumes an essential unproblematised body.

While Bourdieu is useful in understanding the complexity of structure and agent, the limitations of his theory lie in his not giving primacy to human action outside of the dichotomous relations of power. Within such a theory of practice, transformations only work to reinforce capital status in the field, and as such offer little agency outside of perpetuating power relations. There is very little chance to change the field within such a construction of social practice. As it pertains to this work, Bourdieu's theory does not allow one to examine the iterativity in the relationship between teachers and teaching beyond the expected or anticipated, because dispositions are already necessarily assumed.

The metaphors invoked in Bourdieu's theory, those of 'playing the game' and knowing the 'rules of the game', assume a linearity and orderliness of social action that do not offer ways of examining rules as both regulative and constitutive.

This study therefore needed additional theoretical tools capable of explaining why some teachers reported on seemed less restricted by structure and were thus able to act differently. In fact, I needed to explain why some teachers act differently from the way prescribed; why they subvert the given discourse and reinsert a different one, and how they do this. Giddens, who understands structures as a resource that both constrains and enables rather than merely constrains, was useful in extending our explanation of human action beyond Bourdieu's framework. His theory of structuration is described in the next chapter.

4 Subjectivity and Giddens's theory of structuration

Giddens offers a perspective on structure and agency quite different from that postulated by other social theorists. For the most part, theorists like Bourdieu have developed frameworks that demonstrate a complex interrelationship between structure and agent, but downplay the agent's ability to transform structures. These frameworks assume that structures operate 'external to human action' and as such constrain rather than enable and constrain (Giddens, 1984: 16). Giddens, however, proposes a different concept of the relationship between structure and agent, in which the latter is positioned as resourceful, and structures are seen as resources to draw on rather than solely constraining mechanisms.

Three key elements constitute Giddens's theory of structuration: 'structure', 'system', and 'duality of structure.' To him structures exist as rules and resources that people draw on in order to map out the plans of action in their daily lives. Structures, however, do not function outside of the individual but rather act as "memory traces, and are 'instantiated' in social practice" (Giddens, 1984: 25). Giddens suggests that while this might be the case, structures comprise typical features or what he calls "structuring properties", which are able to withstand the confines of time and space (Giddens, 1998: 25). Structures are durable not because they pre-exist outside the individual as Bourdieu suggests, but rather because people in their day-to-day actions repeat them, thus making them *seem* durable and permanent. According to Giddens (1984: 25–26):

> The reification of social relations, or the discursive naturalization of the historically contingent circumstances and products of human action, is one of the main dimensions of ideology in social life.

Because institutions, rules and discourses are available outside spatial and temporal confines, they have the propensity to make people repeat the same performances or activities over time. Their resilience and repetitive nature is inherent. In other words, people draw on structures in order to enact a social practice. But structures do not work to constrain only. Rather, structures work to constrain and enable.

Characteristic of Giddens's description of structures is their disassociation from the subject (Giddens, 1984). In other words, people do not have to be present for a structure to exist. However, and at the same time, the attributes of structures are apparent only when one observes the actions of people in a particular space and time. Structures, therefore, are embedded in a space and time and manifest in agents' instantiated practices.

Social systems are the regularised practices firmly embedded in time/space and are rooted in interdependency. Giddens (1984: 17) puts it this way:

> Systems are the 'patterning of social relations in time and space involving the reproduction of situated practices, and a paradigmatic dimension, involving a virtual order of modes of structuring' recursively implicated in such reproduction.

Structuration refers to the conditions governing the continuity or transformation of structures and, therefore, the reproduction of systems (Giddens, 1979 in Cheal, 2005). According to Giddens, agents draw on the "modalities of structuration in the reproduction of systems of interaction, by the same token reconstituting their structural properties" (1984: 28). So, in structuration theory, the moment an agent produces an action, this is also simultaneously "one of reproduction in the contexts of the day-to-day enactment of social life" (1984: 26). Put simply, agents draw on the rules to enact a social practice but, at the same time, reproduce the structuring features of the practice. This duality of structure presupposes "knowledgeability" by agents, that is, the ability not only to reflect on a social practice but also to reflect on the reflection (Giddens, 1984).

To Giddens agents are knowledgeable about their daily life. They possess noticeably large amounts of knowledge about their lived experience, which they can clearly articulate. However, this 'knowledgeability', what Cheal (2005: 163) calls "gaining and using knowledge about the self", is complex since it is embedded in "practical consciousness" and capability (Giddens, 1984: 163). He describes 'practical consciousness' as that which "actors know about social conditions, including especially the conditions of their own action, but cannot express discursively" (Giddens, 1984: 375). In other words, practical consciousness enables actors to continue with the activities of daily life because it affords them tacit knowledge of its modes of operation. The complexity, in part, derives from agents being occupied primarily with getting on with life, and therefore being more concerned with conduct in their daily routines. And so, while agents are able not only to describe their actions, but also to give reasons for these when requested to do so, their attention is primarily focused on their conduct rather than on the reasons for the conduct. More often than not, though, they are able to rationalise their action when asked to do so. This does not happen routinely. Rather, questions are usually posed when there is an apparent discontinuity between routinised action and what is observed (Giddens, 1984).

People do not engage in social life with explicit motives; they live and act reflexively; people use rules and resources iteratively thereby producing patterns of practice. Practices become routinized only because rules and resources are available over time. Giddens puts it this way: "Routine, psychologically linked to the minimising of unconscious sources of anxiety, is the predominant form of day-to-day social activity" (1984: 282). He describes such reflexivity as an agent's ability to "monitor continuously the flow of activities and expect others to do the same of their own; [they] also routinely monitor aspects, social, physical, of the contexts in which they move" (1984: 5). To him agents continue in their day-to-day practices but at the same time have a mental picture (what he calls a theoretical understanding) of why they engage in these practices. As already articulated, the reason is not the motivation for the action since, as he says, one should not conflate understanding the action with "the discursive giving of reasons for particular items of conduct, nor even with the capability of specifying such reasons discursively" (Giddens, 1984: 5–6). Understanding routinisation in practices is therefore a key element in Giddens's theory since it highlights the duality of structure and agent. It is in the "enactment of routines [that] agents sustain a sense of ontological security" (Giddens, 1984: 282). Therefore, to him all action is constituted in space and time and as such involves the complex intersection of conscious and unconscious, what he calls "unacknowledged conditions/unintended consequences" (Giddens, 1984: 282).

Social systems are sustained only in as much as they are continued in and through social practice "fading away in time" (Giddens, 1984: 83). All social interaction, therefore, is expressed at some point in and through the contextualities of bodily presence. Social actors are positioned in time and space while at the same time holding a social position that is constituted within relations of power, legitimacy, signification, and domination (Giddens, 1984). Social position, therefore, signifies the distinct identity an agent holds within a network of social relations. Positioning, according to Giddens (1984), takes on different meanings. At one level it can mean the position of the corporeal body with all its gestures and expressions in a situation of co-presence with others. Positioning can also mean the "seriality of encounters across time-space" (Giddens, 1984: xxiv). The significance of this differentiation lies in the intersection between these position modalities, that is: every human being is immediately positioned in everyday life situations while simultaneously in the lifespan of his/her existence; and in the "duration of institutional time, the supra-individual' structuration of social institutions" (Giddens, 1984: xxv). Understanding subject positioning, Giddens asserts, is at the heart of understanding structuration theory. He states:

> All social interaction is situated interaction – situated in space and time. It can be understood as the fitful yet routinized occurrence of encounters, fading away in time and space, yet constantly reconstituted within different areas of time-space. The regular or routine features of encounters, in time as well as in space, represent institutionalized features of social systems (1984: 86).

In shedding light on subjectivity and subject positioning, Giddens borrows two concepts from Goffman (1959) that are important for this work, namely, the notion of co-presence and framing. The explanation below becomes significant when, in the analysis, these concepts are used to describe teachers' self-surveillance practices or the way membership of a group or a number of group works as a resource teachers draw on to 'discipline the body' in teacher behaviour. Co-presence (also see Foucault's [1976] notion of the panoptic gaze, which he constructs along similar lines to Goffman's construction of co-presence) is one component in which the bracketing of time-space is both a condition and an outcome of human social association (Giddens, 1984: 36). Giddens invokes Goffman's (1959; 1973) use of the term to describe social interaction and communication with others, sometimes in face-to-face interactions but importantly, often absent in time and space. Co-presence, therefore, is that interaction which holds groups together even in the absence of contiguity in time and space. So, while a distinguishing feature of co-presence is conversation, many other activities may act as the catalyst in holding the group (and/or individual) in a situation of co-presence (Giddens, 1987). Goffman (1973) also distinguishes between co-presence and encounters, the latter of which by definition requires actors to be in a face-to-face relation within the same physical context. In Goffman's work, while all interaction is purposeful, it is not always focused, since in some instances the interaction that holds the group together may be an activity (for example a soccer game) that does not require face-to-face relations. Focussed interaction accordingly shares features that are similar to those found in small group interactions. These include "a division of roles, provision for socialisation, capability for collective action, and sustained modes of connection with the surrounding social environment" (in Giddens, 1987: 115). During encounters, however, other features are present. These include "embarrassment, maintenance of poise, capacity for non-distractive verbal communication, adherence to a code regarding giving up or taking over the speaker role, and allocation of spatial position" (Giddens, 1987: 115).

Framing is associated with control relations and as such, has to do with power. Goffman's definition of framing, as Giddens sees it, suggests that actors "seemingly move in a pre-structured world, in which they must take account of their actions, but which they play no part in bringing into being or perpetuating" (Giddens, 1984: 88–89). Goffman's interpretation of framing, therefore, renders the subject powerless since he proposes a pre-structured social reality in which subjects are predetermined.

Giddens makes the point that paying attention to the reflexive nature of conduct in our daily social lives does not mean a denial of the significance of what he calls the "unconscious sources of cognition and motivation" (1984: 44). The consequence of this discussion, however, lies in the acknowledgement that the concept of self is not stable or fixed, and that the emergence of 'self' and 'me' incorporate an understanding of the shifting nature of 'I'. This means going beyond only understanding the complexity of the linguistic engagement, to requiring a "ramified control of the body and a developed knowledge of how to 'go on' in the plurality of contexts of social life" (Giddens, 1984: 43). Also, it means paying some attention to the distinguishing features that separate 'conscious' from 'unconscious'. In addition, and in understanding the unconscious, it means encompassing an understanding of *memory* as more than a recollection of the past or reference to previous experiences or aspects of the past that have remained dormant in the human being. Giddens suggests that the present is unrecognisable and cannot be written without it "fading into the past" (Giddens, 1984: 45). Relatedly, *perception* is understood as much broader than merely a "set of temporal devices, shaped by, yet shaping, the movements and orientations of the body in the contexts of its behaviour" (Giddens, 1984: 46). Rather, perception is what human agents do; it is integral to their temporal and spatial situated activities (Giddens, 1984).

Unlike Mead's conception of the 'I' as the nucleus of agency (thereby making its inception always concealed), Giddens's (1984) description of 'self' as a 'me' can only be understood when the 'I' is understood in relation to the discourse of the 'other.' According to him this occurs through the acquisition of language, but, as he emphasizes, the 'I' has to be linked to the "body as the sphere of action" (Giddens, 1984: 43). In linguistic terms, the 'I' is not stable or permanent, unlike in Enlightenment beliefs where the notion of the 'self' as a permanent, unchanging, reliable, unifying object (Flax, 1990) is upheld. Giddens (1984) suggests that social positioning determines who is an 'I' in any conversational engagement. What he draws attention to is that the 'I' is not reflective of, nor does it necessarily encompass individual and private features of our experience. It has no meaning in and for itself; its meaning is derived only in conversation or in relation to the 'other'. In other words, 'I' takes on some meaning when there is a 'you'; when 'you' is conscious of being an 'I', and so forth.

It is the interrelationship between these three modes of positioning that provides insight into subjectivity, and that is what is significant here. Understanding teachers as individuals (life-cycle); as agents in a school classroom (time-space); as members of a profession and of one or more communities (relationally positioned) is key to the work reported on in this book. As Giddens (1984: 85) suggests, "only in the context of such intersection within institutionalised practices can modes of time-space positioning, in relation to the duality of structure be properly grasped."

Giddens maintains that all social interaction is positioned interaction and is situated in time and space. He further suggests that the common or recurrent characteristics of encounters, in time and space, "represent institutionalised features of social systems". Routine is embedded in "tradition, custom or habit" but to consider these as unproblematic and simply "repetitive forms of behaviour" is simplistic. Giddens draws on Goffman to suggest that the "routinized character of most activity is something that is worked out continually by those who sustain it in their everyday conduct" (Giddens, 1984: 86).

In summary, intentionality (medium) and unintended consequences or the outcome of social practices are inherent in Giddens's theory. Because agents draw on rather than have rules pressed upon them, they have the capacity to modify and even transform rules. At each point of structural reproduction, there is the potential for change and rupture (Giddens, 1984). Second, drawing on structures to produce action is only one aspect in understanding processes of reproduction; it is not the whole story. The availability of structural resources makes it possible for actors to repeat actions and to engage in routine and recurrent practices in a way that makes them seem natural and reified. Importantly, because there is a visible pattern in routinised behaviour, it is linked to highly generalised forms of motivation; that is, the need to maintain an ideal self – a feeling of being 'at home' within oneself and the world which is also associated with maintaining manageable levels of anxiety.

Before explaining how Giddens's theory of structuration contributed to the analysis of teachers' subjective experiences, I briefly outline its limitations, with a view to shedding light on why, as will become clearer in the final section, in its application, it was insufficient to explain what actually happens in Lifeskills classrooms.

Limitations in Giddens' theory of structuration

Giddens, unlike Bourdieu, does not offer an explanation of how structures are constituted, particularly since he suggests that structure has no reality except in so far as it is 'internal' to agents in the form of memory traces. Agents call 'structure' into being, but at the same time, it is structure which produces the possibility of agency. Such a stance does not account for external power that operates outside the self, that is, regulatory power that forms the subject in the first place. This omission leaves open questions about power and social positioning, since Giddens does not comment on how discourse is made within unequal relations of power.

He does not confront questions about who speaks, who can modify and how modification is understood within a complex set of social relations.

In summary, what I do briefly below is combine the discussion of the previous theories and constructs to highlight how Giddens's theory, in conjunction with Bourdieu's theory of social practice, was useful in developing an explanatory framework to be used later in the analysis sections (Chapters 9, 10). Applying Bourdieu's theory enabled me to do two things, as indicated earlier: namely, to describe the material and social conditions as well as trace the dominant influences on teachers' lives. In so doing, I was able to identify the dominant institutions, rules, and discourses that act as broad frames of reference, structuring the world in which this cohort of teachers operates. Bourdieu thus offered a frame or shell, so to speak, within which I could situate the group of teachers; a particular discursive space. While identity for Bourdieu might include the possibility of multiple positions and choice, the dominant idea is that identity is pre-scripted through the *habitus*. Choice in his theory is only possible within the confines of particular structures; in the case of South Africa, these include race and class (Hetherington, 1998).

What his work, though, was unable to shed light on is (a) how people navigate their way (or how they draw on structures to plan action) in the everyday beyond a prestructured reality shaped by the *habitus*, and (b) how they position themselves outside the normative script. It was here that Giddens's theory became helpful in that he offered a way of examining the interrelationship between past and present and its significance in enabling teachers to map out their day-to-day actions beyond a pre-scripted set of structures. To Giddens, as is common to social theorists working within contemporary frameworks, "the structures of the lifescript are seen as less fixed and certain, the possibilities for producing conventional narratives about work, family, and locality are thought to be no longer possible" (Hetherington, 1998: 23). Giddens's description of structures as embodied, therefore, offered a nuanced way to understand how teachers use institutions (structures), rules, and discourses as resources to plot out their plans of action, while simultaneously being structured (resulting from the durability inherent in structuring features) by them. In other words, Giddens offered me a language to (a) account for difference beyond a predetermined script; (b) describe how teachers draw on structures to make meaning of their daily actions, in and outside the classroom; and (c) trace the ways in which teachers are sometimes constrained while at other times enabled in and through structures. Giddens's theory enabled me to explain how teachers come to understand and describe themselves in a way that foregrounds their agency. I was able to map out experiences in a way that positioned teachers as "in the picture itself" (Hetherington, 1998: 23). In essence, therefore, these theorists made it possible for me to use the data to trace the factors shaping teachers' understanding of experiences involving HIV/AIDS. However, what they were unable to do is provide insight into how teachers position themselves and contribute to this shaping beyond instantiated practice. In other words, the contextual and explanatory tools were limited as an analytical framework for animating what identity positions are taken up in the classroom when teachers teach sexuality and HIV/AIDS.

What was needed, therefore, was a theory model that moved from the explanation of social action to its analysis. While the aim of the study was not to advance a theoretical model, I needed an analytical framework that accounted for how identity is constituted by and engaged in practice; one that accentuated subject positions in the activity of teaching in a way that sheds light on the nexus between teacher identity and teaching. At this juncture, I turned to features of psychoanalysis and feminist theory. In theorising the use of power in understanding subjection, domination, resistance, resignification, and identification, the theories I draw on below enabled me to shift from describing and explaining the conditions under which teachers come to understand who they are, to analysing the subject positions they take up in the everyday as exemplified in their classroom behaviour. In other words, using what follows, I was able to move from explanations of subject formation and subjectivity to developing an analytical tool that offered ways of analysing subject positioning. What follows, therefore, is a brief exposition of an analytical framework that relies primarily but not exclusively on Butler's theory of performativity. In explaining this theory, I draw indirectly draw on Foucault's notion of power and discourse, and Lacan's and Althusser's emphasis on the role of language in subject formation. In particular, I briefly comment on what Foucault's notion of power and Althusser's canon on interpellation offer to the discussion. Through highlighting the limitations in their explanations of subjection, I insert Butler's theory of performativity as the framework that offers possibilities for a different reading of subject positioning, resistance, identification, and resignification.

It is only through combining the explanatory framework above with the theory of performativity below that I was initially able to shed light on how teachers take up positions in constructing their life-script in Chapter 10. More importantly though, it was helpful in animating what is presented in Chapter 11, namely, the multiplicity of subject positions teachers take up in the classroom when they teach sexuality and HIV/AIDS.

5 Subject positioning and Butler's theory of performativity

Discussions on subject positioning are often polarized; according to Hetherington (1998: 23), subject positions are either presented as "choices associated with lifestyle, sexuality, consumption or enthusiasms" or as "subaltern positions of marginality and resistance to marginalization." He suggests too, that choice always comes at a price and that speaking about, for example, 'subaltern positions' does not suggest singularity since the discursive space is constituted in competition among various groups. Non-singularity here also means that subjects themselves do not hold the same position but take up different positions depending on the situation. It is, therefore, no longer possible to take for granted or clearly define the centre or the margin since either can be anything at any given time (Hetherington, 1998). Choices are thought of in a way that presupposes multiplicity of and difference in subject positions, and that acknowledges there is no grand narrative from and through which people construct an identity. Understanding the multiplicity and complexity of subject positions has been the result of work by theorists such as Lacan and Althusser, and more recently, Foucault and Butler.

Structuralist theorists like Lacan and Althusser argue that subjectivity is not stable or essential, but rather constituted either in language or ideology (Hetherington, 1998). Althusser gives a description of the way in which the subject is produced through linguistic modes. This process he describes through his notion of interpellation, where he shows that "the subordination of the subject takes places through language, as the effect of the authoritative voice that hails the individual" (in Butler, 1997: 5). Through the well-known example of the passerby being hailed by a policeman, Althusser explains interpellation by describing how the former responds by turning around, recognizing that he is the one 'hailed.' Butler (1997: 5) explains it this way: "In the exchange by which that recognition is proffered and accepted – interpellation – the discursive production of the social subject – takes place". She states that Althusser's concept of interpellation is based on the premise that power rests with the one who hails the subject into being. His representation of the authoritative, she states, "attributes performative power to the authoritative voice, the voice of sanction, and hence to a notion of language figured as speech" (Butler, 1997: 6). The limitation in this construction as she sees it is that Althusser does not describe what makes the subject respond. In other words, by presupposing that authority lies in the authoritative voice of the state, interpellation assumes a subject who, as in Bourdieu's theory of practice, has already assimilated this position into his conscience (Butler, 1997: 6). So while Althusser's work is useful, it is limited in its application since he assumes a subject constrained (spoken for) by state authority (Butler, 1997). Questioning why the passerby responds to the authoritative voice in the first place, what the role is of the conscience in this 'act' of turning, how one accounts for written discourse, and what the implications are of this 'calling up' a social subject, she says, makes Foucault useful.

For Foucault, power forms the subject, but it is also that which subordinates the subject. This process of forming and subordination occurs simultaneously. In other words, in Foucault's thesis, one cannot consider subject formation without describing subordination. Subject formation and subjection, he argues, takes place in and through discourse (Foucault, 1989a). Subject positions are constituted in discourse and are set up within power/knowledge relationships (Hetherington, 1998). Discourses – understood as "ways of constituting knowledge, together with the social practices, forms of subjectivity and power relations which inhere in such knowledges and the relations between them" (Weedon, 1987: 108) – are potentially bounded, embedded, competitive and contradictory, occurring within what Foucault calls "discursive fields." In this regard Weedon (1987: 35) states that these are "competing ways of giving meaning to the world and of organizing social institutions and processes"; they offer a subject "a range of modes of subjectivity." Discourses do not reside in simple binaries or in relations of power and powerlessness (McLaren in Wyner, 1991) but, rather, are "tactical elements or blocks operating in the field of force relations" (Foucault, 1981: 10). Force relations are the fields comprising social institutions that are the location for 'discursive conflict' where regulatory rules exist. They are "contextually situated and taken up through hierarchically constituted relations of class, race, gender, religion, and age" (Weedon, 1987: 110). For Foucault, no entity (body, thought or emotions) has meaning outside the context of the discursive field in which a broader network of power relations is at play. Importantly, the most influential discourses are articulated within established institutions (like education, medicine or welfare), which are in themselves spaces of contestation (Weedon, 1987). The upshot of this is that, as Hetherington (1998: 24) puts it: "[A]ll we can do, it is argued, is use the subject positions in which we are located to write, not life-scripts but little stories, poems, language games, in which we can rearrange our identities and our identifications with others in partial and contingent ways."

Implied in the above is the notion that identity is never complete. Rather, it is always in the process of being produced within a field of competing discourses, in discursive spaces that do not necessarily carry equal weight and/or power. Important, too, is the recognition that even within a particular discourse, there might be more than one subject position (Weedon, 1987). There might be a privileged position of subjectivity within a particular discourse but, by its very structure, it will imply other subject positions.

According to Butler (1997: 2), the Foucauldian notion of power as that which "presses on the subject from the outside, as what subordinates, sets underneath, and relegates to the lower order" renders the subject passive. In his notion, she suggests, the subject is already caught up "in the scene of psychoanalysis", that is, the subject emerges simultaneously with the unconscious and as such there is indecisiveness from the moment the subject is constituted. The two-mindedness at the point of inception presupposes some form of attachment and dependency by the subject. The assumption that the subject is already subjected, as Butler puts it, takes for granted "a specific psychoanalytic valence when [one] consider[s] that no subject emerges without a passionate attachment to those on whom he or she is fundamentally dependent" (Butler, 1997: 7). Foucault proposes that "this situation of primary dependency conditions the political formation and regulation of subjects and becomes the means of their subjection" (Butler, 1997: 7).

Foucault, though, does not clarify how the body "inhabits daily practices" since he only gives an account of power as subordinating and producing the subject (Aleman in Alexander, Anderson & Gallegos, 2005: 149; McNay, 1992). For Butler there is more. To her, power is that which "form[s] the subject as well as provide[s] the very condition of its existence and the trajectory of its desire" (Butler, 1997: 2). If this be the case, then power is not only that which we go up against or resist but is "what we depend on for our existence and what we harbour and preserve in the beings that we are" (Butler, 1997: 2). She proposes a performative subject who is at the same time produced by power and but also relies on power; one who is not only constituted by but also embodies power.

Performativity assumes a "topological complexity" foregrounding "dispersal, fragmentation, uncertainty, difference, contingency, hybridity, ambivalence and multiplicity" (Hetherington, 1998: 25). In other words, non-singularity in constructions of identity is taken for granted in the notion of performativity (Hetherington, 1998). In this instance these not only infer the possibility of many subject positions, each being contingent on location or the discursive space in which the position is invoked, but also the diversity inherent in the acts themselves. It also means the diffusion of centre and margin positions. However, while this may hold true at one level, at another it is not possible to speak in totally non-essentialist terms. We always speak in relation to an 'other', even if the other does not comprise fixed social structures and relations, but is rather in the in-between spaces between "identity and non-identity and in the recognition of that gap" (Hetherington, 1998: 25).

In theories of performativity, identity is constituted through a "combination and mixing of things at hand and an ordering associated with that process of mixing" (Hetherington, 1998: 26). In her explanation, Butler (1993: 12) states that, "performativity must be understood not as a singular or deliberate act, but rather as the reiterative and citational practice by which discourse produces the effects it names." To her, the materiality of the body relies on power at the point of production, rather than in the way Foucault describes it, as forming or subordinating the material body. The materiality of the body is an effect of power on the part of the subject.

In referring to gender and sex, Butler proposes that gender cannot be understood as that which forms the body or signifies its materiality. In order to understand constructions of gender, she says, one needs to consider the regulatory norms that name it in the first place. In this instance, this means understanding the regulatory norms of sex. To her any explanation of sex cannot assume a neat correlation between sex and gender. Sex cannot be formulated as a foregone agreed upon phenomenon, a natural consequence of human *being* upon which gender is artificially inscribed. Sex in performativity, as Butler (1993: 3) sees it, is constructed as a "cultural norm which governs the materialisation of the body." While sex is not the only regulatory norm that materializes the body, it is certainly an important one. In explaining her thesis, she states:

> [...] once sex is understood in its normativity, the materiality of the body will not be unthinkable apart from the materialization of that regulatory norm. "Sex" is, thus, not simply what one has, or a static description of what one is: it will be one of the norms by which "one" becomes viable at all, that which qualifies a body for life within the domain of cultural intelligibility.

Constructions of performativity and the consequence of such a perspective for this work lie in its offering a very different reading of the articulation between subject formation and power than is evident in Foucault's theory. To Butler (1993: 2), performativity is "not the act by which a subject brings into being what she/he names, but, rather, as that reiterative power of discourse to produce the phenomena that it regulates and constrains." This means that the process by which the material body is assumed, or when and how the norm is appropriated or taken on, emanates from a different position. Rather than being formed or subjected by power, in Butler's theory, it is understood as that which the subject relies on in the process of production. To her, the process of taking on a 'sex' is linked to the issue of identification as well as with the discursive apparatus or rules and regulations by which heterosexuality authorizes some sexed identifications and/or denies others (Butler, 1993). It is in and through this arrangement of disavowing and authorising that the subject is formed. Subject formation, according to Butler, necessitates the construction of a field of the prohibited, shameful, "uninhabitable" or "unlivable", a discursive space "for those who are not yet 'subjects' but who form the constitutive outside of the domain of the subject" Butler, 1993: 3). This domain of the uninhabitable demarcates or delimits the subject's field, since the subject is formed in recognition of what it is not or does not want to be recognised as. Put differently, the invocation of an aberrant that constitutes the 'margin' at a particular juncture is central to forming the subject since it is in repudiating the 'abject' that the subject authorises or claims his/her position. Butler (1993: 3) says,

> In this sense, then, the subject is constituted through the force of exclusion and abjection, one which produces a constitutive outside of the subject, an abjected outside, which is, after all, "inside" the subject as its own founding repudiation.

Subject formation, therefore, necessitates identification with the regulatory apparatus and this identification occurs only through denial or a turning back on itself (Butler, 1997: 3). In other words, the inauguration of the subject not only permits the likelihood of that which it disallows, it relies on this difference to constitute itself – "I" is only possible through "that foreclosure, grounded in and by that firmly imagined impossibility" (Butler, 1997: 8). The "I", constituted in ambivalence, is always threatened by the possibility of the 'uninhabitable', which results in the subject unconsciously re-enacting or repeating the very condition it seeks to deny. Butler (1997: 9) puts it this way:

> Through that neurotic repetition the subject pursues its own dissolution, its own unravelling, a pursuit that marks an agency, but not the *subject's* agency – rather, the agency of a desire that aims at the dissolution of the subject, where the subject stands as a bar to that desire.

Fundamentally then, the subject is not only "produced through foreclosure", she/he is "produced by a condition from which it is, by definition, separated and differentiated" (Butler, 1997: 9). Power in such a construction does not constitute the subject, but rather is that which the subject inhabits, the condition on which the subject relies for its existence. Such constructions of power assume that the subject does not only recognize or acknowledge the 'presence' of an 'other' but needs power to exist in the first place.

The formation of the "I" is not possible without reliance on constructions of the 'aberrant', which in turn necessitates the subject turning on itself through reiterative enactments (Butler, 1997: 29). As Butler (1997: 28) says:

> The subject is compelled to repeat the norms by which it is produced, but that repetition establishes a domain of risk, for if it fails to reinstate the norm, "in the right way", one becomes subject to further sanctions, one feels the prevailing conditions of existence threatened. And yet, without a repetition that risks life – its current organisation – how might we begin to imagine the contingency of that organisation, and performativity reconfigure the contours of the conditions of life?

Reiterative enactments or performances are repetitive actions, what Hetherington (1998: 141) calls "ongoing performative repertoires." These "*stylized repetition of acts*" (Butler's emphasis, 1999: 179), which assume an 'act-like status' in the present, are "at once a re-enactment and re-experiencing of a set of meanings already socially established; and it is the mundane and ritualized forms of their legitimation" (Butler, 1990: 178). Sets of norms that, when reified and ritualized, are accumulated over time and taken for granted as 'natural' and 'real' in the social world, become patterns of 'behaviour' or enactments associated with, in the case of Butler (1990), particular gender performances. Their historicity is, however, neither clear nor known and their production is never clear or complete (Butler, 1990). An explanation of identity from such a perspective foregrounds its temporality and spatial situatedness. One cannot assume, therefore, that such enactments result from a 'true' or 'fixed' identity, but rather, it is the other way round. In other words, if identity is established through repetitive enactments that are, in themselves, "internally discontinuous", then what is made visible in the corporeal body cannot be assumed to be 'natural.' Rather, it is a constructed identity, "... a performative accomplishment which the mundane social audience, including the actors themselves, come to believe and to perform in the model of belief" (Butler, 1999: 179). What appears as a 'stable' identity is actually that which is structured through repetitive acts that attempt to come as close as possible to what is assumed as 'true' or 'real' or 'ideal.' However, as Butler (1999) says, enactments are themselves not stable, continuous or linear in their appearance. It is precisely because they are sometimes discontinuous that they reveal their arbitrariness and their constructed nature. It cannot be taken for granted that acts will be produced in precisely the same way each time they are taken up.

Butler's analytical theory, therefore, offered possibilities for the explanation of difference in this work. However, the question I had to answer is: How do I operationalize it to explain how teachers take up positions in the classroom? In other words, how does one apply such a framework to tease out what teachers do in classrooms that illustrates the performative and constructed nature of teaching? It was Hetherington's (1998) explanation of restored behaviour that enabled me to operationalize Butler's thesis in this work.

Briefly, Hetherington (1998) draws on Schechner (1985) to explain performativity in ways that animate the tools that I apply in the analysis. Schechner (1985) suggests that performance is typified by what he describes as 'restored behaviour' (in Hetherington, 1998: 153). Restored behaviour is rehearsed behaviour or what Butler suggested as "stylised acts" or a set of norms that can be (re)membered, replicated and integrated into performances in the present or future (Hetherington, 1998). It is constituted in repetition and consists of performances that are extractable and separated from the actor who performs them. Their significance is only made visible in their rehearsal and through using the past to instantiate present actions. Schechner (in Hetherington, 1998) describes restored behaviour as an arrangement of behaviours, 'particular strips' of behaviour that are appropriated in performance. These performative repertoires are learned due to their iterative characteristics. The strips of behaviour may be arranged and rearranged to make up a performance (Hetherington, 1998: 150), but as will become clearer below, not in a haphazard way.

The notion of restored behaviour is helpful in describing identity since it brings choice, power, and performance in concert with each other in ways theorists in the first two sections were unable to do. This construction presupposes choice and power on the part of the subject at the inception of the performance. Subjects position themselves but they do not do so unthinkingly, haphazardly or with total abandon because of the expressive and reflexive characteristics inherent in restored behaviour. Hetherington, (1998: 154) puts it this way: "[I]dentity, while it can within certain limits be chosen, is not something one attains but something one performs and reflexively monitors by arranging strips of restored behaviour into a distinctive performance." Because restored behaviour draws on the knowledge subjects hold of the behaviour (its historicity), it is always situated and embedded and will always constitute rudimentary components that are familiar, even though the actions may not follow the regimes that are apparent in the everyday. Choice here means that what is expressed is not contextually embedded but is only meaningful in the moment of performance, in a specific situated context. The restored behaviour will "follow the conventions of the occasion" (Hetherington, 1998: 154). The power to invoke rests with the subject and is made visible through the patterns of behaviour the subject brings into play. These distinguishable patterns of behaviour, invoked – as Butler (1997: 8) suggested earlier – through the possibility of the "uninhabitable" of the "aberrant other", are manifest through what Hetherington calls "a continuous process of experiment and rehearsal, involving forms of sociation – assumed personae – which emerge in relation to their spatial setting" (1998: 154).

At stake here is not the constitution of the elements that are taken up to make up the 'strip of behaviour' and then performed, but rather the pattern of enactment that is followed and the nature of the embodiment and expressed corporeality. The possibility of being able to 'learn' or embody strips of behaviour means that "... the totality of the performance is unbounded and can be unscripted while at the same time having a visibly performative character to it" (Hetherington, 1998: 154). The upshot and hence the relevance such a perspective holds for this work is that one can choose the 'strips of behaviour' to constitute an identity at a particular moment in a particular discursive field of practice.

Explanations of restored behaviour enabled me to operationalize constructions of performativity, and therefore offered two possibilities for this work. First, it meant that I could frame or isolate 'strips' of behaviour in the classroom in order to typify their performative nature. In other words, what became possible was the ability to isolate teacher enactments that demonstrate the performative character of teaching and its iterative nature. Second, through the former, it was possible to account for difference and to show how teachers exercise agency in performative teacher enactments. It also became possible to analyse what was actually happening in lifeskills classrooms, through asking questions about whether or not the 'intended outcomes' of creating a 'safe' space for mediating sexuality and HIV/AIDS messages are realisable within such a discursive space. It meant that I could ask questions about what is lost or sacrificed in this process of mediation. This perspective allowed me to bring together aspects of the main question, namely, the nexus between teacher subject positioning, patterns of behaviour that constitute teaching, content, and the mediation process.

In summary, I began this chapter with a brief discussion that situated the study epistemologically. I relied on social theory primarily, but also included aspects of psychoanalysis and feminist theory to develop an explanatory and analytical framework. Using Bourdieu's theory of practice and Giddens's theory of structuration, I developed an explanatory framework that offered an account of subject formation and subjectivity in a way that illuminated the dominant influences on identity. This explanatory framework made accessible the tools I apply later on in Chapters 9 and 10 of the analysis, to situate the respondents spatially and discursively. In Chapter 9 I use Bourdieu's concepts of *habitus* and capital to situate the respondents by outlining the material and social conditions in which they live and work. This description offers the textual landscape that embeds the study in a particular social setting and offers a lens to read what follows in Chapter 10, the description of another level of influence that teachers draw on to make meaning in their lives. In this section I describe the repertoire of resources teachers draw on by recounting their early and current life experiences. Here, I not only use Bourdieu's theory of practice to frame the discussion, but I rely on Giddens's theory of structuration to explain how teachers draw on structures rather than operate within a pre-structured environment. Useful as these frameworks were in enabling me to describe the various levels of influence on teacher identity, they were limited in their application in that I was unable to use them to animate what actually happens in the classroom when teachers mediate sexuality and HIV/AIDS. In the final section of this chapter, therefore, I described an analytical framework by appropriating aspects of psychoanalysis and feminist theory. Through applying Butler's theory of performativity and Schechner's (1985) concept of restored behaviour I was able, in Chapter 11, to report on what actually happens in Lifeskills classrooms.

The conceptual and analytical framework developed in this work was also useful as a frame of reference for me as a researcher. In brief, applying the framework made me aware of my own positionality and situatedness and the multiple positions I embody as a middle class Black woman, an academic, mediator, educator, mother, partner, and most importantly for this work, the position I held as producer of this particular script.

Part III
Limitations in dominant epistemological orientations and research on teachers, teaching and HIV/AIDS

Introduction

The epistemological orientation developed in Part 2 helps to focus what follows in the next three chapters, in which I examine (a) the limitations of dominant epistemological orientations and interpretations on selected research on teachers and teaching; (b) the limitations of dominant epistemological orientations and discourses in influencing the understanding of and responses to HIV/AIDS; and (c) the limitations of dominant discourses and epistemological and methodological orientations in researching HIV/AIDS. Part 2 thus anchors this study epistemologically, methodologically, and analytically.

Since the study sought to examine the nexus between teacher identity and classroom practice particularly where teachers mediate knowledge of sexuality and HIV/AIDS, it was important to briefly locate it within three fields of research, namely research on teachers and teaching practice, on sexuality and disease, and on teachers, sexuality and HIV/AIDS. The next three chapters, therefore, briefly review selected works in this regard. The conceptual and analytical framework developed in the preceding chapters furnished the perspective adopted in reviewing this work. Rather than a general review of the literature, the approach taken is one that highlights the limitations of dominant epistemological orientations that act as interpretive grids in examining teachers and their work, particularly their work in Lifeskills classrooms.

Chapter 6 examines representations of teachers in teacher research, while Chapters 7 and 8 consider (a) ways in which dominant epistemological frameworks and discourses of sexuality, disease and the politics of the pandemic in South Africa shape popular constructions and interpretations; and (b) research on HIV/AIDS, respectively. These chapters offer insight into how, within particular epistemological frameworks, structures and agents are understood as operating in relation to each other, with the former acting as what Bourdieu (1990) describes as 'structuring structures' that press upon those operating in the field of practice and constrain their actions or ability to act differently. Chapters 7 and 8 give evidence for why it is necessary to question the use of dominant epistemological orientations to understand social action.

I end each chapter in Part III with a proposal for the application of an alternative epistemological approach that accounts for and illuminates relations of power as constitutive of and constituted by agents. Such an orientation, I argue, illuminates how subjects (in this case, teachers) are not only positioned but also position themselves. This lays the groundwork for examining the main question that this book addresses, namely, what actually happens in classrooms when teachers mediate sexuality and HIV/AIDS.

6 The limitations of dominant epistemological orientations and interpretations of teachers and teachers' work in the research

Studying teachers' lives and their classroom practice is by no means novel. In providing a brief exposition on representations of teachers and conceptions of teaching in research, this chapter highlights how, in the nexus of the two, particular teacher subject positions are invoked and produced. In particular, the chapter draws attention to ways in which dominant epistemological orientations in research about teachers and teaching often limit interpretations of teachers' subject positions in the act of teaching. This critique is important in that it not only highlights how particular epistemological orientations offer limited understandings of the nexus between structure and agency and its articulation in teaching practice, but also provides the rationale for the theoretical, methodological, and conceptual focus of the study. The analysis of teacher positioning and teaching here lays the foundation for subsequent argument that proposes a more nuanced approach to research on teachers and their work, one that allows for a dialectic rather than dualistic relationship between structure and agency.

What follows is a brief rationale for the focus on teachers, with particular emphasis on the importance of examining teacher identity (and subject positioning) as a critical component in understanding teaching. I follow this with a review of selected research on teachers and teaching. In this, I focus on the epistemological orientations in the selected research, emphasising the consequence such orientations hold for understanding teacher subject positioning and teacher enactments. I use three broad epistemological frameworks, namely positivist, interpretivist, and critical feminist, to structure the discussion. I highlight the limitations of the first two orientations in understanding the interrelationship between structure and agency by demonstrating how each epistemological orientation focuses on either learner achievement or accountability, thus framing teaching as that which teachers *do* to produce learner results. These two orientations, I propose, are premised on epistemologies that understand power as residing primarily in external structures that operate to constrain the subject (teacher). Such stances, I argue, limit our understanding of agency by positing a passive subject (teacher) who is produced by predetermined structures. In proposing an alternative, I introduce feminist and critical theory epistemological perspectives. I argue for a shift in epistemological orientation, from one that positions teachers as mere reproducers (and by implication deliverers of an uncontested body of knowledge) who are produced by predetermined structures, towards one that accounts for the complexities and contradictions inherent in the structure/agency dialectic. Part of this complexity, I argue, revolves around understanding power as both an imposition, as well as constitutive of self. Along this line of argument, structures are understood to be tools teachers draw on, and thus act as constraining as well as enabling discursive spaces. Such an epistemological orientation gives recognition to the presence of an embodied agent who is not only produced through structures, but who relies on power and acts from, within, through, and upon structures to reproduce and transform them. In arguing for a reorientation, I briefly situate the debate within a South African context, showing the limitations of earlier constructions of teacher positioning in offering explanations of what happens in Lifeskills classrooms.

Epistemological orientations towards teaching and teachers' lives in teacher research

Teachers, like any other members of the human family, have a past, a present, and a future. These influence decisions they make about their work at a variety of levels. Programmatically, they shape decisions in planning what to teach and what knowledge to privilege, even in the face of already well-articulated, prescribed curriculum guidelines mandated by departments of education (Baxen, 2005). At another level, they shape decisions teachers make about the act of teaching, that is, about the nature and active process of engagement in the classroom. Importantly too, these influences, when understood as constructed and reconstituted in and through the acts, content and process of subjects, serve to produce effects at the same time as the effects are produced. Reconstructions and interpretations are bounded within situated contexts and those who interpret and act, do so from a position 'in context', and "speak from a particular place and time, from a history and a culture which is specific" (Hall, 1990: 222). Interpretations are, therefore, not neutral but "positioned" (Hall, 1990) and embedded within social and cultural spaces. As individuals and members of a group (or a number of sub-groups), teachers position themselves and are positioned within bounded contexts in and through which they construct, reconstruct, negotiate and reproduce meaning in complex ways.

Benyon (1985: 158) suggests that unless "we first understand teachers we can hardly claim to understand teaching." He alerts us to the manner in which teachers were treated in the past, namely as "cardboard cut-outs." Such a stance, he suggests, disregarded their positionality and ignored the related ways in which they act within their fields of practice. Connell (1985: 4) concurs when he states that many sociological studies "tended to ignore the personal dimensions of teaching and often give an oddly inhuman account of this most human of jobs."

Placing teachers at the centre of research inquiry is not new. Copious amounts have been written about them in research (see Ball & Goodson, 1985; Benyon, 1985; Butt, Raymond, McCue & Yamagishi, 1992; Carson & Sumara, 1997; Fishman & McCarthy, 2000; Goodson, 1992; Green, 1998; Hammersley, 1999; Rummel & Quintero, 1997; Thomas, 1995; Woods, 1996). In brief, this body of educational research encompasses a variety of aims, providing a historical account of the field, generating theory about teacher research, demonstrating the efficacy of teacher research and offering different research approaches and strategies, and providing examples of improved classroom practice or providing tips and ideas on how to improve classroom practice (Fishman & McCarthy, 2000). General speaking, this research has treated teachers as objects of research, or as participants in collaborative projects examining their practices.

During any pedagogical encounter, teachers, as active agents, make choices. These choices are not solely autonomous, as will become clearer below, but are consciously or unconsciously shaped by their own experiences of and responses to the subject content, their own histories, dominant external discourses, as well as the immediate circumstances of teaching. The context of teaching is thus complex. Any attempt to understand teachers' work and teaching consequently needs to include an understanding of the teacher both as an individual and as a member of a group (or a number of sub-groups), working within a discursive field where multiple discourses that are not always complementary, exist. Goodson (1992: 4) suggests that, "in understanding something so intensely personal as teaching, it is critical we know about the person the teacher."

Teachers are central to any schooling endeavour, be it for the implementation of any policy or for school improvement. It would seem, therefore, that centering teachers within research inquiry with a view to understanding their positionality would mean going beyond asking questions about what they teach, to taking cognizance of their identities and how they make meaning of their lives in relation to what they do in the classroom. The latter seems particularly pertinent in as much as it has consequences for understanding teachers' experience of, response to, and engagement with policy, new curriculum reforms, and for our purposes, social issues such as HIV/AIDS.

One argument for focusing on teachers and teachers' lives might be found in conceptions of self and identity (Green, 1998). Ball and Goodson (1985: 18) concur that, "[t]he way in which teachers achieve, maintain, and develop their identity, their sense of self, in and through a career, are of vital significance in understanding the actions and commitments of teachers in their work."

Such an interest in teachers and their work, teacher identity, what happens in schools rather than what schools *do* to identity, and so on, may be associated with two broader but integrally linked trends occurring in sociology, at one level, and education, at another (Woods, 1996). The first, methodological in nature, is embedded in and closely associated with questions within broader sociological debates about the privileged positions held by dominant positivist, scientific constructions of reality. Methodologically, there has been renewed questioning of dominant epistemological and methodological frameworks shaping constructions of social reality in general and of research in particular. From a research perspective, there is growing scepticism about scientific, quantitative methodologies that sought to know *what* was happening rather than *why* and *how* things were happening within particular social contexts.

These debates facilitated (i) a move towards qualitative research, and (ii) a critique of old frameworks and the development (or incorporation) of more ethnographic research methodologies in which different ontological and epistemological questions were posed about the nature of science and the social order (Woods, 1996). Denzin and Lincoln (1994 in Woods, 1996: 8) outline the history of these developments as follows:

- the 'traditional' moment (1900–1950) of classical, realist ethnography, as in the Chicago School of sociology;
- the 'modern' moment (1950–1970), featuring the attempted integration and systemization of qualitative within quantitative research methods;
- the 'blurred genres' moment (1970–1985), marked by diverse approaches ranging from symbolic interactionism to critical theory;
- a 'crisis of representation' moment (1985–1990), querying the classic objectivist foundations of ethnographic knowledge and calling for a more discursive, reflexive turn;
- the 'postmodern' moment (1990–present) in which theories are read as multivocal stories focused primarily on social criticism and critique.

In short, the ontological and epistemological claims of the dominant positivist research methodologies that understood truth as being "discovered in the objective and the observable" (Thomas, 1995: 2) were brought into sharp focus and rigorously debated and critiqued, causing major shifts in the construction, nature, and interpretation of research. These shifts pointed to new ways of knowing, conceptions of truth and considerations of the subject as operating within situated contexts and cultures. Central to these newer methodological frameworks was the idea that individual and collective experiences and social reality could not be understood outside the contexts in and through which they were constructed and interpreted (Denzin & Lincoln, 1994).

The second trend saw the incorporation of sociological constructs more explicitly into the field of educational research. In Britain such a move towards a new sociology of education occurred in the late 1960s and early 1970s (see Hammersley & Atkinson, 1995). Prior to this, sociological research in education gave little attention to issues related to what happens *in* schools, particularly to issues concerning teaching and learning at the chalk-face. Research was, as Woods (1996: 4) states, "largely locked into positivistic and quantitative frameworks." Interest had been primarily limited to issues of social class and to schools as institutions that reproduce and maintain class inequalities (Hammersley, 1999). Paradigmatically, research in and about schools concentrated on systemic issues (the place, purpose, and nature of schooling) and the interrelationship between input (teaching) and output (learning outcomes and achievement). Framed within positivist constructions of reality, quantitative methodologies were usually applied to questions that all too often made simplistic associations between input and output, curriculum content and teaching, teacher and learner, school and teacher, and between teacher and community. As Woods (1996: 4) states, "hundreds of widespread surveys, remote analysis, systematic and statistical methods texts, abstruse theoretical frameworks, and other depersonalized volumes [of books]" were the order of the day. The qualitative methodologies and interpretive theoretical frameworks were among the available theoretical and methodological resources not regularly used in understanding education and schooling (see Morrison & McIntyre, 1969; 1971).

In light of the above, it can be seen that the use of different epistemological and methodological frameworks to understand education, particularly to understand the purpose and nature of schooling, is relatively new. The move towards a critical sociology of education, more particularly the use of ethnographic and interpretative sociological frameworks and critical theory, heralded a new phase in educational research that centred more on what was actually happening *in* schools. This work, geared towards examining and understanding the quality of interaction within schools, presented the school in more discursive terms as a complex space (or field), where linearity in the relationship between variables (as suggested in previous methodological frameworks) was not accepted as given. This paved the way for studies that came to focus, *inter alia*, more specifically on teachers and their work.

Briefly outlined below are the characteristic features of various bodies of research that focus on teachers and teaching. The discussion focuses on shifts in the construction of 'the teacher' and pays attention to ways in which teachers are positioned in relation to their work. In highlighting the limitations of each approach and in briefly introducing emerging work in teacher research, this section provides a rationale for the orientation of the present study. The discussion highlights ways in which each approach foregrounds particular sociological constructions of society and conceptions of schooling, asks particular sets of questions, and thereby serves different purposes. In conceptualizing and examining this body of research, I use categories applied by Peter Woods (1996) to frame the discussion. These, in a way, illustrate the epistemological origins of the research questions and thus provide a way of locating teacher research in general and teacher identity research in particular. Approaches include considerations of teaching as a *science* and an *art*, the latter of which includes understanding the activity as a performance. In concluding this section, I highlight the limitations of such approaches by introducing emerging research that extends notions of teaching as a performance to the idea of teaching as performitivity.

Teaching as a science: positivist orientations towards teaching

The debate about teaching tends to centre on whether it is an art or a science (Woods, 1996). The notion of teaching as a science was largely influenced by traditional positivism which emphasized the anchoring of theories in observation statements, verification, and prediction as the elemental logical components of scientific activity (Giddens, 1982: 13). Teaching in these terms is understood as a "rational activity, subject to general principles and laws that are discoverable through research" (Woods, 1996: 15). Within such a conception, understanding teaching means unearthing its constitutive variables. Simon (1988) suggests that the basic tenet is common acceptance that the process of learning is more or less constant for all human beings,which makes it easy to extract a few general principles. With these in mind, the process of teaching can be systematically itemized, structured, and planned in a rational, almost linear fashion. Examining teaching would, therefore, require an analysis of all identifiable variables, which might include but not be limited to having clearly articulated aims, systematic plans of action, specified outcomes that are measurable, observable, and quantifiable. Accounting for these variables, it is assumed, would ensure success in teaching regardless of the impact of teachers (as subjects) or context. In such a stance teaching is viewed as an objective, rational act, often quantifiable and driven by objectives, outcomes, systematic plans of action and so on. Behaviourist constructions of teaching (see Bloom, 1968, 1976), for example, subscribe to such a conception of teaching. What, then, are the research implications of such a stance? How are teachers positioned within such theoretical orientations?

In the first instance, teachers are positioned as responsive rather than active subjects. They are usually framed as implementers of an already clearly articulated curriculum with specified teaching and learning goals. The underlying premise positions teachers as 'professionals' who function as 'intellectuals' in society (Carrim in Lewin, Samuel & Sayed, 2003). In line with constructions of schooling as a 'mindful' activity (see Hamera in Alexander, Anderson & Gallegos, 2005), teachers in such constructions are 'rational professionals' whose behaviour is understood to be measurable against explicitly expressed sets of practices deemed appropriate to this role. The consequences of such constructions for this study are twofold. First as 'rational, intellectual professionals' who 'mindfully' educate the 'minds' of learners, invoking the physical body through teaching sexuality or HIV/AIDS produces a particular subject positioning not usually invoked in the public space of the classroom. Second, such constructions presuppose power as residing primarily in structures. Consequently, any identifiable problems are understood to be located in either the structure of the school or the curriculum and, as such, outside or independent of the teacher. Put differently, often such frameworks conceal the agentive position of the teacher, thus denying the teacher any agency to reproduce or insert a different discourse. By underplaying the role of the teacher or presenting context as fixed, teacher influence on pedagogical processes and outcomes of learning is obscured.

Anchored within positivist constructions, teacher research has often laid emphasis on simplistic interpretations of the role and influence of teachers on issues related to curriculum, pedagogy, and assessment and school outcomes (see Hope, 2002 as an example). Giving ascendancy to what teaches *do* as distinguishable from *who* they are, has often translated into examinations of their practice as an objective enterprise to which they did not directly contribute. Concerns in research were, therefore, more *about teaching as a clearly articulated field of practice* (the specification being usually defined by sets of 'experts', for example, curriculum planners) rather than about the constructed nature of the *mediation process,* and the constructed identities and roles of *the mediator* (my emphasis). The interrelationship between teaching (as a practice) and the teacher (who participates in and contributes to the practice) seemed absent in this body of research. As Shulman (1986: 12) states, the role of research was to "collect, collate and interpret the practical knowledge of teachers for the purposes of establishing and codifying its principles, precedents and parables."

The great contribution by science to the field of education, in the form of research generated through the use of positivistic epistemologies, is unquestionable (Woods, 1996). However, this approach often had unfavourable effects by placing limits on constructions of reality as they applied to schools and the activity of teaching. The degree of teacher autonomy and, by implication, teacher agency (as a creative subject, constructor, interpreter or reproducer of the curriculum), is not only underplayed but is largely absent from research applying such frameworks. There is an absence, therefore, of what Delanty (1999: 19) calls the "self-legislating power of human reason", which detracts from the construction of the teacher as a "self-legislating and creative" subject.

Criticism emerged of the seemingly narrow "traditionalist positivist positions and their concomitant, circumscribing research methods" (Thomas, 1995: 4) that led to simplistic associations and a distinct differentiation between teacher and practice that, as Woods (1996: 21) states, "hardly penetrate[d] the surface of the complex activity of teaching." To Eisner (1993), schools not only privilege particular forms of knowledge, but consider rationality as natural and mental ability as one of the most important skills. Cognitive ability to memorize and reproduce facts is often rated above other skills that might require non-linear forms of abstraction. Eisner suggests that a positivist orientation does not consider the classroom as a space where meaning is constructed. The upshot of such a position is that teacher education omits alternative perspectives on knowledge and its production in the context of schools. Such criticism, levelled primarily at research, questioned the epistemic foundations as well as the interpretative orientations characteristic of scientific approaches.

The effect of such criticism is evident in shifts at different levels in discourses on teaching. The first is associated with a redefinition of teaching from a science to an art. The idiom shifted from privileging objectivity and mechanistic constructions of teaching and teachers to recognising creativity as a key component of a teacher's work. The metaphor of 'teaching as an art' is rooted in constructions of the subject as having some control (albeit limited) of the environment. Importantly too, an epistemological shift emerged, which allowed the insertion of different sets of questions about the nature of social reality in general and researching teaching in particular. But perhaps the most significant shift was methodological, that is, towards qualitative research frameworks that included the application of various research approaches. Importantly, the latter shift allowed for the inclusion of teachers as not only objects of research but collaborators and key contributors to the research process (Thomas, 1995; Woods, 1996).

Teaching as art: interpretivist orientations towards teaching

The shift to identifying and understanding teaching as an art is embedded in broader arguments about the role and purpose of schooling. Such debates have involved what Hammersley describes as a "radical political questioning of educational shibboleths" (1999: 3). A shift in focus was evident, away from deterministic and reductionist constructions of schooling and teaching, to ones acknowledging the social embeddedness of schools and the socially constructed nature of teaching. Education is now understood as embedded in space and time and, as such, constructed and contextually contingent.

Constructions of teaching shifted to embrace the notion of teaching as an art. Woods (1996: 21–26) identifies four distinct features as characteristic of this notion: "multiple forms of meaning and representation", "expression and emergence", "creativity" and "emotion."

There are many definitions that incorporate this new way of understanding teaching. One such example from Stenhouse (1985: 105) states that it is an "exercise of skill and expressive of meaning"; one closely associated with personal meaning making. Personal meaning making basically involves an ability to communicate clearly. In this instance, it means having the capacity and competency to express learning intentions, explain the nature of learning, and interpret outcomes in a way that makes learning accessible to learners (Stenhouse, 1985).

The activity of teaching as well as the teacher are brought into sharp focus in models of teaching that subscribe to the ways of understanding described in this section. The activity, it would seem, includes subjects who create and produce meaning. The "I" is, therefore, an important element in that it is through the "I" that interpretation of what is taught, because possible. Importantly too, and unlike the perspective characteristic of early scientific constructions of teaching, this "I" or self is invested in the processes of teaching since teachers create and make choices about what tools and resources to draw on and apply. Newer frameworks unmistakably place emphasis more prominently on teachers as acting and thinking subjects who create and contribute to shaping the process and outcome of teaching. Teaching as an art was, therefore, a movement that understood teaching as that which includes a multiplicity of meanings and different teacher subject positions.

Rooted within modernist/postmodernist frameworks, and common amongst such constructions of teaching, is recognition and acceptance of uncertainty and ambiguity as inherent features in the process and outcome of the activity, since one cannot account for a stable or invariable outcome when one is creative, expressive and where interpretations of truth are multiple. Ambiguity and uncertainty, though, are not understood as debilitating. Rather, they are understood as characteristic features that allow for subject positions that are often foreclosed in scientific and/or mechanistic conceptions of teaching. Essentially, when subjectivity is invoked, questions of interpretation, context, emotions and representation become pronounced and as such, produce uncertainty. Accordingly, an undeniable feature of teaching is the element of 'not knowing" (Woods, 1996).

Teachers are acknowledged as significant players in this activity, since they create the enabling environment in which learners learn. Knowledge is understood as produced within creative environments where teachers are intuitive, imaginative, successful, good managers, enthusiastic leaders, expressive, flexible and active (see Carr, 1989; Eisner, 1985; Stenhouse, 1985; Tom, 1984; Tripp, 1993). Carrim (2003: 308) refers to this as positioning teachers as "producers and disseminators of knowledge" and thus performing "intellectual work." Teaching also has "an emotional heart" (Woods, 1996: 26). In addressing the issue of emotion, Mackey (1993) stresses its cognitive benefits while Hargreaves (1994: 12) describes it as being connected to desire, where the latter is associated with "creative unpredictability' and "flows of energy."

Recognition of the centrality of teachers in the pedagogical process has had major implications for the nature and scale of research. Largely influenced by symbolic interactionism, emerging teacher research shifted from concentration on the impact of structures on learning outcomes to the examination of mediating processes, including the role of teachers in learner success (however this is measured). Recognized as a complex activity in emerging research, teaching involves teachers formulating decisions, making choices and actively 'making' the environment. Teachers are recognised as operating within environments in which and to which they contribute. Importantly too, teachers are positioned more firmly as subjects of research, on the ground that they *act* but are also *active* agents who not only construct and produce meaning, but also act to shape and interpret it. Context in this work is discursively constituted as more than geographic location. It includes constructions of classrooms as complex discursive fields of practice where structure and agents interact in producing particular learner and teacher identities and complex intended and unintended outcomes.

Characteristically, social interactionism is interested in how the everyday aspects of our lives are understood and interpreted. In other words, interactionists lay emphasis on "processes, relationships, group life, motivations, adaptations and so on" (Woods, 1996: 48). They are concerned with how people make meaning of their lives and how they are able to exercise agency despite not having access to capital in a particular field of practice. As Woods (1996: 7) states:

> The emphasis is upon constructions of meanings and perspectives, the adaptation to circumstances, the management of interests in the ebb and flow of countless interactions containing many ambiguities and conflicts, the strategies devised to promote those interests, and the negotiation with others' interests that is a common feature of all teaching situations.

Symbolic interaction, as Woods (1996: 48) states, "does have a view on wider concerns – on social structures and system." According to him, this is pronounced within some interpretations of symbolic interactionism (e.g. structural-functionalism and Marxist economic perspectives), where ways in which structures are expressed in people's behaviour is foregrounded. Nevertheless, the attraction of symbolic interactionist orientations lies in their interpretation of people as not necessarily acting responsively to structures. Rather, people make up a response and as such, make sense of the system in relation to their own lives and in ways that may produce a reaction unlike the system's expected response. According to Woods (1996: 49), "interactionism can also approach society and social structures from below" – meaning that symbolic interactionism can take a perspective on social reality starting from a different point of reference, in this case, from the subject.

One such starting point, as it relates to this discussion, is a particular methodological orientation towards teachers' work. This comprises life history, narrative, and biographical research that attempted to understand the complex interplay between the "developing self" (Woods, 1996: 50) and the localised, situated context in which the self constructs, is constructed and makes meaning. The advantage of such perspectives lies in their providing research possibilities embracing an examination of the nexus between aspects shaping everyday life (social, cultural, political, economic practices) and teachers' lives as expressed in the classroom, as well the process of classroom interaction that makes and is made by the teacher.

Shifts occurring in research included, but were not limited to the emergence of small-scale studies that sought to understand teachers and their work within the context of the classroom. Epistemologically, it was possible to pose different sets of questions that sought to understand who teachers are in relation to what they do as well as questions about what was actually happening during interactions between teachers and learners. Interest shifted from what is known and how it could be measured, to questions seeking to understand how meaning is constructed within particular contexts and how within such spaces, meaning is negotiated, contested, produced, and reproduced. The questions that emerged were fundamentally concerned with how we come to know and understand what happens in classrooms rather than *that* we know. Key questions concerned the interrelationship among teacher, context, and outcome, and the extent to which these are linked to what teachers do. No longer were outcomes important in and for themselves. Rather, emphasis lay as much in the production and reproduction of the teaching activity, as it did in the outcomes of the teaching endeavour.

The most significant change, nonetheless, was evident in a changed methodological paradigm that privileged subjectivity as embedded and situated. There was a greater impulse towards more qualitative, ethnographic forms of research, with various approaches providing increased choices in the types of methodological and analytical lenses available for examining teachers and their work. Thomas in his book titled *Teachers' Stories* provides a short list that depicts the range of research "interests and approaches" (1995: 10) emanating from the shift in perspectives on teaching. These range from but are not limited to narrative, autobiographical, life history, action research, and participatory action research approaches (see Carr & Kemmis, 1986; Carson & Sumara, 1997; Goodson, 1991; Rummel & Quintero, 1997; Sikes, Measor & Woods, 1987; Stenhouse, 1975). The significance of the above and the consequences for this study are the extent to which such perspectives advance a different teacher positioning.

Early constructions of teaching as an art are also associated with the notion of teaching as a performance; what Carr (1989: 5) describes as a "practical activity." Stenhouse (1985: 110) suggests that teachers' artistry is expressed through performance. In this regard he states:

> There is in education no absolute and unperformed knowledge. In educational research and scholarship, the ivory towers where the truth is neglected are so many theatres without players, galleries without pictures, music without musicians. Educational knowledge exists in, and is verified or falsified in, its performance. (Woods, 1996: 23)

Eisner (1985) and Carr (1989) elaborate on the performative quality of teacher engagement by arguing that teaching is more than a mechanistic activity. To them, teaching incorporates processes of engagement in which teachers have continually to construct meaning and make informed choices within environments characterized by complex sets of expectations, situations, and processual demands. Eisner (1985) describes this performance as the teacher's ability to reason and act reflexively, and Carr (1989) agrees that teachers need to think and make many decisions spontaneously when called upon to do so. Decisions, however, are not neutral, but rather filtered through teachers' own values and a tacit or sometimes explicit understanding of what is expected of them as educators. When viewed as a performance, teaching is understood as dynamic, "expressive and emergent, and cannot be set up in advance through, for example, objectives" (Woods, 1996: 23).

Acknowledging teachers as subjects who think, feel, and act to constrain and transform what happens in classrooms is clearly articulated in research alluded to in this section. Its limitation, though, lies in its application and interpretation of teacher subject positioning. Described below are some general patterns that emerge in this work when one examines ways in which subject positioning is framed.

First, and by far the most common, is a body of research that positions teachers as acting *upon* an environment where the latter is understood as already structured and thus inflexible (e.g., the systems of examinations and learning outcomes). The emphasis here is usually on what teachers do as creators of an enabling environment for students to learn. The success of the pedagogical encounter is therefore measured or interpreted according to the extent to which teachers are able to change outcomes for students through what they do; be it through normative measurable improvements in academic results, creating a supportive environment, or motivating learners and so on. The results of this research have been used in establishing professional development programmes as a way of improving practice, leading to effective teaching and successful learning outcomes. The 'effective teacher' discourse common during the 1980s and 1990s is one such manifestation of a focus on teachers as actors or performers upon environments.

Another body of research reflects on the influence of past and present teacher (hi)stories on teaching practice (see Ball & Goodson, 1985; Goodson, 1992; Green, 1998), and examines teacher beliefs and attitudes, as well as social and cultural practices affecting teaching and orientations towards the profession in general. This body of research suggests an articulation between personal histories and teaching practices. Consequentially, the research is concerned to examine how such (hi)stories impact on teaching practice, teacher motivation, commitment and career trajectories. Primarily though, the significance of such an articulation is interpreted in terms of its influence on learner behavior and the outcomes of teaching and learning. Expressed differently, the outcome of this body of research focused on understanding how teacher history produces different sets of teaching and learning outcomes. Its emphasis lay in understanding transformations in learner behaviour and outcomes, rather than on the extent to which this history is instantiated in teacher behaviour and concomitant sets of teacher practices. The upshot, as it relates to understanding teacher positioning, is that there is no account of how the teacher produces or is produced during the teaching activity.

Yet another body of research, largely influenced by critical and feminist theory, is concerned with reproductions of power and agency. Unlike the above, emphasis in this work is on teachers perceived as active agents whose choices transform rather than respond to the environment. Transformation is here associated with awareness (on the part of the teacher as agent) of the power to transform. The focus of such research is twofold. In some instances, it examines the impact and/or influence of factors such as race, sexual orientation, class, and so on, on teaching practice and the power of teachers to transform learner experiences (see Daniel Tatum, 1997; Donaldson, 1996; Edelsky, 1999; Goodman, 2000; McCormick, 1994; Neito,1994; Porter, 1999). The second trajectory of enquiry addresses the paucity in research on women and girls (see Acker, 1989). Results emanating from this work have influenced subsequent orientations in research by expanding the range of research; from questions concerning the impact of the sociological structures of race, class, ethnicity on groups in society in general and schools in particular, to a focus on their articulation in classroom practice and allied learner success. Such work has also contributed to raising concerns about relationships between researchers and the researched. Hammersley (1999: 7) suggests that this work "highlighted the importance of reflexivity, of the ways in which analysis could involve presuppositions that the analyst was unaware of, which significantly shaped the account produced". Power, expressed in the role of the researcher, was brought into sharp focus, thereby raising questions about the ethics and interpretations of research.

Contributions by feminist theorists in advancing research discourses in general, and research on subject positioning in particular, were important to understanding classrooms as complex fields of practice. While feminist theorists produced work in the field themselves, their contribution to discourse in social theory was distinguished by their use of insightful theoretical frameworks. Critical orientations toward social reality, particularly work on race, gender, class, sexuality and notions of the body were important contributions made by feminist theorists. These new perspectives were taken up in social theory research in general and educational research in particular (Hammersley, 1999). Closely associated with criticisms "against overly cognitive conceptions of the human body" (Hammersley, 1999: 7), feminist theorists inserted a discourse in sociological research that de-emphasised dichotomised constructions of the body (e.g., mind/body) and the disassociation of agent and context. Instead, emergent discourses privileged an understanding of subjectivity as embodied. Building on the work of symbolic interactionists, subject positioning in this body of work assumes a nuanced and complex interrelationship between structure and agent, where structures are not merely conduits from which agents speak, but are open to transformation, since they are only present when instantiated in the actions of agents (Giddens, 1984).

Studying micro aspects of schools provided a glimpse into the complexity of schools as systems and classrooms as dynamic discursive spaces in which hosts of influences work in complex ways to produce intentional and unintentional outcomes. The influence of this body of research in advancing understandings of education and what actually happens in schools is obvious in shifts made in teacher research. While criticism exists of this work, a detailed discussion of its character is beyond the scope of this study (see Hammersley, 1999). The significance of this work cannot be overemphasised since it provides the platform for the discussion in the next section.

Nevertheless, in the main, research concerned with teaching as art/performance in which teachers are positioned as performers offers limited possibilities for teacher agency. The research results often privilege the range of ways teachers exercise agency either in the delivery of curricula (changing teaching strategies), changing learner behaviour or in improving their practice (see Carr & Kemmis, 1986; Goodson, 1991; Hammersley, 1999). Often, research reports on ways in which teachers reflect on and improve their practice to produce better teaching results and ultimately, better learning outcomes. Emphasis thus rests upon examining the external outputs of teaching and the externalized attributes of the teacher, often defined (or conceptualized) as the accountable subject upon whom power is imposed to produce observable outcomes. Much of this work offers perspectives on change in practice as measured against learner performance or learner success. 'Success' in this research is interpreted through indicators that measure an externally accountable teacher whose agency is determined by the dominant discourse of schooling (curricular expectations and outcomes, testing, etc). Teachers' power to *act* (to produce, signify, and transform meaning) is minimized. Personal and professional identities are dichotomized and held in polarized positions, suggesting that detachment from the personal results from assuming a professional identity that is decontexualised and disembodied. When reference is made to the personal in research, it is often in relation to its influence on the observable features of teaching practice. Questions are not asked about ways in which the act and activity of teaching produce the teacher and teacher behaviours, and vice versa. There is no commentary on the reflexive nature of teaching performance beyond its impact on learners. Few questions are asked about how teachers embody structures and how structures are instantiated in social action through dynamic and dialectic relations of power. Embedded primarily in structuralist perspectives, this work offers little possibilities for transformation by agents since power is understood as residing in structures that operate external to the subject, and to which agents respond rather than act upon. Conceptions of the subject as constitutive of and by power and through a complex interplay between structure and agency are under-developed in this work.

While 'art' and 'performance' are accepted metaphors in describing teachers' work in this body of research, positioning the subject as a thinking and acting contributor and within a dynamic context is left largely unattended. Rather, change is reflected as occurring in and to the researcher (see Woods, 1996; Carson & Sumara, 1997; Hammersley, 1999) rather than resulting from the actions of subjects.

Teaching as performative: critical theory and recent feminist orientations towards teaching

More recent trends in teacher research shed light on new ways of thinking about teacher subject positioning and classroom discourse. This emerging body of research (see Alexander, *et al.*, 2005; Pinar, 1994) extends conceptions of performance. Alexander, Anderson & Gallegos (2005: 1) suggest that the term is used "in many variations, permutations, and applications in a process of excavating, cultivating, and illuminating even newer ways of seeing the potency of performance as a theoretical lens in education" (2005: 1). This work draws on a range of performance theory (see Bakhtin, 1986; Goffman, 1959, 1973; Schechner, 1985; Scott, 1990; Pollock, 1998), and thus does not rely on one definition. Rather, performance is defined in many ways that include but are not limited to:

> [...] the strategic and the often aestheticised engagement of bodily activity with the intent of knowing through doing and showing, performance as systems of physical training in dance correlated to the habituated ways in which student bodies are cast and controlled in the classroom, performance as a strategic rhetorical construction

> of social influence, performance as it relates to cultural practice and the materiality of the body-hence a displayed enactment of ideology and enfleshed knowledge-influenced and motivated by the politics of race, gender, power, and class in the forms of folklore, ritual, spectacle, resistance, and protest; to performance as a mechanism for measuring outcomes and effective. (Alexander, *et al.*, 2005: 1–2)

This body of research embraces conceptions of the performing or theatrical teacher who is creative, responsible, and accountable in establishing environments that ensure learner success, as well as conceptions of teaching as performative and collaborative, brought together through the interaction of a number of mutually dependent characteristics (of which 'self' is key). The work includes the associated notion of performativity, a term used in two ways. The first draws on the work of Judith Butler (1992), who defines performativity as "the stylized repetition of acts that are socially validated and discursively established" in Alexander, *et al.* (2005: 2). According to her, it is "a reiteration of a norm or a set of norms" (Butler, 1992: 12). The second definition reflects Lyotard's (1984) conception of the term in Alexander, *et al.* (2005: 2) , where performativity is understood as "maximizing efficiency by controlling outcomes and creating a culture of accountability", a conception more closely aligned to descriptions of teaching as art detailed in the section above.

It is Butler's construction of performativity that is of interest in the study reported in this book since, epistemologically, it offers a lens to analyse and understand the nexus between teachers and teaching. The difference in Butler's work to previous conceptions of subject positioning and its relevance here lies in its emphasis on power, not as that which "presses on the subject from the outside, as what subordinates, sets underneath, and relegates to the lower order", but as that "forming the subject as well as providing the very condition of its existence and the trajectory of its desire" (1997: 2). The subject in this epistemological orientation is not only constituted by, but depends on power for its very existence. Teaching here is understood as "a *performance event* as well as being a *performative event* – the difference and link being teaching is 'doing', but it is also the repetitive act of doing that manifests its existential and practical presence" (Alexander, *et al.*, 2005: 4). Research in this work is premised on an understanding that the process and outcomes of teaching cannot be explained outside an understanding of the constitutive nature of the subject as well as the complex, dialectic interrelationship between teacher and teaching. This relationship, as critical theorist

McLaren sees it, suggests the presence of 'an audience' even when the audience includes the individual in dialogue with the 'self' (in Alexander, *et al.*, 2005: xv). Such dialogue is constituted in relations of power that, as Butler states, are "subordinating as well as producing" (1997: 2). Describing teaching as performative offers the possibility of inserting an epistemology that "helps to locate and describe repetitive actions plotted within grids of power relations and social norms within the context of education and schooling" (Alexander, *et al.*, 2005: 2).

The utility of such an epistemological orientation lies in its emphasis on the centrality of agency. Subjects are not merely constituted in relations of power, a stance that functionalists and structuralists privilege; they use and rely on power for their existence. One cannot take for granted, then, that fields of practice will reproduce themselves in the way that Bourdieu suggests. The social site here becomes a field for competing discourses, with subjects taking up positions rather than being defined as already positioned. Such an orientation puts what Alexander, *et al.* (2005: 3) call the "dynamics of any social site" under the spotlight and focuses attention on actors as the main players.

Defining and describing teaching as performative provides different analytical tools for reconceptualising the role of teachers in relation to their work and highlights, "the extent to which people enact assigned *assumed-to-be-natural* roles, and the degree to which they enact counter roles or modify existing ones (Alexander, *et al.*, 2005: 4). It puts under scrutiny pedagogical practices as they have come to be understood within the dominant discourses, revealing the "contradictions and power relations that undergird the practice of education" (Alexander, *et al.*, 2005: 10). Teachers, in this orientation, are described as fundamental to producing the discourse and, by implication, have the power to act in subversive ways to disrupt, transform and/or insert a different discourse (in as much as they are constituted by it). While, at one level, power forms and by implication subordinates them, teachers at the same time depend on power to constitute their identity. This orientation, unlike those previously mentioned, offers possibilities for understanding teacher agency beyond an ability to produce predetermined outcomes. It offers a point of reference for understanding teachers as those who are not only constituted by the iterative act of teaching but who, in the production, transform the discourse.

In its emphasis on teachers as active agents who produce and reproduce in complex discursive spaces, this body of research demonstrates how in the reiterative acts of teaching teachers are not only constituted, but also how the acts in themselves become the very condition they rely on to produce, reproduce and transform the practice (and by implication, directly and/or indirectly, the outcomes of teaching). When applied to what teachers do in the classroom, such an epistemological orientation places teachers centrally as those who 'call into being', through instantiated enactments of teacherly behaviour, that which constitutes teaching, the very condition required to invoke 'the teacher' in the first place. As such, the theory of performativity becomes an analytic tool that can be used to ask different epistemological questions about classrooms as sites of reproduction constituted within dynamic relations of power. The theory offers the potential for examining teachers' work from the premise that what they do is complexly intertwined with who they are. Rather than classrooms being viewed as spaces where teachers deliver an uncontested body of knowledge or a place where teachers create enabling environments in which children learn, classrooms become discursive sites for the production of contestable bodies of knowledge; where productions, constituted in relations of power, are themselves conflictual. When teachers are placed at the centre of the teaching endeavour, understanding what they do becomes contingent on understanding who they are. The corollary is that what they do cannot be viewed merely as that which they are expected to do; that is, mediate an 'uncontested' body of knowledge. They can no longer be positioned as mere creators of a seemingly neutral enabling environment where predetermined outcomes are realised. Rather, the knowledge they mediate and the meanings they transact, as well as the process of mediation they set in motion, are open to contestation and negotiation. As acting agents, teachers make choices; they act to produce and reproduce while at the same time being produced within complex discursive spaces of social action. Within such a perspective, therefore, assumptions cannot be made about teachers, content or processes of mediation. It cannot be taken for granted that because teachers have a learning programme, this qualifies them to teach and indeed deliver the 'expected' outcome.

This perspective becomes particularly useful when set against the dominant frameworks that have been used to understand teacher identity in South Africa, where much of the work followed patterns similar to those described earlier on in this chapter. It, too, was largely premised on functionalist or structuralist epistemological orientations, in which the teachers were positioned as either 'professionals' who serve the function of 'intellectuals' in societies, and/or 'workers' who are competent, accountable, capable and able to produce predetermined outcomes (Carrim in Lewin, *et al.*, 2003: 306). But, this work was also significantly different, as the following brief discussion suggests.

Perspectives on teachers and teaching in South Africa

As indicated in the earlier descriptions of research teachers and teaching, South Africa followed much the same routes in terms of the epistemological and theoretical orientations of research done, but it was also different due to the particular political and educational history of the country.[11] Briefly, the particularity of context in this instance was based on the use of race and class as key classificatory determinants in structuring schools and positioning teachers. Characteristically, and unlike in other parts of the globe where positioning teachers as 'professional intellectuals' tended to assure them middle-class status, in South Africa this was not a foregone conclusion for all teachers. The separatist policies of the country along racial lines produced differentiated experiences for Black and White teachers. White teachers, for the most part, were more qualified, worked in well-resourced environments, earned reasonably good salaries, enjoyed good benefits (medical aid, housing subsidies, etc.), and were more practised in rules that regulated and assured them a middle class professional status. Black teachers, on the other hand, were more often than not ill-prepared for the world of the classroom. Many were not only under-qualified but unqualified; they did not enjoy the same benefits as their White counterparts and worked in under-resourced and poor environments (Carrim, 2003). These categories of differentiation were further accentuated in ways that distinguished between female

11 The history of Education under Apartheid South Africa is well documented. For a comprehensive discussion, see Wolpe, 1988; Christie, 1986; Hartshorne, 1992; Jansen, 1991 Nkomo, 1990.

and male, positioning them differently across economic and class divides. This gendered configuration cut across the racial divide, making all female teachers vulnerable and thus less able to exercise their agency in schools. Characterised as 'permanently indefinite', they could not hold permanent teaching posts once they married. They did not obtain housing subsidies unless they were single and had to resign when they fell pregnant (no maternity leave was granted) (Carrim, 2003). Thus, while the dominant epistemological and methodological orientations in researching teachers were applied, in South Africa their application took on a very particular trajectory. Although much of the research in broad terms followed the trends already articulated in the foregoing sections, there was a greater awareness amongst researchers of the situated nature and particularity of this context as a unique environment that produced particular and differentiated teacher identities. The difference here too, as in feminist research, was emphasis on understanding how these categories produced difference and particular teaching outcomes rather than on what happens with and to teachers, or the inherent complexity in the structure and agent relationship. Much of the research focussed on how teachers *are positioned* within the dominant discourses of, for example, race and class, and the consequences this held for understanding their work. Little, if any, of this research focused on how teachers were positioning themselves and how they, as active agents, might have been complicit in reproducing the Apartheid script of differentiation. Thus, little research focused on teachers who were not only positioned but were positioning themselves (based on acceptance of the status quo), and, were thus able to reproduce, modify and sometimes subvert the dominant discourses.

In sum, any attempt to understand what teachers do when they teach sexuality and HIV/AIDS in a South African context must face two issues that the work has thus far pointed towards. The first relates to the supposedly and taken-for-granted easy fit between constructions of the professional teacher who is able, capable and competent to mediate sexuality and HIV/AIDS messages, and conceptions of schools as neutral discursive spaces where mindful bodies are privileged. The second is associated with limitations in epistemological and methodological orientations that obscure the complexity in the relationship between structure and agency, particularly the role of the teacher. The questions this work poses in relation to the above, therefore, centre on the teacher positions that are invoked when none of the above can be held up as truth. What happens in classrooms when a physical and sexualised body is invoked? How do teachers position themselves? What are the resources they draw on during such encounters? What is the interplay between structures and agency in these particular discursive spaces that are pre-mapped along racial and class categories? It is the nature of these questions that makes studying teachers and their work in teaching sexuality and HIV/AIDS fertile ground for examining teacher positioning through applying an alternative epistemology that pays careful attention to educational performances. Through the application of a framework in which the performative nature of teaching is foregrounded, one can begin to tease out what actually happens in Lifeskills classrooms and attempt to respond to the broader questions of whether or not schools are the best sites for mediating sexuality and HIV/AIDS. This approach brings into question constructions of schooling as neutral discursive spaces and teachers as mere deliverers of uncontested bodies of knowledge. The application of an alternative epistemology in this work will be demonstrated later in the analysis. The emphasis is in keeping with Alexander's views, and depicts iterative actions chartered inside a complex network of power relations and "social norms within the context of education and schooling" (Alexander, *et al.*, 2005: 2).

The next chapter analyses the dominant epistemological frameworks as well as dominant discourses from and through which meanings associated with HIV/AIDS are read. These, I argue, act as durable structuring mechanisms (Giddens, 1984) shaping not only attitudes, beliefs and meanings associated with the pandemic, but also influencing the nature of research. The consequence of this becomes clearer in Part IV, where I outline how these discourses first, influence the process, nature and outcomes of research, and second, become some of the "durable structuring properties" shaping classroom discourse (Giddens, 1984), and thus of importance to this work.

7 The limitations of dominant epistemological orientations and discourses in influencing understandings of, responses to and interpretations of HIV/AIDS

Introduction

At the end of the previous chapter I stressed that teachers are central figures in any pedagogical endeavour because they are not mere deliverers of an uncontested body of knowledge, nor are they unquestioningly responsive. They act to produce structures and discourses in as much as they are acted upon by these. Part II emphasised the notion that teachers do not operate in a vacuum, outside the socially constructed world in which they make meaning of their lives and their work in the classroom. Structures and discourses influence actions but at the same time are produced through the enactments of agents operating in particular fields of practice. Actions and their associated meanings, therefore, are integrally linked to the context in which people act. Those who interpret and act do so from a position, from a particular context that is at the same time both historically bound and instantiated through the actions of actors who operate in different fields of practice (Hall, 1990). In reviewing selected literature on researching teachers and teaching, I highlighted how dominant epistemological and methodological orientations do not offer perspectives on teachers that foreground either the situated contexts in which they live and work or their agency thereby failing to offer insight into the complex interrelationship between teachers and their work. I proposed an alternative epistemological framework that positions teachers centrally as those who act and contribute rather than merely respond to contexts in which they find themselves. Teacher subject positioning, therefore, continues to be a key consideration in examining their understanding and experience of teaching sexuality and HIV/AIDS because, as constructors and by implication modifiers and transformers, they carry or take up the discourse through their daily performances (instantiated actions). As a way to understand the particularized context of this cohort of teachers, what follows in this chapter is an analysis of dominant political, sexuality and disease discourses that have a major influence in shaping responses to and interpretations of HIV/AIDS. As dominant 'structuring properties' (Giddens, 1984), these discourses act as the prevailing frames of reference inscribing meaning onto the pandemic. By implication, therefore, and in the case of this work, these discourses become interpretive frameworks influencing pedagogical content as well as teacher behaviour in and outside pedagogical contexts. In addition, I provide evidence to suggest that such discourses privilege particular epistemological and methodological orientations and put limits on the nature of HIV/AIDS research; orientations, I argue, that propose particular intervention and prevention models which do not question the relationship between content and context in general, and more specifically, the interrelationship between teachers and their work.

In an attempt to understand factors shaping teachers' understanding and experience of sexuality and HIV/AIDS, and hence their teaching on these topics, I introduce this chapter with a brief review of sexuality discourses that shape (Western) constructions of the term. I begin with a brief historical overview and then follow this with a discussion on the frames of reference used to understand and interpret its meaning.

Following on from this, I briefly situate HIV/AIDS within historical discourses on disease. By tracing the similarities in response to disease through time, such a discussion highlights the complexity of meanings associated with the pandemic. Positing it as a modern disease, this section provides some perspective on modernist constructions of HIV/AIDS. The argument here is that this disease is not merely a disease, but rather a signifier, a symbolic bearer of a host of meanings deeply associated with individual and collective identities that teachers implicitly (or explicitly) embody and take up in classroom discourse.

In the third section, I locate the discussion more firmly within a South African context by giving a brief commentary on the political discourses surrounding HIV/AIDS. The controversy surrounding HIV/AIDS in South Africa is not new. As a key discursive space, the political debates regarding HIV/AIDS act to produce specific scripts from which the South African HIV/AIDS text is read and interpreted. Discourses in this highly contested space are riven by contradictory meanings, indicative of how social action is constituted in particularized contexts that produce, sometimes generalized but often, particular sets of meaning in and through the actions of those operating in these social settings.

The final section of Part III brings Chapters 6, 7 and 8 together by reviewing selected literature on HIV/AIDS. Rather than a general review, this section follows the same approach taken in the previous chapter, where emphasis was placed on examining limitations in epistemological and methodological orientations that influence research on teachers and their work. The focus here, though, is two-fold: dominant discourses and the research agenda. I do two things in developing a concluding argument. First, I present an argument that traces how discourses described in this section act both as epistemological filters in constructions of the HIV/AIDS discourse in general, and as points of reference that shape research agenda in particular. I point out that these discourses act as regulative structures from and through which not only meanings and interpretations of HIV/AIDS are constituted, but also from which research agenda are developed. With regard to the latter, the argument is that as regulative structures, they act to constrain the nature of research and the type of epistemological questions asked about social action. In the case of this work, such orientations limit questions about the complex interaction among discourses, structures and agents, and thus offer no insight into this network of relations in the case of teachers and their work. This section, therefore, concludes with a brief comment on how the three section work in concert to provide the conceptual, analytical and methodological framework for the study.

Orientations towards sexuality: implications for HIV/AIDS discourse

Sexuality is at the core of our being; the most natural thing about us, yet also the most difficult to explain (Weeks in Phillips & Reay, 2002). As a phenomenon that touches the heart of who we are, it often works as a producing and interpretive script from and through which social, political, and moral acts are read and sometimes produced and reproduced. As discussed below, issues of sexuality (and by implication HIV/AIDS) run deep in discourses about social life and social action.

Societies over time have tried to find ways of restricting sexual behaviour through prohibitions and other regulatory mechanisms, but it has continued to be something difficult to restrain. It is little wonder, therefore, that HIV/AIDS has become what it is, a symbolic bearer of a host of meanings, because it invokes that which is so deeply private yet at the same time so public: our sexuality (Weeks, 1989). While one would not wish to underestimate the very real and devastating effects of HIV/AIDS on many countries around the world, the perspective taken here is that constructions, material and symbolic meanings and practices ascribed to sexuality are where HIV/AIDS is produced, interpreted, and read. HIV/AIDS is as much about sexuality, morality, politics, social marginality, dominance and power as it is a disease. Or rather in as much as it is a disease, HIV/AIDS also amplifies issues of sexuality, the sexual self and associated meanings and interpretations. Any investigation into HIV/AIDS has therefore to consider its locatedness and associations with the broader discourses of sexuality. Phillips and Reay, in describing the significance of taking a historical perspective on sexuality, state that it "forces [a] rethinking of a wide range of topics already established as subjects for historical investigation, including marriage, family, concepts of sex and gender, roles of men and women, class relations, race relations, religious ideologies, and relationships between the state and individuals" (2002: 4). In the same vein, consideration of sexuality forces a rethink of HIV/AIDS, its associated meanings, and its symbolic significance not only as a disease but also as a script from which identities are produced and reproduced. This discussion therefore examines the influence of epistemologies of sexuality on discourses of HIV/AIDS, and traces the extent to which these have acted and continue to act as interpretive grids from which the pandemic is understood in society and in research. It highlights some of the limitations such a stance holds for the nature of research, on the one hand, and classroom discourse on sexuality and HIV/AIDS, on the other.

It is not my intention to provide a comprehensive overview of the history of sexuality (see Irvine, 2003; Parker & Gagnon, 1995; Weeks, 1989). This notwithstanding, constructions and understandings of sexuality are historically bounded and some historical account is unavoidable. A history of sexuality is also, at the same time, a history of identity. So, while the aim of this section is briefly to outline dominant trends in constructions and interpretations of sexuality, and to show how these are 'imported' and used within HIV/AIDS discourses, I also lay the foundation for the argument later in the chapter that calls for different frames of references for understanding and interpreting the discourses of sexuality and HIV/AIDS in the classroom.

Traceable in this history, are broad themes that Irvine describes as "the denaturalisation of sexuality and its origin; the historicization of sexuality; the analytic shift from 'deviant' to 'deviance/margins to the centre; the destabilisation of sexual categories and identities and emphasis on the fluid and diverse meanings of sexual acts; and the theorization of sexuality and gender as performative" (2003: 429). Although they are not applied fully in this discussion, the categories are useful in that they provide noticeable shifts in discourses on sexuality.

Social theorists (see Irvine, 2003; Weeks, 2002) argue that even though sociologists have a long history of researching sexuality (through sexuality studies dating from about the mid-seventies), this body of work has been largely marginalised, unless it was done within the confines of 'an acceptable discourse' which in this case meant the 'authorised voices' of religion, medicine, medico-morality, law, psychology and the like (Weeks in Phillips & Reay, 2002: 27). Advances in theorising about sexuality, however, have been spurred on by more recent work in post-structuralism, feminist theory, cultural studies, critical theory and feminist, queer and AIDS activism (Irvine, 2003: 431).

Briefly, the history of sexuality is variable and broad, including discussion of "identities, orientations, work-practices, images, bodies, thoughts, institutions, and systems of power but focused in the constant connection with erotic desire' (Phillips & Reay: 2002: 5). While it may be difficult to offer a comprehensive definition of sexuality, Phillips & Reay (2002), thus insist that sexual desire is the underlying characteristic that distinguishes discourses of sexuality from discourses that might be about sex. As they state, "even if manifestations of desire (e.g. arousal, sex acts) are not present, associations with sexual desire are necessary to make an identity, a practice, or a thought sexual" (2002: 5). As such, they posit that it is necessary to distinguish between those experiences that are associated with desire from those which are not.

Early constructions of sex defined it as a 'natural drive', essentially in opposition to civilization, culture, or society. Underpinned by scientific positivist epistemologies, in these early constructions of sex, the sex drive was described as internal to the individual, with societies and cultures playing a responsive rather than proactive role in shaping the nature and context of sexual development. Largely influenced by science and religion, and associated repressive discourses disallowing sexual freedom, constraining sexual behaviour and punishing sexual deviance, such constructions were premised on anatomical differences and the acceptance of males and females as naturally different. As such, sex difference was understood to be the result of natural biological determinants along constructions of femininity and masculinity (Weeks, 1989; Parker & Gagnon, 1995).

It was only from the nineteenth century onwards when discourses of sexology introduced terms like *'heterosexual, homosexual, bisexual, masochist'* that 'sexuality' as a term we know today, came to be used (Phillips & Reay, 2002). This is a period when the move by science and medicine into the "sexual arena meant in effect that something called sexuality was located and defined, boundaries were set up, and deviancy was mapped out" (Phillips & Reay, 2002: 13).

Sexuality, particularly in the West, was usually defined along the binary of heterosexuality and homosexuality (Phillips & Reay, 2002). Premised on moral and religious discourses on sex, heterosexuality is privileged in its identification as that which is 'normal' and 'natural' as opposed to homosexuality, which is defined as 'deviant' and 'unnatural' (Parker & Gagnon, 1995; Phillps & Reay, 2002). Theories privileging the naturalness of the male/female distinction premise constructions of sexuality on male, patriarchal discourses, and largely from heterosexual descriptions, practices, and traditions (Parker & Gagnon, 1995).

Phillips and Reay (2002) suggest that historically, gender was often a defining feature in patterns of sexuality with, for example, "the pattern of dominant, masculine men desiring passive, feminine women" (2002: 3). This pattern of hierarchy precedes even the move from what Lacquer (1990) calls the 'one-sex' to 'two-sex' model. He suggests that it was only in the 1800s that sex as we know it, was 'invented', that is, when Western societies moved from what he calls a 'one-sex model' to a 'two-sex model' of sexual difference (Lacquer, 1990). Prior to that, women's bodies were not considered different from men: the difference being only in the arrangement of body parts (Moi, 2005). Thus, it was accepted that women were no different from men because they possessed all the parts men have. But the anatomical arrangements (exterior versus interior; inverted versus erect) did imply a hierarchical privilege with men exercising power in social and cultural settings. Historically too, other determinants including social status, class, and age, also acted as classificatory frameworks from which sexualities play out. But gender conflated with sex has for sometime written the script from which male and female bodies are read and positioned.

It is only very recently (in the last 30–40 years), that discourses have emerged that do not accept such binaries, but rather recognise a range or multiplicity of sexualities. In describing modern sexualities Giddens, for example, suggests that one of its distinguishing features is "its malleability" (1992: 14–15). To him, these binaries have obscured the way sexuality "functions as a malleable feature of self" (ibid). Such shifts in discourse of sexuality, from polarised conceptions to ones including notions of choice about sexual preference and desire are, therefore, relatively new. They mark the move from sex being defined as naturally determined to one which considers it as socially constructed and contextually bounded. As Weeks (in Phillips & Reay, 2002: 39) states, "it is no longer possible to see sex as caught in the toils of nature, outside of history." This development was influenced to a large extent by Foucault in his work on the *History of Sexuality* (1978), in which he presents the "genealogy of the Western apparatus of sexuality" (Weeks in Phillips & Reay, 2002: 28). This work marked the beginning of a different way of understanding sex and sexuality. The position Foucault takes is that sexuality should be understood as historically and socially constructed. He (Foucault, 1976: 105) states:

> Sexuality must not be thought of as a kind of natural given which power tries to hold in check, or as an obscure domain which knowledge tries gradually to uncover. It is the name that can be given to a historical construct: not a furtive reality that is difficult to grasp, but a great surface network in which bodies, the intensification of pleasures, the incitement to discourse, the formation of special knowledges, the strengthening of controls and resistances, are linked to one another, in accordance with a few major strategies of knowledge and power.

It is in this work that he denounces widely-held assumptions about Victorian societies as repressive. He meticulously describes them as neither sexually repressive nor reticent. For him, while regulatory mechanisms of control were present, Victorian society was far from silent about matters of sex. Expressions of and debates about sexuality were in the public eye; through discussions, research, public debates, medical advice; a sexuality outwardly expressed but falling short of following through with the sexual 'act' (Bailey in Phillips & Reay, 2002). Foucault's work offered new insights into the history of sexuality, destabilising sexual categories.

But it is the work in women's studies, feminist and queer theories, and gay and lesbian studies that prompted not only an expansion of thinking around sex and gender (see Rubin, 1975, MacKinnon, 1982; Butler, 1990), but also a questioning of the epistemological foundations underpinning constructions of sexuality. This work queried the ways in which dominant frameworks were applied in research and problematised questions of who conducted research and for what purpose (Parker & Gagnon, 1995). It also signalled a move away from biological deterministic constructions of gender and sexuality, and from examining and understanding sexual behaviour as an end in itself, to scrutiny of the social and cultural rules and practices that govern, name and shape constructions and behaviour, where the latter was not constrained within binaries of heterosexual/homosexual, mind/body/, masculine/feminine and their essentialist notions. Deconstructing these binaries allowed for questioning of the nexus between gender and sex and made possible the insertion of discourses characterizing such a connection as unstable, fluid, and complex. This work also propelled a resurgence of research on the body, shifting discourses from naturalist constructions of the body to understanding the "corporeal body" (Butler, 1990): a body in, through, and upon which meaning is read, produced, and reproduced. In this work, the body is understood as an embodiment of the material, symbolic, emotional, and social: a lived body (Weeks in Phillips & Reay, 2002, does caution, though, that this work is as much political as it is about expanding the discourse).

The discussion above is instructive in two ways. First, understanding shifts in discourses of sexuality is as much about understanding identity and positioning the human subject in social relations as it is about sexual identification. And so, as will become clearer later, this discussion is not only about sexuality, but also about the intimate interrelationship among sexuality, subjectivity and subject positioning. Second, this discussion is useful for understanding the interpretive lenses through which HIV/AIDS discourses are constructed and reproduced. Theoretical advances in discourses on sexuality, it would seem, have not always found expression in the methodological and epistemological frameworks used in researching sexuality. Since the associations between sexuality and HIV/AIDS are assumed, the limitations to understanding the latter through 'old' and un-nuanced lenses are traceable in research on HIV/AIDS, as Chapter 8 will show.

This discussion in some way highlights the resistance of dominant epistemologies to shifts even in the face of rigorous and prolific struggles by marginal discourses that have since moved from the margins to the centre, metaphorically speaking. But, along with the meanings ascribed to disease through time, as the next section will show, notions of sexuality set boundaries to understanding the material and social impact of the disease.

What follows is a brief discussion that embeds HIV/AIDS within the broader discourses of disease. This discussion is not intended as an overview of the historicity of disease. Instead, it highlights meanings, metaphors, and interpretations associated with disease, and traces the nexus between other diseases and HIV/AIDS, with a view to emphasising how, as seen in the foregoing discussion, the meta-scripts become lenses through which HIV/AIDS, as a modern disease, is constructed.

Orientations towards disease: implications for HIV/AIDS discourse

As a disease, responses to HIV/AIDS seem consistent with ways in which societies around the world have reacted to disease in the past, that is, mainly by explaining their materialization as the will of God. Often disease was associated with judgement for wrongdoing, or indicative of God's wrath upon an evil person or group of persons. Such interpretations are evidenced in the metaphors used to describe and give meaning to diseases like the Black Death, small pox, cancer, syphilis and tuberculosis (Sontag, 1988). Metaphors often bear moral judgements and interpretations and as commentaries, can be indicators of the moral state of a society. The underlying assumptions associated with such metaphors, as Weeks (1989: 2) suggests, "insensibly infiltrate medical theories and responses, and in turn shape and reshape popular attitudes." The view that diseases are moral judgements inflicted on society pervades consequent action. For example, diseases such as syphilis, tuberculosis, and cancer carried significant symbolic meaning, because they connected "individual fault, social marginality and moral inadequacy with a tendency to acquire one or other of them" (Weeks, 1989: 2).

Diseases affect the material and social conditions of people at various levels of the social strata in particular ways, and HIV/AIDS is no exception. Common to all diseases is their social, political, and ethical situatedness. Of social significance are the meanings and interpretations people give to the root causes of disease and illness. Following this line of thought, of greater consequence is the *manner* in which such meanings and representations find expression through "a host of differing, and often conflicting and contradictory social possibilities" (Weeks, 1989: 1), which shape subsequent responses and possible actions.

A cursory analysis of discourses on HIV/AIDS indicates patterns of moral inflation similar to those traced in responses to other diseases. A more critical analysis, though, reveals distinct differences, which as Weeks (1989) suggests, are characteristic of modern society and embedded in notions of modernity. Delanty defines modernity as "the pursuit of autonomy in many different areas in life, of which three can be highlighted: the autonomy of the political subject, the autonomy of culture and the autonomy of the social" (1999: 17). To him, often the pursuit of autonomy is characterized by what he calls a "central conflict" that is, tension between "integration and differentiation"; be it:

> democracy versus capitalism, liberty versus discipline, the individual versus society, differentiation versus integration or cultural ideal versus social reality- and argued, moreover, that in the most general sense this conflict is related to the problem of reconciling the autonomy of the political Subject, who is essentially free and self-legislating, to the demands of social order. (Delanty, 1999: 17–18)

Modern society is described by Giddens as "those modes of social life or organisation emerging in Europe from around the seventeenth century, and which subsequently became worldwide in their influence" (1990: 1). To him modernity is a phase in human history that has changed modes of life in the most overwhelming ways. These transformations are exponentially more pronounced, qualitatively different and unlike anything experienced during times that are more traditional (Giddens, 1991). Modernity, he suggests, has created shifts from more traditional forms of social order to ones that bring together what he calls the "two extremes of extensionality and intentionality: globalising influences on the one hand and personal dispositions on the other" (Giddens, 1991: 1). Characteristically, modernity brings with it different modes of social ordering, key features of which are uncertainty and choice. Associated issues of trust and risk take on specific meanings, details of which, while important to understand, are beyond this discussion. Suffice it to say that HIV/AIDS as a modern disease invokes the characteristic features of modernity in distinct ways, accentuating issues associated with choice and uncertainty: security versus danger and trust versus risk.

As a modern disease, the metaphors associated with HIV/AIDS present it as the "disease of all diseases" (Weeks, 1989). HIV/AIDS is understood and interpreted through the use of "plague" – as its central metaphor – and is, as such, projected as constituting "the highest standard of collective calamity, evil scourge" (Sontag, 1988: 44). Second, together with diseases such as leprosy, syphilis, and tuberculosis, HIV/AIDS is understood as shameful in that it not only has fatal consequences, but also changes the body and makes it abhorrent. Its association with what in many communities is accepted and tacitly understood as sacred (Durkheim, 1952; 2001) exaggerates its calamitous status. In as much as it 'marks' the individual, it acts as a signifier of particular aspects of identity, particularly sexual identity, in a way that other diseases have not always done (Sontag, 1990). The difference, too, lies in HIV/AIDS being seen as a plague that is "collectively invasive", a disease "incurred by (and revealing of) people both as individuals and as members of a risk group" (Sontag, 1988: 45). Unlike other diseases, HIV/AIDS exposes the social vulnerability of both the individual and social group in that it not only infiltrates the body, but also becomes the property of an entire group (Sontag, 1988). In this way, it comes to be a marker of identity. Even in instances when the definition of 'risk group' may have changed as HIV/AIDS penetrated different regions of the world, its identification and signification as a marker of identity remains pronounced.

At another level, HIV/AIDS makes us question science, particularly medical science and the notion of technological advancement. At a time when, predominantly, medical experts seem to have produced successful responses and answers to many challenges (natural, environmental, social, etc.), the virus seems to pose a challenge that so far, has brought with it more questions than answers and/or successful treatment (Sontag, 1988; Weeks, 1989). Fear, anxieties and tensions that arise from the non-treatability of HIV/AIDS, on the one hand, and advancement on the other is, as Small in Weeks (1989) suggests, linked with modernity.

Most importantly, though, HIV/AIDS is perceived as the script from which competing, conflicting and sometimes contradictory messages of self-interest and freedom, indulgence and consumerism, on the one hand, and self-improvement, self-discipline, self-management on the other, are written, read and interpreted. It can be viewed as the text for a deeper examination of personal and societal norms and values. As Weeks (1989: 2) argues, HIV/AIDS has become the "symbolic bearer of a host of meanings about our contemporary culture: about its social composition, its racial boundaries, its attitudes to social marginality; and above all, its moral configurations and its sexual mores." HIV/AIDS has become the symbolic bearer of identity. Nowhere is this more evident, as the next section shows, than in the political debates about the pandemic in South Africa.

The politics of HIV/AIDS in South Africa

HIV/AIDS affects all people directly or indirectly in South Africa. The pandemic permeates the everyday lived experiences of many communities, families, and individuals. Many communities in the country have experienced an increase in the number of deaths, orphans, and in some places, an increase in child-headed families and high incidences of rape.[12] In communities where such occurrences are common, the pandemic has had a direct effect on households and communities in material ways, influencing income and expenditure, and shaping and reorganising social arrangements and family structures. Implicitly, HIV/AIDS affects civil society in different ways, for example, through imposed government policies that seek to address its impact, changes to health care systems, and the like. HIV/AIDS is writing itself into the economic, political, and social conditions influencing the day-to-day practices of the South African population, however removed from the 'problem' some consider themselves to be.

12 In some communities, an increase in rape cases can be connected to myths about HIV/AIDS which include, amongst a host of others, a belief that sleeping with a virgin cures the disease.

Vociferous debates on HIV/AIDS abound at many levels in the public space and, as such, are part of the daily public life of South Africans through media coverage – television and billboard campaigns encouraging particularly the youth to consider minimising the risk of infection through safe sex practices – and through public debates between, for example, health care administrators and advocacy groups. Often, the primary focus in health care, economics, social welfare, and education rests on how to manage systems or how systems will manage in response to the effects of the pandemic. In some instances debates centre more on the effects of the pandemic on the lived experience of those infected and affected. In such instances the emphasis becomes an attempt to understand the day-to-day experiences of people and how this pandemic does or does not affect who they are and how they make meaning of their circumstances.

Debates between politicians and civil society have become common, with each contributing to constructing a volatile, contestable discourse about the pandemic. The ex-State President[13], cabinet ministers, advocacy groups, corporate companies (e.g., pharmaceutical companies), religious organisations, and the like, all share a space in the public sphere and offer varying perspectives on the pandemic. Each group not only offers possible solutions to the dilemmas imposed by the pandemic but also responds and makes meaning of the pandemic from a particular position. While the specifics of the debates are not important for this discussion, these interactions point to the constructed nature of the pandemic, on the one hand, and to the highly contestable and uncertain environment in which these various groups compete, on the other hand. In as much as these debates are largely about HIV/AIDS, they are more than merely about a disease that infects the body; they are about the social organisation of life – the meanings we give to it and the positions from which we speak. Devastating as its effects are, this pandemic does offer a lens from and through which to examine aspects of human interaction and social action.

13 The controversy surrounding Mr. Thabo Mkeki, the State President of South Africa's and the Minister of Health's stance on a range of issues pertaining to HIV/AIDS have been the focus of numerous popular and scholarly articles and are thus well known (see Crewe, 2000 and McCafferty, 2003).

In summary, this chapter has put forward the argument that constructions of the pandemic are largely influenced by dominant discourses of sexuality and disease, and in the case of South Africa, by the public debates resulting largely from the controversial stance taken up by the President and Minister of Health, on the one hand, and advocacy groups and civil society more generally, on the other hand. It has also revealed another layer of influence, namely ways in which epistemological and methodological orientations locate constructions of the pandemic within health and medico-moral discourses that serve to constrain more hermeneutic understandings of the pandemic, as the next chapter illustrates. These layers of influence act to structure the meanings and interpretations people associate with the pandemic, and position people in distinctive discursive spaces where neither the message not the messenger are stable entities. Importantly, though, this section drew attention to the resources that subjects in this study draw on to position themselves in relation to the pandemic.

8 Limitations of dominant discourses and epistemological and methodological orientations in researching HIV/AIDS

In Chapter 6, I described how the application of particular epistemological and methodological orientations in researching teachers and their work produces particular understandings of their positioning in relation to their work. Through a critique of selected teacher research, I developed the argument that these dominant orientations act restrictively as interpretive frameworks and as such, offer limited perspectives on the dialectic relationship between structures and agents and, in the case of this study, between how teachers are positioned (or position themselves) in relation to their work. I offered a combination of Foucault's concepts of power and the panoptic gaze and Butler's theory of performativity as epistemological tools that help unpack this dialectic and offer ways of understanding the complexity in the relationship between teacher identity and teachers' work. In pedagogical enactments in the classroom and as an 'embodied self', the teacher does produce 'the self' through a "turning back upon oneself or even turning *on* oneself" (Butler, 1997: 3).

Chapter 7 put forward the argument that constructions of the pandemic, largely influenced by dominant discourses of sexuality and disease, are framed within particular epistemological and methodological orientations that limit the nature of research on HIV/AIDS. As a way of bringing the discussions in the previous chapters together, what follows is a review of selected literature on HIV/AIDS. Rather than offer a general review, the position I take in what follows below is one that examines (a) limitations in this research in understanding the complex interplay between structure and agent; (b) ways in which the dominant discourses articulated above find expression in this body of research in particular ways; (c) limitations of the dominant epistemological and methodological orientations in expanding understandings and researching the pandemic; and (d) the implications of this work for understanding researching HIV/AIDS in education in general and teachers and their work in particular. Briefly, the body of research reviewed, generally embedded in particular epistemological orientations and particular discourses, often seeks to find out *what* is known about the disease rather than *how* and *where* knowledge is produced and how we come to know. These discourses, I argue, privilege particular types of research and place limits on the kinds of questions asked. In the main, such discourses not only shape general responses to the pandemic, but also frame the HIV/AIDS and sexuality script in the classroom. I put forward the argument that such frames of reference provide particular lenses through which the pandemic is interpreted and researched, in a way that often disallows more nuanced ways of understanding its effects. The review draws attention to the gaps in research that result from an application of particular epistemological and methodological frameworks, and as such, offers a rationale for the epistemological and methodological orientation of this study. Together with the previous two chapters, this one contributes to the conceptual and analytical framework and anchors this study within the broad arena of educational research on HIV/AIDS.

Researching HIV/AIDS: global perspectives

HIV/AIDS research around the world is well documented. Voluminous amounts have been written about the disease in reports, journal articles and books in the last twenty to twenty-five years, as an in-depth library search indicates. While it was beyond the scope of this study to provide a comprehensive critique of this literature, a cursory review reveals two issues that are pertinent here. The first is a consideration of the dominant epistemological and methodological frameworks within which research has been and continues to be located. The brief commentary below demonstrates how, for the most part, these frameworks account for and shape the research agenda, the nature of inquiry, as well as interpretations and responses to the pandemic. The second relates to *ways* in which epistemological and methodological frameworks work restrictively (and often unintentionally) in disembedding the discourse on HIV/AIDS in general and classroom content in particular.

Driven by discourses on sexuality (medico-moral) and disease, and thus a need to understand the biological nature of the disease, early trends in research for the most part, were aimed at developing and providing a medical explanation of the disease.[14] Importantly and rightly so, research during this period was geared towards finding a cure for the disease. Located within health and medico-moral discourses, much of this research laid emphasis on understanding how the disease affects and infects the individual biologized, physical body, as opposed to considering a corporeal body that is constituted in social relations. Three factors seem to account for this limit in focus.

The first may have had to do with who first displayed symptoms of infection and their positioning in communities. In other words, early detection of the disease in the United States and other Western countries was mainly limited to already marginalised members within communities, namely gay men, intravenous drug users and commercial sex workers (see Singhal & Rogers, 2003; Ulack & Skinner, 1991). Since the disease was identifiable amongst particular marginalised members in modern, urban communities, responses could be localised and contained. Even when the spread of the disease resulted in infections being traceable amongst heterosexual men and women in distinguishable mobile communities (e.g. truck drivers and mine workers, through practices that included men sleeping with other men and associations with commercial sex workers), affected populations were usually poor or those perceived as 'high risk', and thus already marginalised and silent or silenced.

The second, related point is that in stigmatising and thus 'othering' the disease as something infecting only 'deviant' and/or 'promiscuous' members of society, a second discourse was invoked. In as much as diseases like cancer[15] and tuberculosis, as described earlier, were understood as resulting from some kind of self-indulgence or the consequence of an unhealthy lifestyle, HIV/AIDS too was characterised as resulting from the weakness of the flesh. But unlike the former diseases, which Sontag (1990) suggests were perceived as resulting from over-indulgence or hazardous practices largely associated with legal drugs or chemical abuse, HIV/AIDS was judged as more than mere weakness or indulgence

14 For a review of this literature see MEDLINE 1966.

15 For example, over-indulgence resulted in cancer of the lungs for smokers; cancer of the oesophagus for alcoholics.

of the 'flesh'. Rather, HIV/AIDS was viewed as a disease of deviance and 'unnaturalness.' With diseases like syphilis, cancer and tuberculosis, communities could in some way attribute their origin to public/explicit/exhibited manifestations (illegal chemicals in the case of drug users, or to sex considered deviant with regard to sexually transmitted cases) and thus rationalise punishment as justifiable. Unlike these diseases, HIV/AIDS seems judged differently since, as Sontag says, "the sexual transmission of this AIDS is understood as a disease not only of sexual access but of perversity" (1990: 114). Making moral judgements of the infected, therefore, produced an artificial boundary between infected and uninfected, in terms of which the latter did not need to reflect on the direct effects of the disease on their everyday practices. While there may have been stigma attached to its contraction, this was obscured by the deeper silences associated with dominant constructions of sexuality (and the perception of HIV/AIDS as resulting from deviant, abnormal, promiscuous sexual behaviours), on the one hand, and the positioning of marginalised groups experiencing infections within communities, on the other.

The third aspect may have had to do with the relatively low numbers of infected cases and the low number of reported deaths during the early phases of the disease, in comparison to how the disease is playing out today.

This discussion is not intended to be a comprehensive history of the origins and changing nature of the disease. Rather, it is useful only in as much as it foregrounds ways in which epistemological and methodological frameworks worked to produce certain meanings and particular ways of understanding and interpreting the disease. Therefore, while anxiety about the origin and nature of the disease exists, as will become clearer below, locating the discourse within health, medical and moral discourses highlighted the individual character of the disease, thereby masking broader issues related to its relational and socially embedded nature. Even when as early as the 1990s, social scientists began discussions about the disease (Ulack & Skinner, 1991),[16] these were still largely influenced by early medico-moral conceptions and interpretations of the

16 In the preface to this book, based on the symposium entitled "AIDS and the Social Sciences: A Public Symposium on Research Agendas and Application", there was an acknowledgement that it was the first time that social scientists had paid attention to AIDS in the United States.

disease. So even in instances where different methodological frameworks and methods of data collection were applied (interviews, observations, etc.), the fundamental research questions remained relatively stable. These questions always seemed to relate to the number and particular group infected (who and how many), with geographic context, gender and sexual orientation being only some of the variables signalling difference in the actual research.

Rarely (see Ulack & Skinner, 1991 for some exceptions) in this early research were questions posed that sought to understand the hermeneutic nature of the disease, beyond numbers, and its systemic effects on health, social welfare and the economy. In instances where social issues were the focus, these were placed within a social justice framework (see Stockdill, 2003) that campaigned against stigmatisation, marginalisation, and discriminatory practices that often prevented access to healthcare for those infected. In instances where gender, for example, was identified as an influential factor, simple solutions (for example, assertiveness training for women) were suggested as a means of eradicating the power imbalances, particularly within heterosexual relationships. Often, too, recommendations included the provision of *more* knowledge to 'vulnerable' and unaffected (for example school-going youth[17]) communities, on the assumption that this would lead to the creation of an informed populace who would be in a position to make *individual* choices to protect themselves against infection. In cases where cultural practices were identified (see Kalipeni, Craddock, Oppeng & Ghosh, 2004), these were often mythologised and exoticised, thereby making change seem implausible.

Questions were seldom posed regarding the largely positivist epistemological and methodological frameworks or medico-moral discourses, which not only situate the research agenda, but also influence responses to the pandemic, as reflected through the types of policies and plans of action adopted by governments (see McElrath, 2002). More importantly, and of consequence for this study, few questions were asked relating to the social and cultural practices as well as the regulative discourses operative within communities. Few questions were posed regarding the constitutive nature of social action and how, within and through social relations people understood, responded to, and experienced the disease.

17 See Health Education debates of the 1980s and 1990s.

The epistemic and methodological frameworks therefore (un)intentionally limited the discourse and left investigations and considerations of the disease to 'hard science' to produce as yet unavailable solutions. Such approaches had, for the most part, obscured ways of understanding the manner in which this pandemic invoked aspects of individual and collective identities. A book edited by Barbour and Huby (1998) has gone some way towards addressing this, by providing insight into the development of theoretical frameworks that began to shift the epistemological and ontological framework away from the positivist paradigm to ones more firmly embedded in contemporary social theory.

The importance and major contribution this early research has had on understanding and responding to the disease is not in question here. There is little doubt that its dominance is traceable in research as well as in interpretive frameworks, responses, and even curricular orientations. The problem, however, relates to the generally unquestioning transposition/transference and application of epistemic and analytical frameworks across geographic and discursive spaces where experience of the disease bears little or no resemblance to the initial research sites discussed earlier in this section. The pandemic today is prevalent in continents like Africa, South America, and Asia where HIV-infections are highest amongst heterosexual populations, with youth and women in some countries being the hardest hit (McElrath, 2002; UNAIDS, 2006). The changing nature of the pandemic induces different concerns, and therefore requires and creates the need for different epistemological and ontological frames of references for its interpretation and understanding. However, this has not been the case, as the brief overview of research conducted in Africa in general and South Africa in particular, below, illustrates.

Researching HIV/AIDS in Africa

Research on HIV/AIDS in and pertaining to Africa and South Africa has proliferated only in the last ten years or so. For the most part, this work followed the trends outlined above in its orientation to the models, research agenda, analytical frameworks, and epistemological questions. While the research output is too large to detail, work reported, for example, in AIDS-ANALYSIS-AFRICA (which includes reports, journal articles, books; Retrieved on 13:08:05 from MEDLINE 1966 – Present: http://olc3.ohiolink.edu) attests to the phenomenon. In short, research on the continent has generally followed four trends that are consistent with descriptions in 4.5.1.

The first includes projection studies, which sought to map out the impact of the disease within and between countries and within sectors such as the economy and health. This included measuring or projecting the impact of the disease on countries in general and marginalised populations (e.g., the poor, truck drivers, commercial sex workers, women, mineworkers, prisoners, and the like) in particular. The second trend sought to gauge knowledge and perceptions of the disease within various communities (often here too the target was those perceived as vulnerable), with a view to providing education that would lead to informed decision making and rational choices regarding sexual behaviour. The third form of research was intended to develop some understanding of the impact of the pandemic on infected and affected populations. In this regard, research emerged that focused either on the experiences of people living with the disease or on those who suffer the consequences of the pandemic (for example, orphaned children and women). This included, amongst other things, attention to the way in which these members of communities were experiencing stigmatisation and how they often suffered double-marginalisation or double jeopardy, in regard to their infected status as well as their perceived moral behaviour. In cases where children were the focus, the catastrophic nature and devastating consequences of the disease was often the main unit of analysis. Where women (and by implication issues associated with gender) were the focus, they were often either positioned as victims of male dominance and as such 'powerless' to change circumstances, or as carriers of the virus and as such to blame for its spread. The fourth, a focus on intervention programmes and their impact in changing sexual behaviour patterns, emerged together with a proliferation of training programmes geared mainly towards women and youth.

The result of this work was helpful in as much as it alerted governments and compelled them to acknowledge the scale of the problem and develop systemic plans of action. However, the research was limited in its application beyond providing on understanding the scale of the problem and as a result, it could not respond to questions about the hermeneutic nature of the pandemic. Earlier discourses of sexuality and disease still prevailed in structuring understandings of and responses to the pandemic. In addition, this research followed global trends in the use of the same epistemological and methodological frameworks and as such posed similar research questions, despite this being work conducted in environments that are qualitatively very different.

The next section directs the discussion more closely towards research on HIV/AIDS in South Africa and traces ways in which similar paths to those described above have been followed, also without much interrogation of the epistemological or methodological orientations. This section highlights the consequences such a stance has for educational research on HIV/AIDS, a field that up until very recently has been on the periphery of research on the topic.

Researching HIV/AIDS in South Africa

In South Africa, health and economics were some of the first sectors active in researching the impact of the disease. As regards the former, understanding the epidemiological nature of the disease and its impact on the physical body took precedence. Controversial as this research has been (see Crewe, 2000; McCafferty, 2003; Willan, 2000), it has led to responses by government that have included, amongst a range of others, an emphasis on education and the development of policies and implementation plans aimed at minimising infection and providing adequate treatment and care for those infected and affected by the pandemic.

Within the economic sector, projective studies abound. These have been consistent with global trends in tracing the probable impact and effects of the pandemic on economic security in general and on human resourcing needs in particular (see Dorrington, *et al.*, 2002). Positioned within catastrophic discourses and using frames of reference outlined in the previous sections, such studies have been vociferous in predicting significant human loss and the subsequent negative impact this would have on the economic well-being of the country (see Johnson, 2000; Simbayi, *et al.*, 2005; Barnett & Whiteside, 2002). These studies, much like the research described in the two previous sections, have unquestioningly and uncritically applied the same dominant analytical and methodological frames of references used to shape earlier research work on the pandemic, and have not taken into account the extent to which these newer contexts produce different complexities and challenges, thereby producing a need for different sets of questions and the application of different epistemological and methodological frameworks. For the most part, the dominant epistemological questions remain those paying attention to the non-hermeneutic consequences of the pandemic.

The relevance of this brief discussion is twofold: the first is the serious consequences such work has for ways in which the pandemic is framed within everyday discourses, and the second relates to the nature of research within sectors like education, that have until very recently remained on the fringes of research debates. As the next section demonstrates, these too have unquestioningly followed the dominant research trends leading to limitations in interpreting what is at the core of this work, the inherent complexity in the relationship between structure and agency – in this case, teachers and their work, as the next section illustrates.

Researching HIV/AIDS in education

Research on HIV/AIDS in education has adopted much the same paradigmatic orientation as that already articulated in the sections above. Baxen & Breidlid (2004) highlight three trends that support this argument. Briefly, the first focuses on research aimed at examining the knowledge base or attitudes of different groups within school communities (for example teachers and youth) (see Harrison, Xaba, Kunene, & Ntuli, 2001; Levine & Ross, 2002; Peltzer, 2000; Peltzer & Promtussananon, 2003; Wood, Maepa, & Jewkes, 1997). This research often includes investigations into whether learners and/or teachers have adequate knowledge about HIV/AIDS transmission and prevention as well as their attitudes towards those infected with the virus. The dominant research strategies include the use of questionnaires and large-scale surveys.

Another trend includes research that projects the impact of the pandemic at the systemic level and the catastrophic consequences this might have for education systems. Through applying modelling and projective techniques, some of this research maps out the potential loss in capacity and delivery of quality education as a result (see Barnett & Whiteside, 2002; Human Science Research Council, 2005; Johnson 2002; Shisana, 2002; World Bank, 2000). Other researchers in this field project the consequences of the pandemic (through the illness and morbidity of teachers and learners), and how this would potentially affect planning for quality education. These researchers describe, often without accurate data, the devastating effects of the pandemic and the consequences these hold for human resource development, financing education, and the demand and supply of teachers at national, district and school levels (see Cohen, 2002; Kelly, 2000; Kelly, 2002; Coombe, 2000).

The third pattern includes studies measuring the impact of training, with a particular emphasis on the impact of training youth and teachers (see Bloomberg, 1993; Hopson & Scally, 1981; Kelly, 2000; Sliedrecht, 1996). Impact here is often interpreted as a change in attitude towards those infected, or an increase in knowledge about forms of transmission and prevention. Survey data and questionnaires are often the primary forms of data collection. The results consistently suggest that these groups have adequate knowledge about transmission and prevention and hold empathetic and supportive views towards the infected. However, reviews like the one by Kaaya, Mukoma, Flisher & Klepp (2002) analyse these studies and question interpretations of 'impact'. They point to the methodological and interpretative limitations of such studies.

Variations in the patterns of research have included some work that focuses particularly on youth, with a view to examining the nexus between education and sexual behaviour. This body of research asks why, in the face of the many prevention programmes geared towards education against prevention, youth are still reported as the population group whose rates of infection show the greatest escalation (see Hartell, 2005; LeClerc-Madlala, 2002; Scorgie, 2002; Wood & Jewkes, 1998).

Emerging research has gone some way in attempting to insert a different discourse from that described in the previous sections of this chapter. This research, also with a focus on youth, has begun to acknowledge the social embeddedness of the pandemic and as such, has begun to examine some of the social and cultural practices that add complexity to issues associated with infection and prevention (see Campbell, Foulis, Maimane & Sibiya, 2005; LeClerc-Madlala, 2002). In addressing the paucity of research that goes beyond knowledge about HIV/AIDS amongst youth, LeClerc-Madlala (2002), for example, expresses the need for new research trends that "shift from an emphasis on *more knowledge* to enabling youth to understand constructions of self and sexual identity in contexts in which issues of gender, power, sexuality are deeply connected to constructions of safe-sex and negotiation within relationships and HIV/AIDS knowledge" (Baxen, 2005: 59). A limitation of this emerging work, however, lies in its not necessarily questioning the underlying dominant epistemological and methodological discourses. Thus, and inadvertently, the recommendations produced are similar to outcomes that sometimes make simplistic associations between knowledge, behaviour, and training (see Campbell, *et al.*, 2005; Hartell, 2005). This notwithstanding, these studies have gone some way in illuminating the complex issues at hand by beginning to ask different sets of questions that require a shift away from positivist constructions of the pandemic to grounding the discourse in different epistemic and ontological roots (see Baxen & Breidlid, 2004; Baxen, 2005).

While not claiming to be comprehensive in detailing each study, what the brief review given above highlights are two key issues that have implications for locating this study. The first is an apparent absence of questioning the dominant discourses that inform responses to and understandings of the pandemic. The second is the paucity in the literature that points to responses, interpretations and understandings of HIV/AIDS at the school level, and particularly of what happens *in* schools, namely, *in* classrooms to teachers, between teachers and learners, and between teachers and the text.

The studies reviewed in this section are instructive in highlighting how dominant discourses work to influence and frame understandings and interpretations of HIV/AIDS. Fundamentally, the dominant discourses of sexuality and disease that have framed interpretations of and research into the effects of the pandemic in the health and economic sectors have been the same frames of reference applied in the field of education. These frameworks, as the above indicated, produce particular approaches to and interpretations of the disease in everyday life and in research. In the main, they limit the kinds of questions to those that seek to explain ways in which the disease either affects the system (structure) or infects the individual (subject). At one level, such frameworks dichotomise and delink these two aspects and at another, they disembed the subject from a context that includes a complex interplay between structure and agent. The influence of dominant discourses and epistemological and methodological frameworks that seek to find out *what* we know about the pandemic is, therefore, traceable and indeed undeniable in this work.

The relevance of this review for the present study lies in its highlighting the paucity of studies that focus particularly on what happens at the chalk-face in schools. In cases where studies exist, these have been primarily concerned with either making recommendations on what *should* be done in classrooms (see Coombe, 2000) or how different methodologies could be applied to improve the knowledge base of learners (see Mirembe, 2002). Thus, and linked to research on teachers in Chapter 6, the focus of these studies has usually been on the improvement of learning outcomes, with simplistic associations being made about relations between teachers, learners and knowledge. No studies pose questions about *who* mediates or what happens during the mediation process. In fact, in a South African context, no studies investigate what happens *in* Lifeskills classrooms when teachers mediate sexuality and HIV/AIDS knowledge. In particular, there is a shortage of work that focuses on teachers, either as mediators within the intervention process or as subjects and objects of research (Baxen, 2005). Where teachers have been subjects of research (see Akoulouze, Rugalema & Khanye, 2001), they have often been, as Baxen states, "positioned as deliverers of an uncontested, already negotiated and agreed upon 'body' of HIV/AIDS knowledge within schools and institutions that are not presented as discursive, complex and negotiated spaces" (2005: 60). The results of such research usually emphasise teachers' lack of *knowledge and skills* to teach lifeskills or sex education programmes effectively (Baxen & Breidlid, 2004). Implicitly, assumptions are made that teachers are able, willing and in the best position to mediate sexuality and HIV/AIDS knowledge. Explicitly, through clear specifications in the Revised National Curriculum Statements (Department of Education, 2003) of what knowledge has to be taught at the different levels of the General Education and Training Band (GET), teachers are positioned as those who can mediate the 'deeply private' in the public arena of the school (Baxen, 2005). The upshot of this is that the outcomes of such research often lead to particular responses and plans of action that more than likely include *more* teacher training and the provision of *more* knowledge, without questions about by whom and how the knowledge is understood, embodied, mediated and reproduced. Other studies (e.g., Coombe, 2000) have attempted to describe teachers as more "vulnerable" and, therefore, needing more special attention than the rest of society, citing mobility as a key indicator. Others, like Paul Bennel (2003), have sought to repudiate this assumption by providing evidence that makes the argument of teacher vulnerability unsustainable (Baxen & Breidlid, 2004).

No literature to date, therefore, considers teachers as individuals who operate as producers, reproducers, interpreters, mediators, and purveyors of knowledge on sex, sexuality or HIV/AIDS, and who work from and within discursive fields where knowledge is negotiated and contested rather than taken for granted as 'truth'. Where gaps in research exist, the suggested response includes examining ways of providing teachers with more effective training and/or programmes to implement the proposed new curricula (Akoulouse, *et al.*, 2001). Some studies, like Rivers and Aggleton (1999), imply a need to consider teachers as sexual beings who themselves might have difficulty teaching sex education. However, the recommendations include reductionist orientations that assume a "linearity about the relationship between knowledge and skills and between training and teaching that, on the one hand is devoid of context and culture and on the other hand, underplay teachers as active agents" (Baxen, 2005: 60). Studies examining the dialectic relationship between structure and agent as it plays out in the classroom when teachers mediate sexuality and HIV/AIDS have yet to emerge, even in the face of a wide acceptance of schools as locations for preventive messages and by implication, the importance of teachers as mediators of these messages (Gallant & Maticka-Tyndale, 2003; Kelly, 2000).

In sum, the dominant discourses of sexuality and disease remain those framing HIV/AIDS in health and economics, discourses deeply embedded in positivistic frames of reference that favour conceptions of a medicalised and/or moralised body which operates in a socially detached way. These constrain constructions of the disease and have inadvertently confined interpretations to those that understand the disease as located *in* the corporeal body, infecting the individual[18] with little regard for the more hermeneutic challenges it produces, such as the social consequences of the pandemic for individual and collective identities. With

18 The scale of the pandemic is almost always numerically and not discursively presented.

reference to what teachers do in the classroom, using medico-moral discourses as interpretive frameworks disallows the insertion of a discourse that traces the intricate set of interrelationships among sexuality and gender and the body as text; one upon and through which meaning, interpretation, and responses to the pandemic are read. Such an omission not only places limitations on the type of content offered in Lifeskills classrooms, but also, importantly, on the associated meanings and frames of reference from which subjects in the mediation process speak. In fact, within such frameworks, the subject is already spoken for.

In the same vein, the dominant epistemological and methodological frameworks applied in the research under discussion is much the same as was the case in Chapter 6, where teachers were often positioned as predetermined and responsive to structures (that is, deliverers of an uncontested body of knowledge or teaching to achieve predetermined and clearly articulated outcomes), rather than as individuals who operate and live in social contexts that shape them but, importantly, contexts in and through which they make meaning and to which they contribute. Few if any of these studies, as was the case in researching teachers and teaching, account for teachers as embodying the social and cultural practices shaping communities in and through which identities are produced and reproduced in the first place. No studies describe teachers as those who exercise choice or agency, who position themselves or who contribute, modify and transform discourses as they make them up.

In applying the dominant epistemological and methodological frameworks, the reviewed literature on HIV/AIDS in education, therefore, produces much the same outcomes as that in health and economics, and offers little insight into the particularity of subject positioning and the specificity of context, where meaning (in general and HIV/AIDS in particular) is constructed and produced within a complex arrangement of structure and agency. While methodologically there have been qualitative and quantitative shifts in the nature of research, for example from only quantitative to more qualitative research methodologies, as well as in number (large and small scale), in 'target' populations (away from 'marginalized' populations to including various respondents across the social spectrum), and in responses to the pandemic (e.g., away from training only about the disease to including training for the affected), such modifications in the *presentation* of the disease have not systematically found expression in noticeable ways through revised research frameworks or in national, systemic, or local responses. Responses have, by and large, remained limited to those making simplistic associations between knowledge and practice, with little or no consideration of situated contexts as discursive spaces where such knowledge is produced and contested.

The discussion so far, therefore, highlights a range of issues that are critical in considering teachers and teaching and raises concerns regarding challenges teachers face in teaching sexuality and HIV/AIDS. For example, locating the disease within a moral and/or religious discourse makes delivering messages of safety problematic, in the sense that encouraging people to practise safer sex using condoms may sometimes be interpreted as condoning illicit and/or pre-marital sex. Such discourses also contribute to the construction, development and implementation of curricula and educational programmes that emphasise discourses of prevention, treatment, and care, without considering the social and cultural practices within which the disease is embedded. Inadvertently, such perspectives make claims about individuals as operating independently, rationally, and autonomously. While at one level this may be true, at another, such a discourse obscures the relational nature of the disease and the complexity of social action. The upshot as it relates to this study is that the dominant educational response is often one that lays emphasis on the impact of the disease on a physical, medicalised, decontextualised body rather than one that operates relationally, always in response to itself, or to an 'other.' "Relationally" is in this instance is interpreted as interpersonal interaction as well as the relation between structure and agent.

Bringing it altogether: subject positioning and HIV/AIDS

Positioning teachers as the embodiment of structures and thus both carriers *and* mediators is an attempt to expand current epistemological paradigms to include frameworks that insert more hermeneutic ways of understanding HIV/AIDS discourse and its articulation in classrooms. This is done through examining the nexus between teacher identity and classroom practice from the premise that teachers operate within complex situated contexts by which they are not merely produced but to which they contribute. Second, such a focus offers the possibility of redefining schools as charged environments where structures and agents operate in complex ways to produce particular subject positions.

Part IV
Dominant factors shaping teachers' lives

Introduction

The next three chapters that comprise Part IV present the empirical evidence of the study. The first two offer insight into the different layers of influence shaping teachers' understanding of themselves as individuals and as members of various groups within communities. Importantly, too, these offer a framework for understanding the discursive space from and within which the teachers in the study are positioned and position themselves, as well as from and within which sexuality and HIV/AIDS discourses are mediated and interpreted. These two chapters situate subjects as operating in a particular space and time and offer perspectives on the specificity of context as a critical indicator for the understanding of social identity, subject formation and social positioning. They anchor what follows in Chapter 11, namely, descriptions of practices that are embedded and situated in a specific discursive space from which subjects speak and act. What the following two chapters do is describe the textual landscape from and through which one might situate the group of teachers reported on in the study. They also serve to demonstrate that context is discursively constituted by structures and discourses that are only visible through their instantiation in the actions and daily practices of social actors. In the case of this study, this is exemplified in what happens in classroom when teachers mediate sexuality and HIV/AIDS.

I begin by developing a description of the contextual landscape in Chapter 9. Using the set of analytical tools gleaned from Bourdieu's theory of practice, and drawing from documentary evidence, interviews and observational data, this chapter describes the *material and social conditions* that act as dominant structures, bringing into play past and present histories and shaping the lived experiences of the teachers and the communities in which they live. I begin with brief descriptions of the aesthetic, economic, and social landscapes of the two provinces from which the sample is drawn. I proceed with descriptions of the regions and communities in which the schools are located. Here I briefly describe the material and social conditions, highlighting similarities and differences between communities across provinces and beyond the racial classifications used to separate communities during the Apartheid era prior to 1994.

This section is followed by a summary account of the HIV/AIDS prevalence rates in the respective communities. I outline the provincial, municipal and district statistics and signal how the pandemic plays out in different sections of the population. This is in preparation for the discussion later in Chapter 10 that shows how only paying attention to provincial profiles obscures the actual experiences of the pandemic at the local level. I briefly comment on the consequences such a discursive space holds for the subjects in this study. Chapter 9 ends with descriptions of schools and the conditions within and through which teachers make meaning of themselves and their roles as mediators of sexuality and HIV/AIDS messages. Such a contextual description, I argue, is fundamental to understanding the factors shaping teachers' understanding and experience of teaching sexuality and HIV/AIDS because it offers insight into the particularity of the frames of reference from which these teachers speak and act.

Using interview data primarily, I proceed in Chapter 10 with an analysis of the *early and current experiences* shaping teachers' social identities. Here I analyse the influences (structural and discursive) shaping individual and collective experience. I foreground this section with questions about who these teachers are and what it is about themselves that they bring into Lifeskills classrooms. To do this I draw on Giddens's theory of structuration to frame the position I take in describing teachers' experiences. Rather than presenting their experiences as fixed and thus determining, I present them in terms of dominant social and cultural practices that act as conditions within and from which teachers speak, that is, as structuring properties that teachers draw on in making 'the self'. Chapter 10 introduces the main players in this study: the teachers. In concert with the previous chapter, Chapter 10 anticipates the discussion in Chapter 11 that examines the interrelationship between these influences and classroom practice, more particularly, the nexus between teacher behaviour and classroom practice.

Chapter 11 brings together what has been the main focus in this study, namely, understanding the nexus between teacher identity and classroom behaviour. I do this by examining what happens in the classroom when teachers mediate sexuality and HIV/AIDS. Through an examination of the practices of some teachers who typify distinct teacherly behaviours, I focus on a central feature of this study, the dialectic relationship between structure and agency. Mediating sexuality and HIV/

AIDS, as I have argued, invokes a physical, sexualized body that is not usually visible in the everyday practices of schools. Such an invocation produces particular subject positions that illuminate the performative quality of teaching. I provide evidence of how teachers draw on the repertoire of attitudes, beliefs, and teacherly behaviours accumulated over time to take up and, sometimes, reposition themselves in ways that are often counterproductive to the intended outcome. This section provides evidence that teachers are active rather than passive in respect of the pedagogical script. Importantly, Chapter 11 offers a glimpse of the complexity in the relationship between structure and agency and provides evidence of the deep struggle teachers endure in their attempt to reproduce a different script.

Diagram 1, below, illustrates the interrelationship between the layers of influence shaping teacher identities. It draws attention to the dialectic relationship between structure and agent that will become clearer as the discussion proceeds.

Diagram 1: Layers of Influence on Teachers' Social Identity and Discourses on HIV/AIDS: Understanding the Context

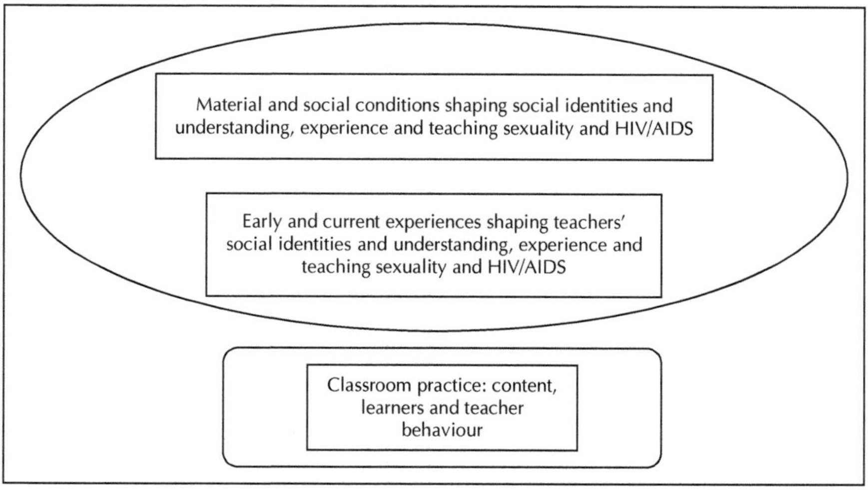

9 Social and material conditions shaping teachers' lives

As a disease, HIV/AIDS is contextual. Through applying Bourdieu's notions of capital, field and *habitus* as broad frames of reference, the contextual portrait here describes past and present histories that have shaped and continue to shape the lived experiences of the communities from which schools and teachers in the study were drawn. These histories, as I show below, act as the dominant discursive space shaping the lives of the school populations across and beyond the artificial categories of race, class, geographic location and gender, or any other social stratification. I provide this contextual narrative as a foundation for understanding the locatedness and social embeddedness of HIV/AIDS on the one hand, and the influences on social identity on the other hand. The descriptions set the scene for the subsequent argument that seeks to engage with essentialist notions of lived experience and to demonstrate how the conventional categories of race, class, geographic location, and so forth are often unhelpful in understanding the political, social, psychological, economic and deeply gendered landscape in which the cohort in this study make meaning of themselves. As the discussion will show, this discursive space produces multiple lenses and a complex arrangement of structure and agency in and through which these teachers take up subject positions in relation to the pandemic.

Social and material conditions of provinces, communities and schools

This section begins with a brief profile of the two provincial sites at which the study was conducted. I follow this with a more explicit demographic, social and economic description of the regional and municipal sites from which the schools are drawn, as well as a description of the communities from which respondents are drawn. Following on from this, I give a short description of the HIV/AIDS prevalence rates in the respective communities. Through this textual account, I situate the teachers within specific contexts. I argue that developing a contextual familiarity is critical for understanding subjects as situated and bounded within particular discursive spaces. Each section, therefore, offers insight into the various levels of influence and, in so doing identifies factors shaping understandings, experiences and the teaching of sexuality and HIV/AIDS.

The Provinces

Geographic Location, Economic and Social Landscape

The Apartheid history of South Africa is well documented (see Davenport & Saunders, 2000; Thompson, 2006). The sample of teachers in this study was drawn from two of the nine provinces[19] in South Africa, namely, the Western Cape[20] and Mpumalanga.[21] These two provinces, as this discussion will show, differ dramatically across a whole range of factors. While they by no means encompass the diversity of South Africa, they certainly offer a representative sample of some of the most critical political, economic, and social features of the country.

The Western Cape, with a population of about 4 524 335, is situated at the south-western point of Africa. It is geographically arresting with sprawling mountains and magnificent beaches. Its natural beauty and the excellent facilities available make it a popular tourist destination nationally and internationally. In 2003 alone, the tourism sector generated 13.0% of the total Gross Domestic Product (GDP) of the province (*South Africa Year Book*, 2003).

19 The other seven are Kwazulu-Natal, Northern Province, Free State, Gauteng, North West Province, Eastern Cape, and Northern Cape.

20 The Western Cape is geographically located where the sun sets. Metaphorically then, it may be called 'Shonalanga, that in isiSwati means 'the place of the setting sun'.

21 When translated, Mpumalanga means 'the place of the rising sun'.

The Western Cape has clothing and textile, printing and publishing, agriculture, fishing, forestry and mining and quarrying industries. The agricultural sector contributes more than 55% towards South Africa's total agricultural export output and 23% of the national agricultural GDP. As the largest money spinners in the province, the real estate, finance and business services (magnate insurance and petroleum companies located in this province) contribute about 26.6% towards the provincial GDP (Census, 2001). With growing economic opportunities created by the above, this province, with an economic growth rate of 14%, boasts GDP rates higher than the national average (South Africa Yearbook, 2003).

The Western Cape's industrial market creates employment for a large number of workers. Results of a study conducted by the Graduate School of Business suggest that new developments such as the Cape Town International Convention Centre that opened in 2003 have the potential to create as many as 47000 new jobs over a ten-year period (South Africa Yearbook, 2003). From a national perspective, therefore, and with only 12%[22] of its people currently unemployed, this province has the lowest rate of unemployment in the country (Labour Force Survey, 2001).

This province also has the highest adult literacy rate in the country. According to the Census of 2001, only 5.7% of the adult population (20 years and older) has not had any schooling experience. Year by year, the matric[23] (Grade 12) pass rate is one of the highest in the country. English and Afrikaans are the dominant languages, even though isiXhosa is also an official language in the province.

What seems unaccounted for and thus not accurately represented in census descriptions is the ever-increasing migrant population[24] found in informal settlements along the highways and the periphery of the metropolis. This population is an integral part of the geographic configu-

22 This is the reported official rate but the experience in communities might be very different.

23 Matric is the final external examination written by all school leavers at the end of 12th grade. This examination is often used as a filter for entry into tertiary institutions and access to the job market.

24 While the majority of this population comes from the Eastern Cape in search of employment and a better quality of life, there is a growing population of people from outside the South African borders who too, are forced to live in these informal settlements.

ration of this province but more importantly, it marks this landscape geographically, economically, socially, and politically.

It is from this geographically appealing and supposedly economically stable, primarily urban environment that seven schools (three primary and four secondary) were purposively sampled. From the above provincial profile (comparatively low levels of employment, many employment opportunities, world class tourist amenities and the like), one could easily be lulled into believing that communities in this province constitute and inhabit relatively stable environments where children go to school, parents work and where there exists, by whatever social index we might choose to use, optimism and relatively high levels of social comfort. What emerges, however, as described in more detail in the next section, is a picture of immense complexity and contradiction. Many communities exist in stark contrast to the bright and glamorous tourist portraits. While all the communities and schools on which this study reports, are situated within a 50-kilometre radius of the Cape Metropolis, their proximity to the city does not necessarily translate into equal access to the political, economic, social and cultural capital available. So, while for some proximity means enjoying the privileges that a modern society has to offer, for the majority of the participating communities and schools in this region, proximity serves to draw attention to the stark inconsistencies in individual and collective histories and experience.

Mpumalanga, on the other hand, is situated in the northeast of South Africa. It is flanked on its east side by two independent countries, Swaziland and Mocambique, with Guateng, one of the nine provinces, on the west. The independent borders create both an opportunity and challenge for this province. The Maputo Corridor, a transport route that links Mpumalanga with Maputo and Guateng, is one such economic opportunity. However, an emerging challenge is the growing number of illegal immigrants that flee their home countries (particularly Mocambique) to settle in the region for one or other reason (poverty, unemployment, hopes for a better future).

Mpumalanga is one of the smaller provinces geographically, yet it has a population of 3 122 990. The Census Report of 2001 suggests that more than 27.5% of its adult population has never been to school (South African Yearbook, 2003). The province also struggles educationally, having had the lowest matriculation (Grade 12) pass rates in 2003, 2005 and 2005. isiSwati is the most common language and is spoken by at least

30.8% of the population in the province, with 12.1% and 26.4% speaking isiNdebele and isiZulu respectively (South Africa Yearbook, 2003). Unlike in the Western Cape, English and Afrikaans serve as second, sometimes third languages for the majority of the population in this province.

The geographic landscape ranges from majestic mountain peaks to deep valleys and canyons. Mpumalanga also incorporates extensive tracts of the Kruger National Park, one of the largest national game parks in the southern hemisphere. Thus, like the Western Cape, it attracts a large national and international tourist population. Unlike the Western Cape, though, the economic benefits of, for example, the tourist and coal industries, are not evident in the province's economic GDP rate. While manufacturing, agriculture, forestry, coal mining, dairy and sheep industries offer employment opportunities for thousands of people in the region, according to the Labour Force Survey of 2001, this province has an official unemployment rate of about 16.5% (in South Africa Yearbook, 2003). Unofficially, and the same could be said for the rest of the country, the figure is probably significantly higher.

Unlike the urban, largely built environments of the Western Cape, the geographic landscape of Mpumalanga is expansive, with lots of open land between towns and cities. Most of the cities, towns and villages were established as a result of the existing natural resources and concomitant industrial activity. For example, Witbank was developed as a result of the coal reserves in the area, while Secunda developed as a result of the petroleum-from-coal installation activities. Sabie and Graskop are towns that developed around forestry plantations, while Barberton is known as one of the country's oldest gold-mining towns.

Nowhere is the apartheid-orchestrated plan of separate development more starkly in evidence than in this province. The general configuration of the cities, towns and villages was and is such that White dwellings are close to the town, as are places of employment and industrial business centres, all with well developed facilities (roads, hospitals, clinics, schools, etc.) and suitable amenities (water and electricity). The majority of the Black population, on the other hand, are settled in townships and villages in outlying rural areas far from modern centres. Deliberate plans were developed to relocate Black populations as far away as possible from Whites so as to minimise the perceived 'Swart gevaar' (the Black threat). As a consequence, Black people spent and continue to spend long periods of time commuting to and from work. The lack of proximity to the industrial and economic centres combined with the lack of a good public transportation system compounds the problems these people face in Mpumalanga. Moreover, while the province boasts some of the finest highways, toll roads and main interlinking roads in South Africa, many of the interlinking roads between towns, business centres, villages, and townships in outlying rural areas, from where most of the respondents were drawn, are less well maintained. Some of the damage to the tarred roads has been the result of inclement weather but generally, local people believe, it is the result of shoddy work supplied by ill-trained and inexperienced contractors.

From this largely rural environment, eight schools (four primary and four secondary) were purposively selected. All the schools were drawn from Khabokweni, which falls within the Mbombela municipality in the Ehlanzeni district. This district is located in the Lowveld[25] region. All the schools are between 25 and 30 kilometres away from Nelspruit, the provincial administrative capital. While on the surface the distance from this city may not seem significant, for these schools and communities, the lack of proximity to an urbanised environment has had far-reaching consequences for their individual and collective psyches.

Understanding how the inscription of apartheid on the geographic landscape works in constructing the particular collective and individual identities one finds in each area is critical to this discussion. A key feature in this social landscape is the configuration and playing out of particular identities that emerge as a result of the interrelationship between tradition and modernity, as the next chapter will illustrate. Understanding this complexity, I argue, is central to understanding factors shaping teachers' understanding and experience of HIV/AIDS. But what is the HIV-prevalence in these provinces and how is the pandemic experienced? This question is briefly explored in the next section.

25 The province is divided into three geographic regions: Eastern Highveld, Highveld and Lowveld. Each region is further demarcated into municipal districts.

HIV/AIDS prevalence

The Western Cape and Mpumalanga are as diametrically different regarding their HIV-prevalence as they are when geographically juxtaposed. The data below are drawn from the National HIV and Syphilis Antenatal Sero-prevalence Survey of 2002 (Department of Health, 2003). Mpumalanga, with a rate of 28.6%, is the fourth highest[26] in HIV-prevalence in the country. The Western Cape, on the other hand, currently has the lowest HIV-prevalence rate in the country. However, it has the fastest rate of escalation in the country. While Mpumalanga has consistently reported rates within the same statistical range for the last three years (29.7% in 2000 and 29.2% in 2001), the Western Cape has had a dramatic increase from 8.7% in 2000 and 8.6% in 2001, to 12.4% in 2002 (Department of Health, 2003). However, the provincial profiles do not necessarily provide a comprehensive picture of the way in which particular communities are *actually* experiencing HIV/AIDS.

Bureaucratic structures in Mpumalanga made it virtually impossible to obtain specific data on the Ehlanzeni municipal district from which all the schools were drawn. Available reports were only those containing HIV-prevalence information at regional levels. Thus, the available regional data revealed the HIV-infection rate in the Lowveld to be at 34.5%; at least 5% higher than the provincial average of 28.6%.

Data in the Western Cape were more accessible. In this province, schools were drawn from the Nyanga, Tygerberg East, Oostenberg and the South Peninsula municipal health districts. HIV-prevalence indicators of April 2002 to March 2003 confirm that some of these districts have prevalence rates that exceed those of the province by more than half. The rate of infection in Nyanga, (from which two schools were drawn), was 25.9%, while at Tygerberg East, Oostenberg and the South Peninsula, prevalence rates were 9.7%, 10.2% and 6.9% respectively (Provincial Administration of the Western Cape, 2004a). Increases were also evident in all the above-mentioned districts during the January-March 2004 quarter. For this period, the first district's rates of infection increased

26 At 36.%, the province with highest HIV-prevalence is Kwazulu-Natal followed by Guateng with 31.6%, and Free State with 28.8% (Department of Health, 2003).

from 25.0% to 30%, while the other districts show respective increases of 14%, 12% and 7% (Provincial Administration of the Western Cape, 2004b). While these municipal statistics begin to illuminate difference, they do not expose the scale of difference between and within the respective districts.

Deeper analysis reveals that HIV-prevalence rates in some districts is exponentially higher than that of the province or municipal region. During January – March 2004, 1653 males and females were tested in the three clinics within close proximity of the selected schools in the Nyanga district. Five hundred and fifty tested positive, rates that indicate a HIV-prevalence of about 33% (Provincial Administration of the Western Cape, 2004c). The high prevalence rate in these three facilities remained relatively stable for the three years indicated in the report (Provincial Administration of the Western Cape, 2004d).

HIV-prevalence rates in the South Peninsula district were consistently low, a phenomenon that was associated with perceptions of risk in the community. For the most part, members within this district did not perceive themselves falling within a 'high risk' group and as such, did not readily present themselves for HIV-testing. This notwithstanding, the ante-natal data showed an escalation in HIV-rates during the last few years. For example, from April 2002 to April 2004, of the 499 males and females that were tested, 37 presented as HIV-positive, a higher percentage than that indicated by the regional frequencies. In February 2004 alone, 15 of the 40 people tested presented as HIV-positive (Provincial Administration of the Western Cape, 2004e)

In the main, women are most vulnerable to infection with a consistent patterning emerging of increased prevalence across different age categories. Using data drawn from antenatal clinics, both provinces mirror the national results that indicate women between 25 and 29 as those most infected with the HI-Virus. Nationally in 2000, the rate of infection amongst this cohort of pregnant women was 30.6%, with an escalation of about 5% by 2002 (Department of Health, 2003). However, the fastest growing rate of infection is among women in the age range 40 years and over. Infection rates amongst this group of women increased from 11.0% in 2000 to 17.2% in 2002. Similar patterns are traceable amongst 30–34-year old women, whose prevalence rates show an increase from 23.3% in 2000 to 29.5% in 2002. In the same vein, rates of infection among pregnant women between the ages 35 and 39 increased from 15.8% in

2000 to 19.8% in 2002 (Department of Health, 2003), showing overall increases in many categories.

Highlighting age differentiated infection rates is important for two reasons. First, the female subjects in the study fall within the fastest growing HIV-prevalence age range of over 40 years and 35–39 years respectively. As I show in the next chapter, many female respondents who are either married or in long-term relationships, expressed difficulty in negotiating the use of condoms in relationships (with husbands or partners) understood to be stable, even in circumstances where infidelity was evident or openly acknowledged. Second, the reported national rate of teenage pregnancies is about 15%. Many teenagers are still school-going youth, an important consideration when questions are posed about what happens in Lifeskills classrooms when teachers mediate knowledge about HIV/AIDS and sexuality.

What emerges above is a picture, at the municipal and district levels, of very different rates of infection and, by implication very different circumstances and experiences of the pandemic from that expressed in the national statistics. As the demographic profiles portray in the next section, the municipal and district frequencies above emanate from those communities hardest hit by poverty, ones still geographically, economically and socially removed from modern localities such as hospitals and other health support systems. This notwithstanding, the prevalence rates are racially skewed, with poor Black communities still experiencing higher infections. But, as this work sought to illustrate, using the broad sociological constructs of race, gender, class and location alone is insufficient to explain the experience in communities, since it was more often than not difficult to separate the race factor from what was poverty driven.

The communities

Geographic location and social and economic capital

The community and school profiles that follow are derived from a combination of observational data, Statistics South Africa[27] (2004) and the Census (2001).[28] They illustrate the manner in which the history of forced removals and separation by race and class described earlier worked to create different individual and collective identities within and between communities.

The communities and schools in the study are categorized into three economic and social clusters, namely affluent, middle income and poor, as Table 3 below illustrates. Most of the selected schools are from poor communities (four schools in the Western Cape and all eight in Mpumalanga). Only one school was selected from the affluent category and two schools from the middle-income cluster of districts. The reasons for such a skewed population have already been explained in an earlier chapter.

Table 3: Community, Region, Economic and Social Cluster and Selected Number of Schools

Community	*Province*	*Economic and Social Cluster*	*Selected Number of Schools*
Bloukoop	Western Cape	Affluent	1
Gapeng	Western Cape	Poor	3
Gracious Heights	Western Cape	Middle income	1
Joseph Rhodes	Western Cape	Poor	1
Stanton	Western Cape	Middle income	1
Nyalunga	Mpumalanga	Poor	3
Mapagama	Mpumalanga	Poor	1
Elangeni	Mpumalanga	Poor	1
Thokoza	Mpumalanga	Poor	3

27 They include annual household income, employment status, levels of education and occupations in respective communities for the specified period (Appendices D–G).

28 The social topography is derived from data that includes the type of housing, availability and access to basic amenities (sanitation, water, refuse disposal and energy supply), and modes of transportation to work or schools (Appendices H–L).

Communities display vast economic disparities. The figures in Appendix A suggest that levels of unemployment in all the poor communities in this study far exceed those in the affluent and middle class clusters. The poor communities in both regions report unemployment averages of 50% or higher. Uneven levels of education, occupations and annual household incomes (see Appendices B, C and D) served as auxiliary indicators of the disparity that expresses itself economically amongst these communities. But, as (re)presentations of a complex set of circumstances and conditions, these indicators imply another, unspoken dimension. For while statistics are helpful as indicators of general unemployment profiles and associated levels of poverty, at another level they obscure the real or material conditions and experience of poverty. The concealed picture in this instance is one of struggle in the poor communities. So, while a cursory exploration of the numerical indicators points to the clinical reality of unemployment and, by implication, poverty and neglect, the other side of these numbers points to a (hi)story in which members of these poor communities misrecognise the interconnectedness between geographic location, political distance and identity, on the one hand, and, on the other hand, their agency (or lack thereof) in re-inscribing history. Whereas geographic distance and locality were legislated inscriptions on collective and individual identities prior to 1994, the poor communities in this study still seemed unable to transform themselves in meaningful ways. They seemed inadvertently to re-inscribe the poverty script in complicit ways through sustained low levels of education and low matriculation pass rates.

The stark economic inequality amongst communities is exacerbated by differentiated access to centres of employment, trading centres, housing, basic amenities such as water, sanitation and electricity, as well as transportation (see Appendices E–I). The affluent and middle-income communities have quantitatively and qualitatively better homes and well-developed infrastructures, while the poor communities struggle to survive under harsh social conditions. Though, for example, roads in the latter communities are tarred, their condition is poor and neglected, making it difficult for people to commute long distances to work. The most common available shops in the poor communities are those best described as 'house shops' in peoples' yards. In some instances, a converted room of a main house serves as a trading centre. These 'shops' serve as outlets for a variety of commodities which ranging from basic necessities such as bread and milk, to liquor and cigarettes. Often, prohibition laws are not strictly adhered to, leaving the possibility open for underage children to gain access to prohibited products.

Housing in poor communities ranges from owner-built family homes to low cost housing and shacks erected in the backyards of already existing homes or wherever there is available vacant land. As a result, informal settlements are a common and permanent feature of the geographic landscape, often creating pressure on limited resources. Amenities such as toilets and taps are often either shared by clusters of homes, where the tap and a group of bucket latrines would be situated at a strategic location unattached to any homes (commonly called a community stand) or by groups of families where these amenities are in a yard (see Appendices E–G). In other instances, where housing comprises small free-standing homes, semi-detached or high-rise buildings (commonly called flats), the condition of available amenities is said to be poor due to these being shared by more than one family constituting a household. All poor communities in the Western Cape share amenities like clinics and libraries with neighbouring communities, placing a great burden on the availability and access to such spaces.

While the levels of unemployment and general neglect were common features in both regions, the picture that emerged of the poor communities in Mpumalanga was bleaker. These communities are not only far removed from the economic and modern hubs of the province; they are situated in areas that are not easily accessible.[29] Unlike the poor communities in the Western Cape that light the metropolitan night sky (albeit dimly), the former are geographically far-removed and thus affectively concealed. Such concealment worked (and continues to work) in two interrelated ways. First, during Apartheid physical distance was used as an ideological tool to remove 'poor' and 'Black' from the modern landscape, a set of circumstances that continues to mark the collective identities of these communities in Mpumalanga. Concealment though, is more pervasive in that it continues to create particular identities characterised by silence, suppression, and shame. These markers continue to find expression in the everyday experiences of those living in these environments and have seri-

29 Kabokweni, the region from which six of the eight schools were drawn, was the previous homeland for the Ndebele tribe and may best be described as expansive and mountainous.

ous consequences for the way in which people understand and respond to critical issues such as HIV/AIDS.

While the census data reports a large number of families living in 'brick houses on separate structures', the figures belie the reality because the numerical description does not account for the quality and/or nature of these structures. During the observation period in 2002–2004, my impression was that many of the houses were not only self-designed and owner built, but often badly built. As one travels deeper into the interior of the region, the houses become less and less sophisticated with few of them being brick-built.

Running water is a precious commodity in many parts of Mpumalanga. The scarcity of water in the region was particularly noticeable when visiting schools in that, more often than not, flush toilets were inoperable. The lack of water also had serious consequences for schools and communities that attempted to be self-sustaining through the development of food gardens.

Fewer amenities (access to shops, clinics, police, etc.) were available, partly as a result of the expansiveness of the area but also partly because fewer resources are allocated to such rural areas. So, for example, a teacher at one of the more remote schools in the sample reported that it could take a week or more for the police to respond to reported cases, if they did at all. Consequently, community members often refrained from reporting misdemeanours, a situation that had and continues to have adverse consequences, particularly for women and children. Teachers expressed feelings of helplessness in dealing with the larger issues of rape, poor health, abuse and HIV/AIDS.

The picture that emerges is one of particularly poor communities living under desperate social and economic circumstances. Their histories constitute a direct riposte to the official history of the province. Theirs is a story of marginalisation, othering, immiseration, and struggle. In this story are the marks, signs, and symbols of individual and collective identities that are fractured and intensely divided and positioned in complex relationship with the dominant forces of power in the province.

Emerging from the numerical descriptors (Appendices A–J) and the brief contextual profile is a picture of affluent and middle-income communities enjoying better social and material conditions with easier access to amenities. However, relying only on numerical descriptions to explain the complex social conditions and circumstances of the poor is problematic, as indicated above. Numbers, to some extent, offer a semblance of normalcy: they imply that so long as things are measurable, they can't be 'that bad'. Absent in the numerical configurations is the degree and complexity of the struggle in poor communities, which extends beyond economic survival to include social, emotional and psychological survival. These poor communities have continually to confront their past histories in ways that make it difficult for them to create and write a new reality. The social struggle often seems deeply embedded in the collective psyche of its members, a condition which seems to allow little hope for a better, or even a longer life. What emerged in this study, therefore, was a picture of continued compliance that manifests itself through low levels of education and low level occupations and other phenomena such as vandalism.

Factors such as those described above have important consequences for the ways in which people in these contexts understand themselves and experience or respond to HIV/AIDS. These are communities in flux, continually confronting and being confronted by past and present histories in complex ways. Even in instances where the material conditions of teachers had improved, many expressed an embodied self illustrative of the deep rootedness of their past histories, as the next chapter will show.

At one level, it may be correct to suggest that the juxtaposed identifying markers of race and geographic location continue to imprint themselves on the collective identities, lived experiences and present histories of people living within these geographic spaces. Intertwined are past and present historical patterns that are being persistently rewritten and maintained through the sustained unevenness in unemployment rates and status of occupation, levels of education and concomitant occupations and household income, on the one hand, and on the other hand, by the type and availability of housing and access to and availability of basic amenities such as water, electricity and sanitation.

At another level, though, these markers of identity fail to sustain an argument that privileges essentialist forms of understanding experience as being racially or geographically located and defined. For instance, the poor communities in the Western Cape comprise ethnic Black and Coloured groups that are situated in primarily 'urban' settings. The lived experience of members in these communities, however, is not far removed or qualitatively different from that of the poor communities in Mpumalanga. Both suffer deep neglect, lack of access to basic amenities, high levels of unemployment, and both seem to experience difficulty in maintaining children in school (Appendix B). While in the Western Cape, for example, communities are in urban environments, in close proximity to modern facilities, their experience is still one of struggle, whether it be physical or psychological. The Mpumalanga communities commonly described as 'rural' experience similar struggles. So, while in some ways geographic context and race have shaped the collective identities and experiences of these communities, the complexity of this experience may be obscured if these categories are used as the key indicators in any description. As a descriptor, therefore, and in this instance, 'poor' is a more evocative and nuanced organising adjective than race or geographic location for this group of communities since it describes their lived conditions as embedded in material and social conditions that have roots extending beyond racial and geographic configurations.

Demographic identities

All the communities from which schools were drawn are still demographically divisible according to race, as the Census statistics (2001) in Tables 4 and 5 below indicate.

Table 4: Geographic Population Groups: Western Cape

	Black African	Coloured	Asian/Indian	White	Total
Bloukoop (B)	22 545	31 551	317	23 588	78 002
Gapeng (2G)	79 363	899	9	11	80 282
Gracious Heights (S)	487	22 987	320	154	23 948
Joseph Rhodes (BL)	518	23 163	68	38	23 787
Stanton(GP)	555	19 029	456	117	20 157

Table 5: Geographic Population Groups: Mpumalanga

Communities	African Black	Coloured	Indian/Asian	White	Total
Nyalunga	16 473	60	–	–	16 532
Mapagama	12 835	36	3	3	12 878
Elangeni	12 043	41	–	–	12 084
Thokoza	6 352	30	–	12	6 394

Characterised by race, this relatively stable demographic profile was a direct consequence of the Apartheid apparatus that worked to create and entrench differing and separate racial and ethnic identities, and that continues to etch its mark materially and socially on the collective and personal identities of communities twelve years into democracy.

It was not surprising, then, that the demographic profiles of six of the seven participating schools in the Western Cape remained largely unaltered. For the most part, each school still provides educational opportunities for the respective racial populations they were designed to cater for prior to 1994. For instance, while there are large isiXhosa (20 041), English (11 570) and Sesotho-speaking (1 003) populations in the affluent Bloukoop community, as Table 4, below, indicates, the participating school in the sample still attracts learners from the predominantly Afrikaner middle-class population in the area. This notwithstanding, the demographics of the learner population at the school have slowly become more representative while the staff composition has remained relatively unchanged. Observations revealed that there was only one Coloured teacher in a staff of 72, with the rest being Afrikaans speaking and White. The rest of the schools in the Western Cape sample were no different in their demographic profiles. Thus although all the communities from which these schools were drawn displayed a multilingual profile, as Table 6, below, indicates. The schools still provide instruction in the dominant language used prior to their integration from 1990 onwards.

Table 6: Language Profile of Communities in the Western Cape

	Bloukoop	Gapeng	Gracious Heights	Joseph Rhodes	Stanton
Afrikaans	44 749	1 185	4 511	21 575	5 132
English	11 570	229	19 209	2 038	14 816
IsiNdebele	37	17	9	11	16
IsiXhosa	20 041	76 056	107	31	100
IsiZulu	126	329	4	5	8
Sepedi	30	88	–	3	–
Sesotho	1 003	1 552	3	62	8
Setswana	94	400	6	12	8
SiSwati	50	115	–	4	5
Tshivenda	21	30	–	11	–
Xitsonga	130	40	–	23	29

All five communities in this region are in urban environments but geographically removed from the city centre. The reasons for this are as different as the material and social conditions and experiences in these communities. Using racial categories as an organising device for orchestrating and implementing separatist ideologies, the government resettled non-White communities in different areas of the Cape Flats. The coloured communities of Gracious Park and Joseph Rhodes were, therefore, established as a direct consequence of the orchestrated plan of forced removals by the then Apartheid government. In contrast, Bloukoop was established in a geographically appealing environment far away from the 'swart gevaar' and in favourable, modern circumstances.

The Mpumalanga communities, on the other hand, were all drawn from rural environments and have remained demographically unchanged, as Table 3, above, illustrated. While the distance between the communities and Nelspruit, the provincial administrative capital is only about 25 kilometres, these environments are economically, psychologically and physically totally marginalised. Unlike communities in the Western Cape that are visible, albeit dimly, the Mpumalanga communities might as well not exist. So while the communities are in a sense comparably sited, their experiences are very different, thus creating very different social identities for their members. It would seem, therefore, that placing non-White communities away from the public and political eye made it easy for them to be forgotten and neglected.

In both regions, distancing and disconnecting communities from the modern social infrastructure of good roads, clinics, shopping and business centres of employment evident in primarily 'white' communities, translated into marginalisation at the material level. But at a psychological level, distancing translates into communities being marginal in the dominant discourses of modernity, thus creating and recreating particular collective and individual social identities. What is significant for this discussion is an understanding of the deeply embedded and intertwined nature of past and present histories, and particularly of *how* separateness in geographic arrangements has worked and continues to work to produce expressions of difference and inscribe particular identities on communities. Critical, too, for the later discussion is an understanding of how this situated context shapes individual and collective responses to the main question this work poses, namely understanding, experiencing and teaching sexuality and HIV/AIDS.

The schools

What follows below is a composite portrait of groups of schools within each economic and social cluster in the respective provinces. It was less cumbersome to follow this route than to present each school separately. Using observational and interview data, the pattern I follow is one that highlights similarities and differences between schools within and across clusters in the same region. I introduce the names of the respondents from each school as I go along. This is in preparation for Chapter 10 where they are profiled more comprehensively and where I describe the influence of this discursive space in shaping teacher identities.

The description below offers insight into another layer of influence and illustrates the ways in which schools and teachers, as microcosms of each community, experience the social and economic realities. This explanation also sheds light on the way communities are continually forced to confront and work within past and present historical frameworks. Put differently, this account demonstrates the ways in which essentialist categories that divided classes of people neatly into race, class, location and the like, obscure rather than shed light on the complexity of social life in these communities.

Western Cape Schools

Affluent schools

Boshendal Senior Secondary, a dual-medium school in Bloukoop and the only historically "white" school in the study, is situated about 40 kilometres north-east of the city centre. It has expansive grounds and well-kept recreational facilities. The general condition of the built environment was excellent, partly as a result of the high level of sponsorship the school enjoyed from parents and neighbouring business companies, and partly because parents in this community were better educated and in better paid occupations in larger numbers than those in the other four communities in this region. They were able to pay school fees and support the school financially.

This school has a vibrant extra-mural curriculum that includes all the sports codes. More than one sports code had its own fleet of minivans for transporting learners to and from sporting events. It also had a history of successful drum majorette squads, demonstrated by the accumulation of trophies and pictures displayed in the corridors and principal's office. The school possessed facilities like computer laboratories, well-equipped science laboratories and other resources that enabled teachers to concentrate on the core task of teaching. Twenty of the 72 teachers were appointed in what is commonly called 'governing body posts', meaning that they were paid with funds generated by school fees and fundraising activities and not by the education department. More than 80% of the teachers lived in the immediate vicinity of the school. During an interview Kobie, the white male teacher from this school, intimated that most teachers knew the parents of the children they taught very well because they attended the same churches and socialised with them over weekends. As such, he suggested, it was easy to teach 'these' children because he 'knew' their family values. Vera, the white female teacher, suggested that the community was very insular and conservative. She said that members within this community would not easily admit that they knew someone who was HIV-positive, let alone acknowledge that an HIV-infected person might be living in the area. This community she said was "family-oriented and Christians."

Learners at this school were governed by the bell. They were conditioned to know the meaning of each of the many bells that rang to signal either the beginning of school, silence, standing still before entering the classroom, interval, etc. No learners were seen outside classes during designated teaching times. Teachers came to school on time and were at their designated classroom doors five minutes before the first bell before school and as soon as the first bell rang after each interval. While the school had a firmly erected fence and a gate, these did not need to be monitored because parents and any other visitors made appointments to visit the school and had to report to one of four secretaries in the reception area. There was no question that everyone at the school not only knew their place and adhered to the rules, but took for granted why they were there. Teaching and learning was simply 'expected', and as I will illustrate later on, teachers went about their duty understanding what was at stake.

Middle income schools

The selected schools from the middle income communities of Gracious Park and Stanton also had well-built structures and relatively large grounds, but these were overshadowed by the Boshendal Senior Secondary School in Bloukoop. Parktown Senior Secondary, an English-medium school[30] in Gracious Park was about 20 kilometres south-east of the city Centre, and Macadamia Primary School, also English-medium, in Stanton, was about 30 kilometres. Parktown Secondary School attracted the largest number of learners in the area, even though there were two neighbouring secondary schools within close proximity. The school had about 1 400 learners with 44 members of staff in the year fieldwork was completed. Apart from one white teacher, the entire staff and learners were 'coloured'. All the teachers resided in the immediate or surrounding coloured suburbs. The two teachers interviewed, Pauline

30 This school was established as a dual-medium school. Reasons why Afrikaans was phased out were not given.

and Gwen, both held strong views about service to the community through education. They viewed teaching at this school as their contribution to, as they put it, 'giving back' or as serving 'their community'. The entire staff at the primary school was coloured, with 99% of the learner population comprising the same racial group. The rest comprised a handful of Xhosa-speaking learners.

The physical environment at both schools was stark and barren. Many attempts had been made to beautify the surroundings, without much success. Teachers' perceptions of why they had been unsuccessful included over-crowding (too many learners relative to the size of the building), limited financial resources, lack of parent involvement and/or lack of ownership by the respective communities.

The physical environment was not only inadequate in proportion to the number of learners in each school; it was underdeveloped. There were few facilities for extramural activities. Teachers in both schools said that the limited spatial arrangement, particularly in the primary school, restricted the nature of activities in which children could participate. While some learners at Macadamia Primary were creative in their use of confined spaces (e.g., playing variations of hopscotch that didn't require much space), more often than not learners were inactive. This notwithstanding, both schools participated in some regional sports codes. In particular, learners at Parktown Senior Secondary were involved in popular sports codes. They also participated in debating, canoeing and hiking activities that were administered independently, but in close collaboration with the school. Pictures on the walls at the office attested to learner participation in these independently managed activities.

Teaching and time on task in both schools was very noticeable. Few if any learners were seen out of classrooms during official school hours. Discipline was characteristic of both schools. While the secondary school reported some experience of truancy and drugs, the scale of the problem was nowhere near that experienced in the poor communities and schools described in the next section. The principals at the two schools in this cluster were well respected by the staff and community as professionals and strict disciplinarians who had good control of their respective schools. While he was supportive throughout the fieldwork, Parktown's principal was rarely available even for a courtesy call by the researcher, partly because he was required to teach and partly because of the high demand on his time by parents. Parents, more often than not, did not make appointments but expected nevertheless to see him, and in most cases succeeded. His task as principal extended beyond responding to school-related issues, to being a guidance counsellor and mediator between family members and very often, between parents and their children. Macadamia Primary School, where Shahida the only Muslim teacher in the study taught, functioned easily with few interruptions at the office.

Poor schools

The distinction among schools in the Western Cape was most conspicuous when the conditions in the two primary and two secondary schools were profiled. Gapeng, from which Zondi Primary, Vuyani Primary and Mzandi Senior Secondary were selected, and Joseph Rhodes, from which Redhill Secondary School was selected, were communities that comprised black and coloured populations respectively. Both schools remained either black or coloured in their learner and staff profiles. A Coloured principal had been appointed at Mzandi Senior Secondary soon after the election of the first democratic government in 1994. However, he was no longer there at the time of the fieldwork.

Mzandi Senior Secondary was English-medium in a predominantly Xhosa-speaking community. Redhill Secondary School, on the other hand, was Afrikaans-medium in a community that was Afrikaans-speaking. Together with what is described below, language played an important role in not only identifying communities but in acting as a discursive space for the production and reproduction of particular teacher identities.

It was in these communities that past histories continued to etch their mark on the physical environment and everyday practices, features that were acutely visible in the four selected schools described below. Theirs was a history of severe neglect that continued to write itself through the *modus operandi* of schools as well as through a severing of schools from the broader community. Neglect was not only visible; it was imprinted on the buildings and physical space. Moreover, it was deeply embedded in the psyche of those working and using these spaces.

While these two communities were geographically separated, the conditions in the schools mirrored each other. These two secondary schools were both dilapidated with defaced buildings, no windows or dirty classrooms, broken tables and chairs, and broken door handles. Vandalism (by learners themselves and members of the community), gangsterism and theft were common experiences, sometimes with traumatic consequences for teachers and learners. Teachers at Mzandi Senior Secondary school locked their doors while teaching for fear of gang members or vandals who, sporadically and without announcement, entered classrooms. They also locked doors to keep learners in class. Zodwa from Mzandi Senior Secondary reported in an interview that teachers themselves installed the handles and locks at their own expense. While Carol and Paul from the coloured secondary school in this cluster did not lock doors while teaching, they reported disruptions by gang members. Consequently, they were always on the alert and locked classroom doors during interval or each time they left the classroom.

The condition of the surrounding physical environment extended this picture of desolation. The school grounds of both secondary schools were barren, dusty and dry. There were no trees, lawn, plants or flowers. A security fence built around Redhill Senior Secondary literally halved the designated recreational space. As a result, sports activities were non-existent. Only a few learners at this school participated in sports activities. Almost all of these operated independently of the school. Teenage pregnancies, cases of physical and sexual abuse, abortion, gangsterism, absent parents,[31] drugs and other substance abuses – all were common in this school. In particular, many children frequented shebeens,[32] which are called 'yards' in the local community. Paul and Carol, two Coloured teachers who are a married couple and who both teach Life Orientation at the school, attested to there being sixteen shebeens along the periphery and within a one-kilometre radius of the school. Paul, who grew up in this area, suggested that visits to these 'yards' were the main, and sometimes only, form of recreation for children after school and often even during school. Smoking, drinking and sex were commonplace in such places, with some children selling their bodies in exchange for a drink or cigarettes.

Both schools experienced high rates of attrition. While no statistics were available at the time of the fieldwork, Paul from Redhill Senior Secondary sketched scenarios that illustrated the severity of the prob-

31 The two respondents at this school had conducted a survey in 2002 which indicated that as many as 70% of the learners are living with grandparents or extended families and not with biological parents.

32 Shebeens are taverns where locals gather.

lem. He suggested that every year the school began with six classes of Grade 8's (the first year of secondary school), with each class averaging forty learners. Yet each year, the matric group (final year of secondary school) comprised one class only, suggesting a high drop out rate between the first and fourth years. Matriculation results in both these schools remained consistently low and qualitatively poor,[33] even though there was an emphasis at both schools on teaching the matriculants to the neglect of other grades, particularly if the same teacher taught classes across grade levels. Zodwa and Paul both admitted to being 'guilty' of giving more attention to, as Paul stated, "... where it mattered."

Learners at Mzondi Senior Secondary were allowed to leave the school premises during intervals that lasted up to an hour, a practice that had roots in the early Bantu Education system. Reasons for this were linked to poverty and the inability of parents to provide school lunches. The objective was for learners to go home to eat and then return to school. While this may have been the case then, commonly today, children still left the school premises but there was no guarantee they would return. This practice had serious consequences for schools in that it became the breeding ground for all kinds of unsupervised activities.

What emerges in the description above is a picture not just of deep neglect, but one of complicity with the dominant Apartheid script of neglect by teachers, parents and learners themselves. They continued to rewrite the script of neglect through irresponsible sexual behaviour, low levels of education, high rates of school attrition, vandalism, gangsterism and physical neglect of the built environment.

Zondi and Vuyani Primary schools, situated in one of the oldest black townships in the Western Cape, were close to hostels that had been erected to accommodate migrant workers in the early 1960s and 1970s. These hostels remained the bedrock for abuses of all kinds. Gugu, the female black teacher from Zondi Primary School and Xola, a black male teacher from Vuyani, both reported that the hostels posed a serious threat to the wellbeing of the children in the area. Gugu stated that not a week went by without a report of some form of abuse that often involved the children from the primary schools in the study. Even though

33 Very few learners in these two schools take the higher grade stream of subjects resulting in few, if any, obtaining results that are suitable for entrance to university.

cases were reported, these often went unsolved and the perpetrators unpunished. This, though, was not the whole story. Discussions on sex and sexuality were largely absent in these communities, as the next chapter will illustrate. Commonly, therefore, sexual abuse was not spoken about and sometimes not even reported (either to family members or the police). More seriously, though, she stated that children in these communities often experienced difficulty in explaining the abuse. This, she said, was largely due to silence surrounding issues like sex, but importantly, it also had to do with the meanings ascribed to the use of certain language in 'their culture', as I explain later. Gugu gave an example of an occasion when a case involving a learner from the school was thrown out of court because she (the learner) described the incident using colloquial terminology that did not provide sufficient evidence for a rape charge. More often than not, therefore, abuse was met with silence.

The two primary schools were physically a little more appealing than the secondary schools described earlier in this section. Zondi Primary had a large vegetable garden and some flowers at the entrance of the school. The food garden, which fed learners in and out of school, was managed by some parents from the local community. While the garden project had positive spin-offs for the school and immediate community, it took up much of the available physical space, thus leaving a very limited area for recreation in an already overcrowded school environment. Like Mzandi Senior Secondary, this school was also the target of vandalism and theft. Gugu insisted on escorting me to my car each time I visited, not only as a courtesy but also as a precaution against possible mugging or hijacking.

For the most part, all four schools in the two communities operate as alien spaces for parents whose participation in the broader life of the school was either minimal or non-existent. The psychological distance between schools and communities and between teachers and parents, as I explain later on, was exacerbated by a perception of teachers as 'outsiders', since many of them did not live in the communities in which they taught. The limited contact between teachers and parents was confined to school activities such as parent meetings. However, even these activities were poorly attended and often met with indifference.

Mpumalanga Schools

I indicated in the community profile earlier on that all the schools in Mpumalanga were rural, poor, and black. Most of the learners at these schools were Swazi. There was a low number of Sotho and Zulu in some schools.

Since all the communities in this region were characterised as poor in the earlier discussion, I use a different categorising strategy to describe their material and social conditions in this section. First, I clustered the schools into primary and secondary categories. Thereafter, I applied another set of distinctions within each category. In the primary group, I distinguished the two schools that were geographically further removed from the two that were situated closer to main roads and were in more established townships. In the secondary group, I distinguished between old and new schools. Reasons for this distinction will become clearer in the discussion below.

The discussion that follows seeks to illustrate how people within these discursive spaces contribute to, sometimes comply with but often also subvert the discourse to write and re-establish identities not far removed from the formal script of Apartheid. The first part of the discussion below focuses on the four primary schools in the sample, and the second part describes the secondary schools.

Poor primary schools

The four primary schools were situated in townships established in the 1970s as part of the Apartheid government's plan to relocate blacks away from urban areas. While all the schools were drawn from rural environments, Hambani Primary and Mbazani Primary from Thokoza are best described as deeply rural. Their proximity to Nelspruit, the modern urban capital of the province, was not any different from the rest of the schools. However, they were not easily accessible. Roads to the schools were unmarked and their condition was poor. The insularity of these communities was exemplified by what the four teachers reported, namely, that children here rarely ventured beyond their immediate surroundings and thus had very little life experience beyond their present set of circumstances. While this region had experienced a drought for many years, torrential rains that fell during the fieldwork washed away parts of the road making the schools almost inaccessible. I relied on taxi and bus tracks to make my way to the schools when I visited them.

Yiso Primary in Elangeni and Siyabonga Primary in Mapagama, on the other hand, were situated in more established townships closer to main roads. Like the two schools described above, they were also inaccessible, but for entirely different reasons. The two communities from which the school populations were drawn experienced wide scale unemployment, gangsterism and a disproportionately high drop-out rate, particularly amongst young boys. The upshot was that there was a high incidence of crime that included car hijacking and petty theft. Teachers and learners at Yiso Primary, for example, were targets of numerous attacks on the school premises, with gangsters coming into classrooms to rob both staff and pupils. On at least two reported occasions, teachers were held up at gun-point in classrooms and relieved of their cell phones and money. These gangsters called themselves 'tollgates' and usually positioned themselves at strategic locations where they could easily hijack or rob motorists. As a result, teachers resorted to either using public transport or travelling in a hired mini-van rather than risk their lives by using their own cars. During my visit to the school, a police escort was arranged to and from the school to ensure my safety. As a further safety measure I interviewed Jenni, the female teacher, at her home rather than at the school. Despite the challenges teachers faced at this school, they suggested that the material conditions were not a deterrent. Rather, they said that the situation made them more reliant on each other for support and as a result, they were a very tight-knit staff. According to Jenni, their positive attitude was attributable to their faith and the fact that they often prayed together as a staff.

Similarly to the situation that played itself out in the poor schools in the Western Cape, unemployment amongst the poor communities in this region resulted in a complex set of practices that made, particularly, young girls vulnerable. Ester, from Siyabonga Primary, reported that young girls sometimes resort to prostitution, often not by choice but as a result of coercion from adults in the family. As in the Gapeng community in the Western Cape, reports of many forms of abuse in these two communities were not uncommon. Like teachers in the Gapeng community, teachers in the primary schools under discussion also reported reluctance by teachers to report incidences of abuse due to intimidation and/or a lack of support from parents and members of the community. This situation resulted in a strained relationship between parents and teachers, leaving the latter in a precarious position with not many options to help children. As in the case of poor black schools in the Western Cape, the three communities from which the primary schools were drawn were also silent regarding sex in general, and abuse in particular. Dorothy from Mbazani Primary, who said that teachers were reluctant to report cases to police, health or social welfare officials for reasons already given, but also because in their experience, follow-up was tardy and sometimes non-existent. However, when probed, Dorothy suggested that, like their counterparts in the primary schools in the Western Cape, teachers here also felt unable to respond to situations of abuse due to their status as 'outsiders' who live outside the community in which they taught. Their 'outsider' status, as I explain in detail in the next chapter, marked them as 'other', and therefore unqualified to 'interfere' with what was perceived as 'insider' community business. Compliance with the dominant discourse of silence, therefore, was pervasive in these poor communities irrespective of where they were located, an issue closely aligned with conceptions of sexuality, as is illustrated in the next section.

Against the backdrop of poverty and other challenging circumstances, these schools were conspicuous in that their grounds were spotlessly clean and the built environment exceptionally well maintained. All four schools had flower gardens. For example Hambani Primary, where Jabulani taught, had a well-established and economically viable vegetable garden that had won environmental awards for three consecutive years despite the shortage of water in the area. The staff and a few community members had devised plans to save or recycle water to maintain the garden. They had large retainers to save rain water and often made children wash their hands in buckets and, thereafter, used the water for the garden.

This notwithstanding, the lack of water created other challenges for these schools. For example, while all the schools had flush toilets, these did not always function. In instances where toilets worked, their condition was poor, often because, as Jabulani the female teacher from Hambani Primary suggested, seats were stolen or broken by members of the community. Schools were thus forced to build pit-toilets. However, Jenni from Yiso Primary stated that these filled up very quickly because "children use[d] stones to clean themselves." They were also a health hazard because pit-toilets could not be sanitized.

The majority of the school population in these four primary schools spoke isiSwati, with only a few speaking either isiSotho or isiZulu. These schools continued the practice of teaching children through their mother-tongue in the first three grades and, thereafter, switching to English as the medium of instruction in Grades 4 to 7. This practice held serious consequences for teaching sexuality and HIV/AIDS.

The four primary schools were well functioning environments, with a dedicated staff. Administration at the schools was exemplary. Teachers produced daily preparation files that either principals or heads of department monitored every morning. There was no loitering and learners remained in school for the duration of the school day unlike, as I describe in the next section, the experience in secondary schools in this region. During the fieldwork I often heard teachers teaching and learners chorusing in all the primary schools.

Poor secondary schools

The secondary schools in this region reflected many of the characteristics of the poor schools in the Western Cape. Neglect and poverty was written into the environment through decrepit buildings, vandalised school surroundings, high rates of theft, lack of respect for rules (by adults and children), and seemingly little consideration of a future beyond the immediate reality. They were also similar in their experiences of high attrition rates, absenteeism, teenage pregnancy and truancy. While this was the case generally, the schools in Mpumalanga revealed important differences that are instructive in the context of this study.

Four secondary schools were selected. These included two old schools, Hamba and Vuyisile Senior Secondary, and two new schools, Khonzani and Buyisa Senior Secondary. All except Vuyisile were located in Nyalunga, the most established of the four communities in the region. Vuyisile, together with Hambani and Mbazani primary schools described above, was located in Thokosa, a community I described above as deeply rural. The teachers from Hamba Senior Secondary were Lizzie and Sipho. Mzi, a black male teacher, taught at Vuyisile Senior Secondary in the community where he was born. Thandi, an articulate black female teacher taught at Khonzani Senior Secondary, while Volene, who was the only black female teacher whose HIV-status was revealed in the study, and Patricia taught at Buyisa Senior Secondary.

The student enrolment at all four schools far exceeded the designated teacher/student ratios recommended by provincial and national Departments of Education. Unlike Boshendal, the affluent school in the Western Cape, the teacher/learner ratios in the schools drawn from these poor communities were disproportionate. Khonzani Senior Secondary, for example, had 1135 learners and 23 teachers, while Hamba Senior Secondary had 1300 learners and a staff of 30. Most of the teachers reported the difficulties experienced by their respective schools with keeping accurate official learner records since it was a 'common' practice for learners to drop in and out of school. So, while the official records reflected the numbers given above, the reality was very different.

Even though there were many similarities amongst the group of four secondary schools in this region, in that all were geographically marked as rural and poor, and all were oversubscribed, their responses to their contextual realities were qualitatively different. What I do briefly in the next section, therefore, is designate the schools as either historically 'old' or 'new', terms that relate to the length of time they had been in existence. Illustrative in these descriptions was how in each school, past and present histories intersected to create and recreate particular school and teacher identities.

The 'old' schools

Hamba Senior Secondary, where Sipho, a single black male and Lizzie, a black female, taught, was situated in Naylunga. It was the oldest in the group of four secondary schools in the Mpumalanga sample and had been established twenty-nine years previously. On the other hand, Vuyisile where Mzi, also a black male, taught, was built five years later. It was situated in Thokoza, the same region as the 'deeply rural' primary schools. The former school was situated in the heart of a well established township, close to amenities such as hospitals, public transport, post office, clinics, home-based care centres, etc. It was also situated close to all the main routes that led in and out of the township and was, therefore, easily accessible. The area had many more well-built brick homes than any of the sampled poor communities in this region. This school was within walking distance for most of its learners, though a few from other areas choose to attend and thus travelled.

As with the primary schools from Thokoza, Vuyisile Senior Secondary was far removed from the main transport routes and basic amenities such as hospitals, clinics and police stations. While the school had electricity, it was not uncommon for this area to experience power outages. The school did not have running water. I was told that laying water pipes for the school and the surrounding community was difficult because the area was, according to 'authorities', geographically inaccessible. As was the experience of the selected primary schools in this region, scarcity of water resulted in teachers having to bring their own drinking water to school. Learners, on the other hand, walked home during intervals for water and food. Sanitation and hygiene were thus seriously compromised. Staff toilets were used as a storeroom and the learners' toilets were locked to prevent vandalism. Pit toilets were built for learners but, as in the case of the primary schools, their condition was unhygienic.

Both secondary schools may have been beautiful a long time ago. When the visits were conducted, though, their physical environment was poor. Their buildings were dilapidated. Neglect and chaos characterised both schools and a sense of carelessness prevailed. Vandalism, theft and many years of continued neglect had resulted in conditions that can best be described as appalling. Classrooms had windows but no glass, broken desks and chairs, and doors without locks. Some classes did not even have doors. Desks and chairs were chaotically strewn about in many classes. Learners showed little respect for furniture in that they either walked on chairs or toppled desks as they scurried for seats at the back of the classroom. Entry into and exit from classrooms was usually disorderly and loud. Disorganization was exaggerated by learners having to scramble for available seats since the furniture was insufficient for the large numbers in the classes. It was, therefore, not uncommon to have learners standing during lessons. The ceilings of a recently erected building at Hamba Senior Secondary were ripped open. Since the walls separating many classes in this building were not erected right up to the 'ripped out' ceiling, teachers and learners could hear what was taught in adjacent classes. During my visits, this arrangement impeded observation processes and, in many instances, affected teaching and learning. It also resulted in teachers privileging the chalkboard as the primary and sometimes only teaching tool. Many teachers walked around with chalk and board dusters because these could not be left in the classroom. The prevailing picture, therefore, was of schools in dire need of repair and care.

During the fieldwork, there was a permanent 'decoration' of paper along the school 'fences' of both schools. Schools had very limited recreational space because extra classrooms had been erected to accommodate the ever-increasing number of learners. The most recent building at Vuyisile Secondary School, for example, was a computer laboratory that had at least 40 computers donated by an overseas benefactor. The donation was made without training the current staff and as a consequence, the computers were not used, except by a few teachers for administrative tasks. The school was built on a slope, which further limited the development of any recreational facilities. In addition, teachers were either unable or unwilling to coach sports, for reasons that included being involved in transport lift clubs that left directly after school, and a perception that learners were not interested in sports. This notwithstanding, Mzi, the male teacher from this school, said that he was committed to promoting sports and had established a soccer team. Sipho, one of two teachers from Hamba Senior Secondary, merely laughed when asked about extra-curricular activities at his school.

The schools had no auxiliary staff to clean classrooms. As a result, girls were required to take turns to clean classrooms every afternoon. For the most part though, classrooms were only cleaned the next morning, a practice that had major implications for time management and discipline at the schools.[34]

At both schools it was common to find groups of learners loitering on the school grounds or unsupervised classes. Another common practice was for learners to wait until teachers arrived before settling into their respective classrooms. I got the impression that if teachers were late or 'absent', learners interpreted this as a license to remain outside or walk around the school premises. At Vuyisile Senior Secondary the situation was exacerbated by teachers' absence from class rather than from school. So, while they were present in school, some chose to remain in the staffroom for lengthy periods of time. I asked Mzi about this situation and his response was that teachers claimed to be too stressed to teach, and that the nature of the stress was mostly 'financial'! The principals in both schools had little control of such situations and often turned a blind

34 Often, this meant that the first period was used to clean the classroom. The upshot of this arrangement was that teachers and the rest of the learners usually came late to class.

eye. In fact, the principals at both secondary schools were rarely present during the fieldwork.

Latecoming (for lessons) by teachers at Hamba Senior Secondary, resulted in their having to spend time first locating and/or settling learners rather than teaching. On one occasion during the fieldwork, Sipho resorted to combining learners from different classes in the same grade to make up a class for me to observe. Like the secondary schools in the Western Cape, the only space where teaching was sacrosanct, was in the Grade 12 classes. In keeping with the poor secondary school profiles of high attrition in the Western Cape, the number of learners also showed a steady decline between Grades 8 and 12 in these two schools.

Unlike those in Hamba Senior Secondary, learners from Vuyisile Senior Secondary walked long distances to school, and teachers relied mostly on public transport or lift clubs. This notwithstanding, latecoming and absenteeism was a routinized practice amongst *teachers* and *learners* at both schools. Both schools had security gates and fences. However, the fences were broken. Even though the main gates were locked daily by eight o'clock, it was easy for learners to leave the school premises at various times of the day. Together with Khonzani Senior Secondary, a school in the category I describe in the next section, the practice of leaving during interval in these two schools was consistent with Mzondi Senior Secondary in the Western Cape.[35] As in the case of the school in the Western Cape, the unintended consequences of such arrangements included unsystematic and uncontrolled dropping in and out of school, teenage pregnancy, loitering and truancy.

I found, upon my return to Hamba Senior Secondary early in 2004, that the provincial government had restored the fence and placed a security guard to monitor access to the school. This was established not only to curb the incessant problem of absenteeism and latecoming but also as a consequence of the consistently poor matriculation results at this school. While poor matric results were characteristic of this school for a number of years, the situation was perceived as desperate when, in 2003, it obtained the second lowest matric results in the province. The department had to be seen as reacting in some way to improve the situation. As a result, the school was marked as one of the 'high risk' schools

35 While this is a common practice in all the poor schools in both regions, the youngest school in Mpumalanga has revised this practice, as is explained later in this section.

in the province and received daily visits from officials who monitored teacher attendance, lesson preparation and time on task. These measures of surveillance were unwelcome and, as I explain in the next chapter, were seen as unfair and unprofessional. Though Sipho, the teacher from this school agreed that some measures were necessary, he interpreted the current practice as harsh and punitive. Teachers here did not recognise these as either important or necessary for improving the quality of teaching or creating enhanced learning opportunities for learners. In response to questions about the poor matriculation results, Sipho eloquently and smilingly stated that the results were indeed atrocious, particularly since the province already had the lowest pass rates in the country. He reported that teachers were angry about the department's surveillance strategies because, according to him, the children were at fault because they did not want to learn.

The matric results at Vuyisile Senior Secondary had also declined in 2003.[36] Mzi stated, though, that this decline was not a major concern for teachers. According to him the school was 'not too bad' because they were not rated amongst the lowest on the provincial scale, nor were they targeted as high risk.

Practices in these old schools were ritualized and legitimated in ways that made it difficult for those operating in them candidly to question or even consider alternative ways of functioning. Teachers did not recognise their role in recreating this history of continued neglect. Instead, they blamed the government for the poor condition of schools, and learners for their lack of scholastic achievement.

The 'new' schools

Khonzani Senior Secondary was situated less than a kilometre away from Hamba Senior Secondary. It was less than 15 years old. As a relatively new school, it was neat and well maintained. During the fieldwork, for example, learners were seen cultivating sections of the school grounds. Shrubs neatly adorned the entrance to the administrative block.

The grounds of this school were inadequate for the number of students, as was the case in the two old secondary schools in this region. Possibilities for expansion were limited because this school was also

36 From percentages in the 50s down to the 40s.

built on a slope, with a river and the main road as its respective boundaries. Interestingly, this was the only school in the rural sample with a teacher from a different racial group.

Like the old schools, Khonzani Senior secondary school also had no auxiliary staff to clean classrooms. Unlike the former schools where cleaning was left to the girls, at this school, all learners were expected to clean their respective classrooms on Friday afternoons. However, during the fieldwork, I noticed that cleaning began soon after the interval (between 10:30–11:30), with girls doing most of the work.

Loitering at this school was much more controlled. Compared to the old schools, fewer learners were outside classes during official teaching time. There was much more evidence of teaching and learning, and teachers were in attendance in many more classes. Learners responded to the bell as a signal for class to resume and often stood in neat rows at the entrance of their respective classrooms. During the fieldwork I noticed that learners waited to greet the teachers before entering the classroom. Classes were orderly. Desks were placed in rows and these were generally in recognisably good condition. In classes where learners had to share desks, teachers designated seats to learners and managed this process in an orderly manner.

The principal of this school was present on two of the three occasions that I visited the school. He left instructions about my visit on the occasion he was absent. Unlike at the older schools, where my visit was a surprise to the management staff (even though a letter, fax and phone calls had confirmed my visit), this school was prepared. A room was readied in advance for the interviews. The general impression I had was of a school working very hard to reverse the years of neglect and chaos. So, while there were remnants of past practices (some loitering, long breaks with learners leaving the school premises), there was evidence of a material and psychological shift in the practices of this school. The concomitant results were visible in a number of ways. For example, this school consistently produced comparatively good matriculation results. While it was not amongst the best performing schools in the province, its pass rates averaged between 55–65% each year. There were more matric classes, suggesting that retention rates in the lower classes were high. Thandi, the female teacher from this school, reported that the school had a programme that identified and supported vulnerable children (particularly orphans and child-headed families).

Buyisa Senior Secondary, like the school above, had also been established less than 15 years ago. The newest secondary school in this sample of rural schools, it was situated in a poorer part of Thokoza and was at least six kilometres from the two schools mentioned above. While the geographic distance between the three schools was small, access to Buyisa was difficult since it was situated in an area where roads were underdeveloped and in very poor condition. This area had fewer brick houses and many had no running water or electricity. But the school had a very well maintained building. It had a gardener who, at the time of the fieldwork, was in the process of changing the physical landscape of the school.

Many of the current staff had started out when the school was established. Patricia, one of two black female teachers in the study, was one such teacher. She reported that many teachers went unsalaried for months in the first year of the school. She said that this situation did not deter them from offering learners quality instruction.

The practices at this school stood in sharp contrast to the rest of those in the sample of poor schools in both regions. This school locked its gates when the school began and only opened them for visitors who had appointments. It had a permanent security guard who monitored access in and out of the school. Unlike Hamba Senior Secondary where a security guard was appointed by the education department, this course of action was initiated by the school. Teachers perceived such action as central to maintaining order and quality.

Absenteeism was not tolerated at this school. Parents or guardians were held accountable for any learner who was absent. As at Khonzani Senior Secondary, loitering was not tolerated during the designated schooltime. A culture of teaching and learning was evident. Teachers were not only present in class, but they were teaching. The staffroom was partitioned into subject-based zones. Teachers who had administrative periods sat quietly marking in their designated zones. Staff meetings were usually held after rather than during school. Volene and Patricia, the two teachers from this school, both agreed that the management was inclusive and that teachers participated in all decision-making processes. With a very approachable management team, the staff was comfortable, motivated, and enthusiastic, providing learners with the best teaching and learning opportunities under the circumstances.

There were discernible benefits from a disciplined approach to schooling. This school maintained high retention rates across all grades.

Many more learners completed and succeeded in the matric examination than in any other poor secondary school in this study, irrespective of the region. Noticeably, not only were the school's matric results consistently much higher than the norm for the region, but it boasted the best matric results in the Khabokweni region, a mark of distinction held for a number of years. Therefore, while situated in a poor community, it was identified with a different ethos and very different sets of practices.

In summary, the descriptions above provide a backdrop for understanding and situating what appears in Chapter 10, namely, descriptions of the dominant influences on teachers' lives. This chapter has served to embed these experiences within contexts that are spatially and materially complex. While in South Africa a racialised identity was imprinted onto the geographic landscape by Apartheid separatist ideology, what emerged is a description of a context that blurs the artificial categories of race and class. So, while many communities remained racially polarised, they were similar in their experience. Proximity to modern centres for the poor did not necessarily ensure access to the economic and cultural capital available in the field. For the most part, poor school communities continued to rewrite the history of neglect and poverty through particular sets of practices. Change occurred in those schools where teachers, parents and children recognised their role in reproducing the cycle of neglect. The new schools in Mpumalanga are an example of how, in exercising agency, schools were able to reverse the legacy of neglect and produce good results.

These complex discursive spaces, together with what follows in the next chapter, served as sites for the production of particular teacher identities and teacher behaviours that are detailed in Chapter 11.

10 Dominant factors shaping teachers' subjective experiences

The previous chapter provided descriptions of the material and social conditions that act as discursive spaces in which this cohort of teachers make meaning of their lives. Drawing on in-depth interviews, what follows here describes yet another layer of influence, namely, experiences shaping constructions of teacher identity. Initially, I set about developing narratives of each teacher, but this process proved too cumbersome to include in the final work. I opted instead for what I am calling collective narratives. The intention in Chapter 10 is to provide descriptions of the past and present experiences that serve as a backdrop to understanding teachers' lives in relation to their work, particularly as Life Orientation teachers. I outline some of the dominant social and cultural practices that have influenced and continue to influence constructions of their teacher identity and, as the next chapter will describe, their subsequent classroom practice. It is important to describe these social and cultural practices since they are the resources teachers draw on to construct their identity as teachers. The questions this chapter responds to are: who are these teachers and what, in relation to their past and present lived experiences, shaped and continues to influence their individual and collective teacher identities? Put differently, I pose questions about how these teachers are positioned or are positioning themselves within a specifically South African HIV/AIDS hermeneutic space that was and still is deeply raced, classed and gendered. What rules and resources do they draw on to take up positions and produce the 'strips of behaviour' they enact in the classroom? How, within such constructions, do they understand themselves as Lifeskills teachers within a particular situated context? This is in preparation for what follows in Chapter 11, an attempt to understand the articulation between the teachers and the teacherly behaviour or enactments they call up.

This chapter is presented in three interrelated sections, with each outlining factors teachers report as having had an influence on their teacher identities. While the parts are not distinguished as such in the writing, each culminates with descriptions of a distinct subject position that characterised teachers or their subsequent behaviours at a particular point in time. These are not presented as fixed. Rather, they highlight only three of the many distinct positions teachers called up. Holding these positions constant momentarily in this work was helpful in analysing teachers' behaviour, in that it illuminated what they concealed about their identity as well as what was at stake during the mediation process.

Part 1 begins with a profile of the teachers in the study. I follow this with descriptions of their early lives, which have had (and continue to have) an influence on the attitudes, beliefs and values they hold in general. Here I describe the role of politics and poverty, the home and family, education and schooling, role models, and finally the role that religion played in developing their 'teacher identity'. The latter conduced to the identification of four types of teacher position. Teachers were classified as fundamentalists, conformists/traditionalists, nominalists, or unconventionalists. The descriptions in the first part served as the basis for the positions that teachers adopted in the second and third parts. While the process of developing all three parts was by no means linear or distinct, reflecting on them highlighted their difference and how the levels of influence played themselves out through overlap and the reproduction of particular subject positions.

The second part describes the influences on teachers' perceptions of teaching. These include the influence of role models, their deportment, and the whole question of what constitutes a 'teacher'. Here I highlight positions that typified teachers as disciplinarians or nurturers.

Chapter 10 is brought to a close with the third part, namely, respondents' perceptions and experiences of sex, sexuality, and HIV/AIDS; aspects that are fundamental to understanding the core questions posed in this work. I describe various issues associated with sexuality that influenced teachers' conceptions of who they are and what they do. These include constructions and perceptions of and responses to sexuality and HIV/AIDS, the role of language and conceptions of marriage. It is here that issues at the heart of this study come together to illustrate the ruptures in identities in most distinct ways. As will be illustrated later, this group of teachers performed ways of being that were difficult to trace back to their experiences as described in the earlier sections. What the final section highlights, therefore, is the moment of disruption, the discontinuity between the sociology of their identities and their 'teacher' performance in the classroom.

Descriptions of teachers as exaggerators, normalizers, framers, or binders indicated subject positions which served as a basis for understanding what they did in the classroom. I use these to describe how teachers managed the curriculum content as well as the process of mediation. Importantly though, they foreground what teachers concealed or left out about their identities and as such, highlighted the performative nature of teaching. In short, these categories of description served as the analytical framework for describing what actually happens in Lifeskills classrooms when teachers mediate about sexuality and HIV/AIDS.

Diagram 2, below, illustrates the levels of influence described in this section. These intersect at various points, producing distinct subject positions at different moments in time. I illustrate these points of positionality diagrammatically at the end of each section.

Diagram 2: Factors and Four Levels of Influence Shaping Teachers' Subjective Experiences

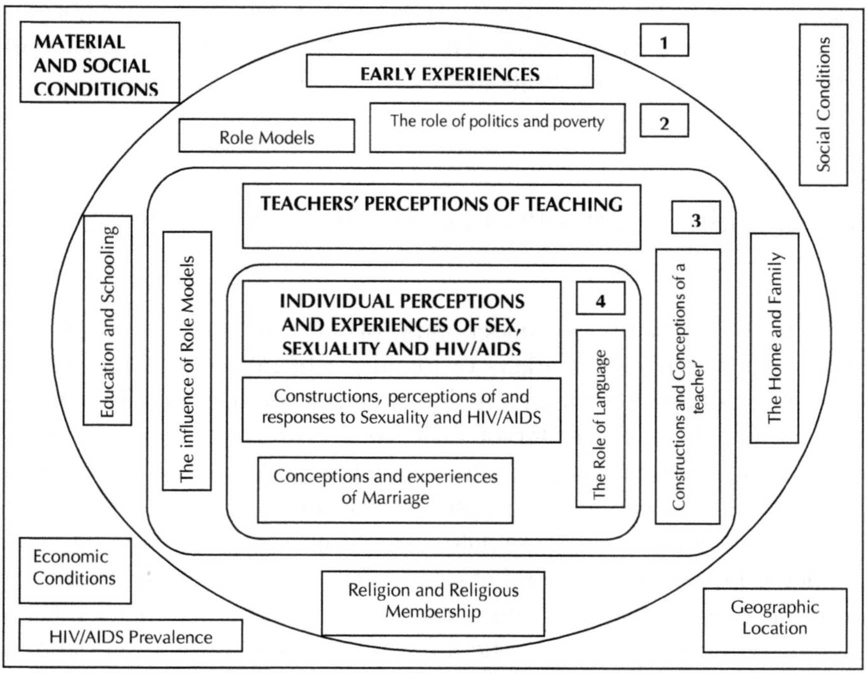

This work takes as its point of departure the notion that constructions of identity are complex, and that "structural properties" (Giddens, 1984) and agents are complexly intertwined within social practice. Using Giddens's theory of structuration as a basis, I work from the premise that "structural properties" (Giddens, 1984), while acting as that which shapes constructions of identity, are at the same time operationalized as rules and resources that this cohort draws from and interprets. Such interpretations and reproductions find expression when instantiated in social practice, in other words, in the actions of people. While they may have a historicity, rules and institutions are given voice and action or instantiated in the present and are thus open to modification and transformation by agents. As Giddens's (1984: 25) suggests, structure does not function outside of the individual but rather as "memory traces", and as "instantiated in social practice." However, when applied in isolation, Giddens's theory proposes subjects who are already positioned in positions that are determined. I use Butler's theory of performativity here to counter this notion because, as the evidence below suggests, teachers take up many different positions, depending on what is at stake. What the data offers below, therefore, is insight into the multiplicity and complexity of teacher subject positioning rather than just evidence of teacher subjectivity.

Social and cultural influences on teacher identity

The codes of description reflect some of the dominant practices that emerged as significant markers of identity. I begin each theme with a description of the general picture that emerged and then highlight differences where they exist. I attempt, however, not to make claims about the fixity of these structuring properties since they are contextually situated and as such are open to modification and difference.

I begin below with a tabulated profile in which I outline the age, gender, school level, race and marital status of teachers. I proceed with descriptions of social and cultural practices in eight broad themes. Each theme comprises categories. The themes are linked to the discussion in Part II where I described Bourdieu's theory of practice. There I detailed the discursive spaces that he suggests shape beliefs, attitudes and values.

These include home and family, schooling, role models, religion, etc. I used these as broad frames of references to develop the themes and categories I present below.

Profile of the respondents

The original sample comprised twenty teachers, five males and fifteen females as Tables 7 and 8, below, illustrate. While I tried to maintain the same number of primary and secondary school teachers, this was not possible. The composition of the sample did not adversely influence the results of the study, since my aim was to examine teacher practices and factors shaping teachers' understanding of HIV/AIDS and sexuality. The unit of analysis, therefore, rested on understanding teachers as subjects of the study rather than on what level they teach within the school system. This notwithstanding, I deemed it important to include the perspectives and experiences of a broad spectrum of teachers across the school system. As a result, the thirteen secondary school teachers selected were those who taught Life Orientation in Grades Eight or Nine and the seven primary teachers were Grade Six Life Orientation teachers (all of them were also class teachers, teaching more than one learning area).

Table 7: Western Cape: Teachers' Profile

Teacher	*Age*	*Marital Status*	*Gender*	*Race*	*School*	*School Level*
Kobie	45	Married	Male	White	Bloukoop	Secondary
Vera	35+	Married	Female	White	Bloukoop	Secondary
Pauline	32	Married	Female	Coloured	Parktown	Secondary
Gwen	35+	Married	Female	Coloured	Parktown	Secondary
Paul	43	Married	Male	Coloured	Redhill	Secondary
Carol	35+	Married	Female	Coloured	Redhill	Secondary
Shahida	40+	Married	Female	Coloured	Macadamia	Primary
Zodwa	32	Single	Female	Black	Mzondi	Secondary
Xola	30+	Single	Male	Black	Vuyani	Primary
Gugu	40+	Married	Female	Black	Zondi	Primary

Table 8: Mpumalanga: Teachers' Profile

Teacher	*Age*	*Marital Status*	*Gender*	*Race*	*School*	*School level*
Mzi	40+	Married	Male	Black	Vuyisile	Secondary
Sipho	35+	Single	Male	Black	Hamba	Secondary
Lizzie	45+	Widowed	Female	Black	Hamba	Secondary
Thandi	35+	Married	Female	Black	Khonzani	Secondary
Volene	40+	Single	Female	Black	Buyisa	Secondary
Patricia	35+	Married	Female	Black	Buyisa	Secondary
Jenni	35+	Married	Female	Black	Yiso	Primary
Ester	45+	Divorced	Female	Black	Siyabonga	Primary
Dorothy	35+	Divorced	Female	Black	Mbazani	Primary
Jabulani	35+	Married	Female	Black	Hambani	Primary

The cohort comprised two white, five Coloured and thirteen Black teachers. All the teachers from Mpumalanga were from ethnic black communities. The black group comprised teachers of Siswati, Zulu, and Sotho ethnicity.

The average age of the group was thirty-seven. All the teachers in the study were not only educated in racially segregated environments, but most of them had also attended segregated teacher training institutions. The majority of the teachers trained in institutions that were designed either for blacks or coloureds. Sixteen of the group trained at colleges of education, some of which were in 'homelands.'[37] Sipho was the only black teacher who completed his initial teacher education at a racially integrated university in Natal.[38] Gwen, the coloured teacher from Parktown Senior Secondary, trained at a historically White university. As was the general practice with people of colour at such institutions, she obtained special permission to train there. Vera and Kobie, the only White teachers in the study, trained at a predominantly Afrikaans university in the Western Cape. Vera, who began her career as a psychologist, returned to university to train as a teacher in the early 1990s. For Kobie,

37 Homelands were 'independent' states within South Africa established by the Apartheid Government as a way of maintaining a racially and ethnically segregated population.

38 Integrated here means that the university comprised Coloured, Black and Indian students.

going to university was taken-for-granted as the expected and accepted. Paul and Carol met at the coloured teacher training college they attended in the 1980s, married and both taught at the same school. Ironically they taught the same subjects to Grades 8 and 9. Paul went on to complete a series of diplomas and his Bachelor of Education (Honours) at a historically coloured institution, the University of the Western Cape. Jenni and Jabulani, who both taught at primary schools in Mpumalanga, also completed degrees in education, the former as a full-time student at the University of Zululand and the latter, part-time, with the University of South Africa. Jenni was in the process of completing an honours degree in psychology, which she hoped would lead her out of teaching into a career in counselling. The significance of the above becomes evident later on in the analysis when teachers describe the influence teachers and college lecturers had, both in the career decisions they made as well as in understanding constructions of 'the teacher.'

Nine of the twenty teachers worked before attending teacher training college. The nature of the work differed, but most worked as unskilled labourers. Ester from Siyabonga Primary school in Mpumalanga, for example, worked as a domestic worker for 18 years while Mzi also from Mpumalanga, worked as a juice-maker. While the situation may have been so, and as will become evident later in the next section, all nine together with at least six others in the group, had ambitions to become teachers and as many put it, to someday 'become somebody.'

Thirteen of the twenty teachers were married, two divorced, four single and one widowed. This status was an important marker of teacher identity.

The majority of the respondents were female. The skewed gender representation was not surprising, for two reasons. First, female teachers constituted the majority within the teaching population in South Africa. Second, while observing and talking to teachers in schools, I noticed a prevailing perception that Life Orientation was a 'soft' subject, one that a female with her supposed natural nurturing disposition was better qualified to teach. As such, female teachers were more likely to be approached to teach the subject. At another level, and particularly in the secondary school context, Life Orientation teachers were, for the most part, previously home economics teachers who were now expected to take on this new role. This often meant that at the participating secondary schools, males teachers volunteered to teach the subject rather than were expected to. Even in cases where home economics teachers were reluctant to teach the subject, they understood their position as having already been established and as such, non-negotiable.

While almost all the black and two coloured teachers came from working class backgrounds, they nevertheless all had middle class aspirations. Poverty was a key descriptor in their experiences, as I detail in the next section. Parents, particularly mothers, put pressure on their children to accomplish something 'better' and 'become somebody'. The primary means by which this could be achieved was, as parents saw it, through education. Middle-class ambitions were often associated with becoming a teacher, a policeman, or a nurse.

Together with the two white and three coloured females, Jenni was the only black teacher from a middle class environment. This notwithstanding, the community in which she lived was predominantly working class and poor, as the descriptions in the previous chapter illustrated.

The importance of the profile adumbrated above becomes clearer in the next few sections, where I provide more detailed descriptions of the teachers themselves as well as the practices shaping their teacher identities.

Teachers, politics, and poverty

A striking feature of the descriptions given by 18 of the 20 respondents interviewed was the absence of any mention of the role of politics as a structuring influence on early experiences or constructions of identity. For the most part, descriptions of early life and current experiences were disembedded from any political, geographic, or racial associations. Absent in such descriptions was (re)cognition, therefore, of the way in which political structures shaped family life, employment opportunities, access to school, housing conditions, and everyday lived experiences. Below, I describe the role of politics and poverty in constructing identities in two interrelated categories, namely, teachers and politics, and teachers and poverty.

Teachers and politics

Most of the teachers showed little (re)cognition of the political conditions which dominated South African life. Eighteen reported that they had not participated in overtly political activities, a striking fact given that most were in high school during the height of the political struggle in South Africa. Pauline, a coloured teacher from the Western Cape, provided a comment typical of this group of teachers. She stated:

> I don't think it really affected me. I was in Std 6 during the 1985 boycott, and it was very confusing for me. You heard little snippets of what was happening but it didn't really affect me as such. The only thing I can remember is as a child going into a restaurant on Cape Town station, and I remember my dad attempting to go in through the front of the restaurant and I walked with my mom behind him, at the time I was the little one and being told you can't, this is for whites only, that kind of thing. But it didn't really affect me.

Thirteen of the 20 teachers, particularly those from poor communities, often described poverty rather than the political system as the key indicator that shaped their individual and collective identities. The role politics played was minimized in teachers' narratives even in circumstances where poverty was not mentioned. For example, the two teachers from the affluent community of Bloukoop accepted their histories of privilege with little questioning. To them, strict family regimens rather than politics or poverty played a significant role in their early experiences.

Only two teachers acknowledged the role of politics in their lives. Paul, an expressive coloured teacher from the only 'poor' coloured community in the Western Cape, described poverty as a result of the political situation. While he also understood the role of politics in structuring peoples' lives, his reasoning was different from the rest of the group. To him, every lived experience *was* political. Every facet of his life, therefore, was interpreted through a political lens. While growing up (and encouraged by his parents), he participated in what he called "subversive political activities." His parents, he suggested, did not ever subscribe to the racial categorisations used by the Apartheid government but rather encouraged him to consider himself as a human being. He states, "[to] be honest I never ever considered myself as a coloured, but as a human being and again my parents taught me that. You're a human being." The description below of a significant event in his life was a poignant illustration of the beginning of his overt political orientation. It described an experience between himself and a White teenager. Briefly, he recalled how this teenager:

> [The teenager] ... took a mothball out of his pocket, and he urinated on it. And then he took it and put it in my mouth. [His friend] ... took my other brother and pushed him around and smacked him around. I was just smiling at that stage because these were two big guys. The evening when we got home our dad spoke to us about what to do [as revenge] ... I took revenge ... at that stage and even at a later stage ....

This event sparked a lifelong commitment in him: the fight against inequitable conditions. To this teacher, the political struggle is still not over. His speech remains charged with political symbolism and imagery. He continued to be the leader of the teacher union at his school. He serves as an ombudsman for teachers even when they act inappropriately. As an example, while I was at the school during observations, a teacher belonging to the union was charged for using corporal punishment. Paul was angry that the principal had made this a legal case. The issue was 'minor' and 'internal', he said, and as such, could have been managed at the school level. He remains vocal about a host of other issues: a perceived lack of freedom, constant surveillance by the principal, appraisal by peers and the like. In these positions, he embodies his 'political struggle persona' and wears it as a key signifier of his teacherliness.

For Gwen, a soft-spoken but eloquent coloured teacher, politics assumed a very different role. Growing up in Gracious Heights, a predominantly coloured middle-income environment, she described how choices made by her parents to send her to a "white" all-girls private school (and thereafter proceeding to a university that required her to obtain special permission for entry) produced unintended consequences and a sense of ambivalence. On the one hand, she considered herself *'privileged'* for having had the opportunity, a word she used often during the interview. On the other hand, though, the ridicule she experienced created alienation from the community and a sense of being different. Interestingly, her ambivalence also emerged in her actions during our interactions. She cried during much of the first interview, even though I offered to continue the interview at another occasion. With many pauses, tears and deep breaths, she insisted that we continue and recalled incidents in which she still "remember[ed] the comments ..." When asked what the comments were, she stated, "[t]raitor! I suppose ... in a nutshell. Because they obviously could see that I wasn't at one of the schools in the area. Of course my uniform said it all."

The reasons offered by this teacher for the choices her parents made were interesting. While she was aware of the benefits, the reasons offered represented community rather than individual gain. She put it this way, "I didn't have a problem with having to have a permit because I knew that I wasn't going to be going to a white school to be a teacher there. I was going there to empower myself so that I could come back to my community to empower other kids."

While I assumed that I would find a more direct correlation between politics and constructions of identity amongst this group, such recognition was not obvious, as I describe in the summary at the end of this section. Instead, as the next section shows, poverty played a significant role in influencing many among this group of teachers.

Teachers and poverty

Thirteen of the 20 teachers, particularly those from poor communities, often described poverty rather than the political system as the key indicator that shaped their individual and collective identities. In this regard, they described poor housing conditions, lack of income, the absence of fathers, and employment on farms during school vacation as descriptions of the way poverty played out in their everyday experiences. The following excerpt by Patricia, a black teacher from Buyisa Senior Secondary, one of the 'new' schools in Mpumalanga, provided what was a typical description of poor housing conditions amongst this group. She states, "[a]ll the seven of us sharing two rooms: two rooms together with our parents. One room was used by our parents, our brothers in one room and we were sleeping in the dining room, sometimes in the kitchen. It was very difficult." It was not uncommon, too, that some families shared their homes with extended family members, a condition which sometimes led to girls being sexually harassed by older members. In other instances, though, having the extended family in one's home served as an extra source of income.

Seven (six females and one male) of the 13 teachers reported growing up without the constant presence of their father, a situation that held consequences for how families functioned and their ability to provide for their children. Reasons for this absence varied. In the main, work arrangements were responsible for separating families. Other teachers reported not knowing their fathers because they were raised by single mothers. Lizzie from Hamba Senior Secondary, the oldest school in the Mpumalanga cohort, was raised by her grandmother. With regard to her absent father, she stated, "I was living with my grandmother and my mother never married, a single parent raised me. I don't know my father ... even today." Xola from Vuyani primary, a school situated in a poor community in the Western Cape, was one of two male teachers raised by a single mother. He stated, "My father passed away when I was two years old. So I was raised up till today by my mother who is about 75 years old today."

Fathers often worked away from home for long periods of time, leaving mothers to take responsibility for rearing families. Gugu, a black teacher from Zondi primary school who was raised in the Eastern Cape, recalled meeting her father for the first time at ten years old, when she was in Grade 4. She said:

> My father was working at Cape Town. It was not easy for my mother alone to take care of us without my father because I was born in 1964 but I only saw my father for the first time when I was in Standard Two. I was ten years old. It was not a good experience for me to see my father when I was ten years. But anyway, that's how it was at that time.

Long periods of absence by fathers sometimes led to the disintegration of family structures because parents seemed unable to sustain long distance relationships. In two instances, such arrangements led to fathers taking other wives in their places of employment, situations that left the families concerned stranded and fatherless. Dorothy from Mbazani Primary School, one of two divorced teachers in this study, stated, "[s]o when I was doing grade ... standard ... form two by that time, my father left us for another woman, so we struggled a little bit growing up."

Another consequence of fathers' working arrangements was that often, financial support proved insufficient to sustain the family even in instances where fathers remained financially (and emotionally) committed to the family. Mothers were compelled to seek employment, a situation that often led to siblings taking care of each other without adult supervision. Such circumstances, as some teachers suggest, led to a lack of guidance on a host of issues including those associated with sex and sexuality (discussed later).

Poverty was commonly depicted as a significant indicator of lived experience even among the six remaining teachers in this group whose familial arrangements seemed more traditional (where both parents remained together). Patricia described it this way: "My growing up has helped a lot because I was from a poor family and my mother was a housewife. My father was working very far away and only came home once a month. So we grew up having nothing."

A common characteristic among this cohort of thirteen teachers is the manner in which poverty was depicted with a 'taken-for-granted' acceptance. What occurred was a situation in which they were caught up in the experience of being poor and seemed unable to recognise the interconnection between politics and poverty. To them, being poor was just the way life was at the time. The following excerpts were illustrative of how most in this group described their early experiences. In describing the conditions under which his family lived, Sipho, a well-spoken male teacher from Hamba Senior Secondary who was the university-trained teacher stated: "... so, *needless to say*, (my emphasis) I was born into a poor family." Patricia pointed out that they were "[from] ... a very disciplined family. Although we did not have anything as my father was the only person who was working. And in that small town ... there were no jobs. But my mother used to go in the kitchen and used to do domestic working."

Gugu, in describing the situation when she met her father for the first time, illustrated a similar sense of inevitability when she stated, "[b]ut anyway, that's how it was at that time."

Notwithstanding this and as I describe in the next section, this group did not consider their early experiences of poverty as pre-determining their future life chances. Instead, and in the main, such experiences led to parents (particularly mothers) placing an emphasis on education as a way out of poverty.

In summary and at one level, irrespective of race, economic status, or class, what emerged was a picture of all but one respondent misrecognising (Bourdieu, 1990) the effect of the political situation on their lived experience. While descriptions of poverty were stark, these were not often associated with reasons beyond those taken for granted as the 'way it is'. Experiences of poverty were thus normalised; the condition one was born into rather than the result of an orchestrated political plan. In instances where poverty was not mentioned as a primary signifier, respondents were unable or unwilling to acknowledge the way in which politics worked to hierarchise and stratify privilege on a racial basis. What was revealed was a picture where 18 of the 20 teachers, irrespective of race, described the political situation as something removed, as an aspect of life of which they were not necessarily a part.

Descriptions of poverty and family were disassociated from politics. In other words, politics was presented as a phenomenon that took place outside the reality of their privilege or poverty. Instead, their early circumstances were associated with an accepted inevitability. In this respect, Bourdieu's notion of habitus was useful for understanding how many act in the present, misrecognising the real reason for the condition in which they find themselves and the degree to which the political structure acted as an apparatus in shaping their collective identities and individual life chances. Such misrecognition was apparent in explanations given by Gwen. Rather than acknowledge the benefits that private school education and subsequent university education offered in creating better life chances, she proposed coming back "to the community" to "empower other kids" as the 'real' reason for pursuing her interests.

At another level, though, and as the following section highlights, such misrecognition was strategic and sometimes even deliberate. While at some level poverty acted as the base structure from which identities might be read and from which most of the teachers in this group made meaning of their daily lives, it also acted as the base from which they were able to exercise agency. As such, poverty was both a disabler and an enabler. It acted as the condition that limited the possibilities for better life chances. Simultaneously, though, it was put forward as the reason why many were able to propel themselves out of dire situations. Put differently, while it determined their early experiences, it nevertheless served as the structuring property (Giddens, 1984: 25) from which modifications were possible, leading for many, to a shift in *habitus* as well as their "remaking" as 'middle-class teachers.' The critical role of education in offering better life chances for this group of teachers is described below.

Teachers and the purpose and role of education

The role that education played was significant in shaping individual and collective experiences among the majority of teachers. The value placed on education by parents had a particular influence on conceptions and the perceived value of, as well as responses to, education. Some individuals understood very early on in life that education would be the means through which they could better their life circumstances. In these cases, their parents linked education with the possibility of a better life. These attitudes were most prevalent among teachers from the poor communities in both regions as well as among the middle income communities in the Western Cape. As I explain below, in the case of the two teachers from the affluent community, education was a predetermined, taken-for-granted activity, which they merely did. What follows is a description of the role and purpose of education as it played out in the lives of this cohort. The descriptions below are grouped in three categories: education as a taken-for-granted activity, a way of becoming, or as a class status identifier.

Education as a taken-for-granted activity

Vera and Kobie, the only white teachers in this study from the affluent community of Bloukoop in the Western Cape, were the only ones who perceived education as something that was guaranteed, something they were born into and, therefore, a taken-for-granted activity. For these teachers, there was inevitability about it; it was what people do. They, for example, described their educational histories with an inherent confidence, with a certainty that suggested a way of being and a way of knowing. There was no question as to whether they would complete school. As members of the dominant group within the field (those who make the rules and have social and cultural capital), these two teachers provide an example of how those with cultural capital act in the field: without much thought and (re)cognition of their privileged status. Schooling was accepted as that which is done 'naturally', as a way of gaining and maintaining symbolic capital (Bourdieu, 1991: 166). As such, these two teachers offered information about schooling in a way that suggested an unquestioning acceptance of the circumstances, experiences, and conditions of schooling. Such conceptions seemed obvious even in circumstances where the female teacher, for example, first married and had a family. The marriage notwithstanding, she understood that the possibility existed and chances remained strong that she would complete some form of higher education (and indeed she did). What emerged in the interview descriptions, therefore, was merely technical information that suggested the educational progression of each teacher. The following excerpt by Kobie illustrates the point: "[I] stayed on a farm until I was about 15 years old and then I came to ... (school) where I completed my matric. And then I attended ... (the university)."

Education as a way of becoming

For the rest of the group, meanings associated with education varied. All 18 teachers recognised the importance of schooling as more than a socializing structure. In the case of four teachers, as I describe in the next section, education identified their class status. For 14 respondents whose experiences I describe below, it was understood as the platform from which they could imagine a better life. For this group becoming educated was not merely what people do, but rather what they were and could become.

Staying in school was a struggle for many. While circumstances and the extent of the struggle varied, all eighteen commented on the sacrifices they, their parents, or their guardians made to ensure that they either remained in or completed school. Reasons for this struggle varied. All 18 respondents, irrespective of economic status, described lack of funds as the primary source of struggle. Such a lack led to some, for example, having to work during school vacations to supplement the family income and to enable them to obtain school uniforms and educational materials. However, in the case of seven female teachers, early teenage pregnancy resulted in their having temporarily to abandon school. While all went on to complete the most basic school-level requirements[39] that would enable them to enter a college of education, their pregnancies meant that they had protracted educational histories. Other struggles associated with their

39 Some teachers entered college with a Grade 10 certificate, a minimum requirement in many Black Colleges of Education prior to 1994. Other teachers went on to complete matric before pursuing a career in teaching.

training included living at a considerable distance from their schools, a situation that meant long separations from their family for some.

Unlike Vera and Kobie, for whom education shaped up as 'taken-for-granted', the role and importance of education took on different meanings among the rest of the 18. Some perceived education as that which would provide them with the possibility of a 'better life' while for others, as I suggested above, it offered the opportunity for improving their class status. Frequently, it was their parents who held a vision of a better life for their children. But in some cases, respondents themselves decided that they needed to 'have an education', since it would offer better life chances.

Eight teachers from poor environments emphasized that their parents were determined that they should have 'a better life' through educating themselves. Volene, a black teacher from one of the poor but 'new' secondary schools in Mpumalanga, encapsulated what was a common view among this group. In describing her mother's sentiments, she stated:

> All that she wanted was for us to be educated one day. And from us as children, me ... myself, and my older brother, we were so enthusiastic, we also wanted to learn so that one-day we (could) enlarge the house because it was so small we could see the situation. But she was always behind us, every step of the way.

In describing her family's stance on education, Shahida, the only muslim teacher in the study who taught at Macadamia Primary School in Stanton, stated, "I come from a family that was very much for education. I have three other sisters who are teachers. We are six sisters together." To her they "are all concerned with knowledge because that is what my father wanted us to be, to educate ourselves. Just to go forward in life, being somebody, ..." When she failed and was reluctant to return to school, she did so at her father's insistence. She stated:

> ... [b]ecause as I said, when I failed Standard Nine, then my father wouldn't have me just lying at home. I didn't want to go back to school because I was embarrassed because all my friends have progressed to the next level, but here I am. He said to me, 'You will go back to school until your teeth grows hair!' I thought to myself that my father wanted something for me and today I can see.

Five teachers, all from poor-income environments, described how, individually, they made the decision to seek out educational opportunities as a way of establishing a 'better life', to 'become somebody'. Sipho gave a typical example when he stated, "[s]o out of that poverty stricken family, I was determined to go and try to start to go my way to the University of ... where I completed my Bachelor of Education in ... Yes, that's when I came back and taught."

Taking steps towards educating themselves sometimes produced unintended consequences for many in this group. These included having to leave home at an early age, going against traditional practices and working against expectations of what women were capable of achieving. Gugu, for example, described how she decided to leave home at an early age to pursue a career. She described the reasons for her choice. She had a child at 18 while completing Grade 10. Initially, her mother took care of the baby. However, she realized that her chances of creating a better life for herself and her baby in the Eastern Cape were limited. She described the path she selected to 'becoming somebody' and make a better life for herself in the excerpt below. She said:

> Oh, when I was doing Grade 11, I decided to leave Eastern Cape to go and look for greener pastures. I said to myself, 'no, [when I was doing Grade 9, 10, 11,] you know my parents are not educated. They were not illiterate but they were not educated. Because they were looking forward to [one] amongst their children ... they need somebody ... who can at least do something. Okay, I said to myself, 'Now is the time. My parents give me everything at their best. So I must try something on my own. I must discover. I must look for greener pastures'. I completed Grade 9, 10 and 11. Now I [thought] there is nothing that I can get now from them. The best way is to go the people that I think can give me something to progress in life. I came to Cape Town.

Characteristically always well-dressed and well-spoken, Lizzie, from Hamba Senior Secondary, provided an example of how she went against a traditional cultural practice to reach her goal of becoming 'somebody.' She described how she "found someone who could take care of me, and take me back to school, at that time I wanted to be somebody, wanted to be something tomorrow." She made the choice to live with 'this man' (as she refers to him throughout the interview) thereby going against the long-held traditional practice of '*lobola*'.[40] When asked why she did that, her response was instructive. She said, "I never thought of that *lobola*.

40 Lobola is a dowry paid by the male to the family of the girl he has chosen to marry.

I only thought of myself ... of being taken care of, of being catered for ... it was not about that *lobola*."

Ester, a shy and soft-spoken divorced black teacher from Siyabonga Primary School in Mpumalanga described how, as a woman, the pursuit of a career produced an unintended consequence for her. She described how initially she had been forced to leave school in Grade 8 because, as she says, "... from there, I have to (pause) to, to have a family and after having a (pause), my three kids." While working as a domestic worker, a position she held for 18 years, she decided to register at night school to complete her matric. This decision bothered her husband intensely. He felt that she was not behaving appropriately for a woman. She says "... that time my husband left me because I was going back to school."

Teachers were aware that education provided a 'better life' and a shift in class status, thus a shift in their *habitus*. The black teachers in the Mpumalanga schools were conscious of what education provided them, namely, an elevated position in the community, but were also quick to admit that it did not 'change' the way they viewed the poor communities in which they worked and lived. Sipho, the single black teacher from Hamba Senior Secondary School, said "[n]o, now I am a 'so-called' middle class worker. However, I still have roots from my, from my background. I do not undermine other people that are less fortunate than me so I also identify myself with the poverty stricken."

But education did not only offer the possibility of better life chances: in the case of the next group of four teachers, it signified class status.

Education as class status

Conceptions of the role and value of education also played out in other ways. In the case of the four coloured teachers, it signalled their class identity. For Paul who taught at Redhill Senior Secondary, situated in the poor coloured community of Joseph Rhodes in the Western Cape, education was a symbolic indicator of his status and class. Unlike the groups above for whom education was either something people *do*, a natural process of socialisation, or what people *become*, these four described education as a marker of a shifted *habitus*: a signifier of a new class identity. In this regard, Paul provided a long but useful description of the importance of education. For him, the educational trajectory of his family was a signifier, a marker of his 'middle-class' identity, and a shift from the working class status into which his parents were born. He provided a short description of his parents' working class background and, thereafter, proceeded with an educational profile of his siblings, signifying what education does rather than what it is. He stated:

> My mother used to work at ... (place) for the white community as a cleaner, a domestic worker for all her years. My father worked for the council as a carpenter. He was lucky to have made it to Std 6, as it was called. Yes, I think they cared a lot for us. *Education was the basis of our upbringing* (his emphasis). My eldest brother has just turned 50. He's qualified as a surveyor although he is into business nowadays. My eldest sister is a senior lecturer at (university). She just came from America now for a month. My other sister, second eldest sister is a teacher. She's got an Honours in Psychology ... My youngest sister is at the, I don't know the company's name now but she is there for quite some time now. She is quite good in the computer business, a programmer ... that kind of thing. She is linked up with Namibia and London. Then, I'm the 3rd eldest of all. I said my youngest brother is becoming a priest but at the moment he is teaching at the school for the blind as Head of Department also. Then it's the sister that is in the computer business, and then it is [I] teaching. I've got a degree in history and psychology in majors. I've got a three year diploma in physical education. I've done little bits of certificates for example all of the new history thing, that certificate I did at ... (university) I did an entrepreneur's course at (university). I did a practical computer course at ... (technikon). I did a nine-week speech and drama course at ... (technikon).

His pronouncements were a marker of a changed and changing identity. In a sense, education was both the condition that produced a change in identity, but more than that, it was a signifier of his middle-class status: an educated teacher with an educated family.

In sum, and for the most part, education played a significant role in shaping identities among this cohort. For the majority, education seemed the condition within, through, and from which modifications in identities were and are still possible. While it may have been constraining, as the next section indicates, it was (and is) the discursive space in and through which this group made and continue to make themselves. Education, as Giddens (1984) suggests, thus played itself out in the lives of these teachers as both the structure and the condition in and through which they acted to modify the *habitus*, thus creating new identities and 'becoming somebody.'

Teachers, teaching and becoming somebody

While it may hold true that, for the most part, education played a significant role as an enabler in the lives of many teachers, it nevertheless also acted as a constraint on what it was possible for teachers to achieve. Even though education in general, and teaching in particular, offered to many the possibility either of 'becoming somebody' and/or the likelihood of a shift in *habitus,* the former also acted as a constraint. Choice in career was integrally linked with early educational opportunities. In the majority of cases in this group, political and economic fields acted as regulative structures that limited respondents' chances of a future beyond 'the expected.' For the most part, the 'expected' included a choice of three options: teacher, nurse or policeman. Jenni, the only black middle class teacher in the study contended, "Ja ... and if you can think back, the only thing you could be was only to be a teacher or a nurse, or a police. So, we had not choice."

Despite this, though, teaching was the career of choice of at least fifteen teachers. For many of them, the possibility of another career choice seemed unlikely. Often, choice (or the lack of) was contingent on and associated with a complex interplay among economic opportunity, parent/family expectations, considerations of the perceived capital gain embedded in the status of 'teacher', the perceived status of the profession and its association with the need to become somebody, as well as a perceived lack of options. The upshot for the majority, therefore, was at one level, acceptance of teaching as a strategic option associated with mobility and capital gain, and as such, a career worth pursuing. At another level, as I describe below, what emerged was a picture in which females felt less able to exercise choice in the way their male counterparts were able to. Not only was the emerging pattern raced and classed, it was also gendered, as I describe below. I use two categories to do this: teachers, gender and choice; and teachers, teaching and status.

Teachers, gender, and choice

Teaching was perceived as one of two career options (the other, nursing) available to the majority of black and coloured female respondents. According to them, a career outside of teaching or nursing appeared highly improbable. For females, choice was perceived as externally determined both by family and/or parental expectations and by social norms associated with what girls do (or can and cannot do).

Those females who, for example, considered alternative careers were unable to exercise choice for two reasons: parental expectations and restricted options. Concerning the former, parents usually encouraged females to pursue a career in teaching, a choice they associated with security, status, and access to job opportunities. Four females, for example, expressed their frustration at not being in a position to fulfil their dreams of becoming something other than a teacher. In describing family influence on career choice, Pauline, a middle-class coloured teacher from Gracious Park, put it this way:

> I think my dad had basically just set very high standards for all of us. His girls had to get into a career and then be secure. And at that time teaching was secure. My heart's desire was to do hairdressing, cosmetology, hairdressing and so on, but according to my dad there was no sense of security for a woman. For that reason, I was kind of, forced to go into teaching.

While teaching was not a first choice, three proposed nursing as their first option, a career choice with a similar political, economic, and social trajectory as teaching. Nonetheless, all four teachers expressed their love for teaching and as Pauline stated, they have "no regrets whatsoever, I love teaching."

The male respondents reasoned differently in that all but one made the conscious choice to become a teacher. While options for three of the five males were limited due to poverty and a lack of opportunity to pursue studies in higher education, they did not seem to experience constraint in the same way as female teachers. While they too experienced limited options, these seemed more internally (what I can and cannot do) rather externally (what men can or cannot do) framed.

Teachers, teaching, and status

Choice of career was also largely influenced by the possibility of a shift in status and class. For thirteen teachers from poor communities, teaching offered mobility, not only out of poverty (as explained above), but into a different class and improved social standing in the community. Though limited by race and gender, it offered modifications in the field (social, class, and teaching) as well as access to some form of cultural capital (improved status, respect, and better housing opportunities). For example, Volene, an articulate black teacher from the 'new' school in Mpumalanga that obtained good matriculation grades, stated, "[w]hen I started as a teacher, it was all about being a teacher, of having a status, wherever you go, you get the respect of a teacher."

Assertions concerning the elevated status of teachers, though, remained mixed. Only seven of the ten teachers in Mpumalanga, for example, made the point that teaching was a prominent profession that offered improved social repositioning. Sipho summed it up in this way, "[i]n the society they look up to teachers, they regard them as people who are above the normal classes you know. They put them in a better position." Teaching gave them prominence in the community, given widely-held perceptions of teachers as role models and knowledgeable, educated persons. The following comment by Lizzie illustrates a common sentiment amongst this group:

> To be educated in the community you become a light, or a bearing light, a symbol, to which people can refer to. People can come for help, whilst, because you are educated, they believe in you. They think that if they come to you, they will get help and advice. Being educated is so important for your life and for the community as well. Because the community, they do rely on you.

While the remaining six recognized the degree to which teaching was the enabling factor for their achievement of middle-class status, they held a different view of their position in the community. For them, as the next section illustrates, teaching no longer held esteem. They felt that teachers' positions were in flux, constantly under threat and open to negotiation rather than taken-for-granted as stable.

The sentiment that teaching no longer holds status was also common among those in other communities. For the coloured teachers, Pauline, Gwen, Shahida, Paul, and Carol, teaching signalled or identified them as belonging to the middle class. Being identified with teaching was for this group a marker of position in a field rather than an enabling condition through which shifts in class or social positioning might be produced (as in the case of the former thirteen). The loss in its status, therefore, held consequences for class positioning and capital gain in the field.

For Vera and Kobie, the two white teachers from the affluent community, teaching offered the opportunity to maintain rather than change the field. Put differently, teaching offered little other than a job opportunity, with little capital gain. In such instances, teaching secured a stable teacher identity, one associated with a field. Consequently, teaching did not necessarily result in a change in status, but rather in maintenance of capital in a field.

In summary, the political effects of education as a structuring apparatus during Apartheid were discernible amongst this cohort of teachers. For the most part, career choices seemed restricted as a result of the nature and quality of education for 17 of them. All those from poor backgrounds and three from the middle-income category experienced its restrictive and constraining nature. This group, however, was deeply aware that the promise of a better life depended on their becoming teachers, nurses, or policemen. They were also alert to how the political and education fields worked to restrict and maintain social order through limiting their career choices.

Limitations in choice, while restrictive, were not perceived as debilitating. Respondents played the political and educational game (Bourdieu, 1990), and modified the rules (Giddens, 1984) from within, thus leading to changes, not only in their own experiences but also in the meanings and the identity 'teacher' invoked in communities and schools.

Being a teacher, teaching and surveillance

Notwithstanding the above, the perceived diminished status of the teacher held serious consequences for work in this field. Teaching, as many suggested, no longer offered natural or unambiguous respectability. For the most part, it had become associated with a lower status (than for example, medicine). Six teachers, for example, recognized that *being a teacher* no longer secured status or privilege in the community. Sipho, an eloquent speaker and the only black 'university educated' teacher from Mpumalanga in this study, stated: "... in the past, you used to get respected by the community when you were educated, but I don't think today you still get the recognition that you used to get in the past." Volene had a similar view:

> I would say that the teaching profession has dropped tremendously. The respect towards teachers has really dropped a lot. They see teachers as, most of the time, they look at you, those days, they used to respect you, whatever you say, and the way you walk. We were presentable to most of the community.

Interesting though, is what teachers identified as the consequences of this reduced status. A significant consequence involved increased surveillance in school, such as the erection of fences and placing guards at school, monitoring by members from the district department of education, developmental appraisal, and peer assessment. Safety for learners and teachers was the reason commonly offered for the new structural surveillance arrangements by the education department. However, teachers ascribed different meanings and interpretations to these. To them, it seemed primarily associated with monitoring teaching and learning behaviour. Moreover, the arrangements were interpreted as being mechanisms for monitoring and controlling behaviour. What I describe below are ways in which surveillance was experienced and the consequences this held for teacher status and behaviour. I do this in two ways. First, I describe the ways in which surveillance worked in and out of school, and second, I frame the discussion around conceptions of role modelling and its effect on constructions of what is and is not allowed or accepted as teacher behaviour.

Teachers and working and living in glass houses

Some teachers explained how surveillance conduced to a reduced social position. Sipho was very vocal about this, saying that he felt his lowered status even though he is still recognised as a 'so-called' middle class teacher. He offered an articulate description in this regard:

SIPHO: (Long pause) People used to take teaching as a profession. Ja ... like comparing [it] to like doctors for instance. So that's why I ... so I do not see any parallel in that. Because a doctor [does not] need someone to guide [him/her] in what to do, to do this and that, while teachers are being voluntarily watched whether they are doing the correct steps.
RESEARCHER: So you think there's a difference between doctor's work and teacher's work?
SIPHO: Ja. I think that there is.
RESEARCHER: So, I like your analogy and the differentiation that you make. Do teachers still have to be looked after in a way?
SIPHO: Yes
RESEARCHER: Tell me about that. They still need somebody? Tell me about it.
SIPHO: Ja. I think actually ... I usually see them at school after some time. We are subjected to supervision from our superiors and so on and so on. [So] I have never heard or seen doctors being followed in such a manner, although there is a council, which may impose a ban on a doctor who performed badly.

While on the one hand the teacher above acknowledged the manner in which teaching offered him improved status, he recognized its diminished capacity to do this and the consequences concomitant with this. What Giddens (1984) describes as the duality of structure is exemplified in this example. In this instance, a reduced status acted as the structuring device that framed action and produced the unintended consequences of surveillance and discipline. Simultaneously, surveillance acted as the site of production that, in some way, reproduced the teacher's lowered status (Giddens, 1984).

Experiences of surveillance, however, extended beyond the confines of school to include the scrutiny of teachers outside the school gates; taking a variety of forms and producing differing kinds of meaning and experience. Critical in understanding surveillance as a construction is the manner in which individuals themselves operate under what Foucault describes as 'the gaze'. Teachers were not only supposedly monitored but also monitored their own behaviour. Such 'self-monitoring' is best explained through applying Goffman's (1959) notion of co-presence and Foucault's panopticon lens, the latter of which is explained as "drive to self-monitoring through the belief that one is under constant scrutiny" (Wood, 2003: 239). These two concepts seem relevant in an understanding of teachers' experiences of surveillance.

Teachers, role modelling, and surveillance

In general, teachers were positioned as role models. Significantly this was taken for granted by teachers themselves. In all the interviews teachers confirmed this as an important marker of being not merely a teacher, but a *good* teacher. It was apparent that this self-description served to produce censorship and self-monitoring. To many, being a role model was an important part of who and what a teacher was: a role many believed extended beyond the school building to include exemplary behaviour in the community and in their private lives. Many were expressive about their attempt to be just that: role models. Jenni provided what seemed a typical response. Teachers *had* to be accountable for their actions at all times. They *were* role models by virtue of *being* teachers. Importantly too, they had to monitor their own behaviour. She stated:

> For instance, I cannot just go to any place being a teacher. I cannot go to a shebeen, being a teacher. I think that, that is immoral and is degrading me as a teacher. So I have to see, to ... to have choices, I won't just, not that I'm trying to segregate other people, but I have a choice of people whom I go with. I must know the places where I go to, not a shebeen as I have already said.

Kobie expanded on this by suggesting that his behaviour ought to be exemplary in his "personality and my conduct and also in my life." Model behaviour, therefore, was what teachers perform in and out of school.

However, for some respondents, this positioning (teacher as role model) created tension in so far as it made it difficult for them to act without considering the consequences. Tension arose between how they understood themselves as fallible human beings, and the expectation that they always behave in an exemplary fashion. For this group, the distinction between public and private and the personal and professional seemed blurred, causing discomfort and eliciting feelings of being under constant surveillance, feelings of unfairness and sometimes even anger. The sense of being under constant scrutiny meant that they had little privacy in and out of school, which restricted their behaviour, particularly in their private lives. In explaining how teachers' actions always seemed under scrutiny, Volene stated:

> … But whatever we do as human beings, as teachers as well, but people look at us. It's natural when someone is a teacher, something happens and it goes off a blow, you know. They take it because … Oh! She's a teacher, because he is a teacher, that suddenly the news flashes all over. But if a person is working for a factory or so on, it tends to be just a talk for a few days [and] then it's off. But once you are a teacher, fair enough I understand we are the children's guardians, we are second parents. They look at us to be perfect people. They look up to us to be exemplary, as trying to live a perfect life, I will say. But you know, we are human beings which is a lot of things. We talked about teachers in general, but at the same time I would say yes of course we have our faults as well as teachers. We do things as human beings … but because of the fact that you are a teacher and you are expected by the community to have a very low profile [when it comes] to relationships.

In sum, teachers associated experiences of surveillance not only with reduced status, but also and more importantly, with group membership (of a number of groups or fields), as the next section describes. Awareness of their position in a group and the rules and regulative practices that held particular groups together or that operated within the field of practice were traceable in the teacher interviews. All the teachers seemed keenly aware of what communities valued and expected from them. *Knowing and awareness of 'the expected'* produced experiences of being under constant scrutiny. Interestingly, too, *knowing* also worked as a self-monitoring device, where, as already discussed, teachers monitored their own behaviour. Important to note was what produced self-monitoring (the structure that acted to produce) as well as the way (the condition in and through which) it manifested in teachers' actions. Group membership thus worked as a structuring device in and through which subjectivity was produced. Community and group membership here is discursively rather than constitutively defined.

Teachers and membership

Experiences of co-presence through group membership were traceable in teacher interviews. Membership (co-presence, being aware of and/or the panoptic of the self) included belonging either to a specific community or location, ethnicity, gender and/or religious denomination. It worked in interesting ways to produce and construct lived experiences amongst this group. Importantly, too, it worked as the discursive space from which teachers invoked particular subject positions. Membership was sometimes ethnically determined, while in other instances it depended on whether or not a teacher lived in the community. Sometimes, membership was attributable to religious and linguistic associations and at other times it depended on whether or not one was male or female.

At one level, teacher behaviour was regulated by the co-presence of the desired 'self' or the panoptic of the desired 'self', but at the same time, teachers regulated their own behaviour in (as the next chapter will illustrate) and outside of school. In many instances, teachers were aware of what they were or were not *allowed* to do in their conduct and speech.

At another level, co-presence regulated behaviours during teaching and learning encounters, as the next chapter traces. In the case of many teachers, behaviour in the classroom seemed regulated by a host of competing discourses which included, amongst others, considerations of membership in a group, parent expectations, and curriculum content demands (what and how, as well as the time/space/span in which teaching has to be completed).

Overall, productions and reproductions of teacher identity through co-presence and the panoptic of the self were complex and multi-layered. Membership here is understood as discursive rather than constitutive. The following three analytic frameworks afford descriptions of how co-presence was experienced by this cohort: teachers, gender, and membership; teachers, ethnicity, and membership; and teachers, religion, and membership.

Teachers, gender, and membership

Experiences of co-presence were particularly exaggerated among female teachers. For males, being a teacher or a role model was primarily associated with what they did in school. The general perception amongst many teachers was that it was excusable for male teachers not to exhibit exemplary behaviour outside of school. Male teachers were also able to give logical reasons and normalised excuses for their behaviour when these were called in question. In many ways, their 'inexcusable' behaviour was taken for granted as something males/men do anyway. Xola, a black teacher from the Western Cape, illustrated the point when he said,

"I like to teach, to let people learn from me, to let people gain from me, to let people walk from my footsteps, to lead by example, to let people follow me, to let people know that although you make mistakes, at the end of the day you have to look for your mistakes and don't do your mistakes again." The mistake he referred to here was having contracted the HI-virus. His behaviour was pardonable and did not 'disqualify' him from his group membership. Instead, he was not only able to disclose his status but also to reconstruct his identity as 'an HIV-positive survivor who can teach others.' He was now recognised as an AIDS-survivor; an HIV-positive male leader who was invited regularly to funerals, civic meetings and other activities in his community to educate people against infection. His experience was unlike Volene's, who remained silent about her HIV-status for fear of stigmatisation and ridicule. In her case, non-disclosure and silence resulted not only from a complex interplay of discourses from competing group memberships (ethnic, professional, female, etc) but, importantly, also from how she understood herself in relation to these discourses. In other words, not only were restrictions imposed by group membership, but by Volene herself through her own silence about her status.[41]

As opposed to their female counterparts, male teachers seemed better able to maintain a definite separation between what they did in and outside of school and, as is traceable in classroom behaviours in the next chapter, to distance personal identities from the content they mediated in the classroom.

Teachers, community, and membership

The majority (17) of teachers did not reside in the communities in which they taught. While some had grown up in the area where they now teach, they nevertheless no longer lived there. These spatial arrangements had consequences for teacher experiences of co-presence or surveillance, which it would seem, took many forms and operated on many levels.

On one level, the black teachers who shared a common ethnicity with their learners seemed to be more readily accepted as insiders who knew the practices, irrespective of whether or not they stayed in the

41 In 2005, three years after the fieldwork was conducted, Volene declared her status.

community. For nine respondents, experiences of surveillance were associated with belonging to the same ethnic group. In the case of these respondents, insider knowledge of the rules associated with the group acted as the lens from and through which they acted and made pronouncements about themselves. In other words, teachers knew that as members of a particular community, they were expected to be the bearers and protectors of the practices communities revered. They could, therefore, be trusted to maintain and uphold these practices. Mzi, who was a male teacher from the same ethnic group as those he taught, also came to teach in the area where he was born. He provided an apt description:

> You know when I grew up, I had a liking for being of assistance to the community, more especially realising that in the area where I am staying, there are no people who are role models so to say for the community it is good for a person to be of assistance to his community. So, in a way, to encourage those who are younger than me to see the value of getting an education, was for me to become a teacher. This is why I even opted to work at the place where I grew up because some of them, their fathers, and their mothers were my classmates in about Standard four and Standard five, and I know them. And they also know this was my father's friend when they were at school because they talk about this at their home.

Living in the community, however, did not always secure membership. Teachers who transferred from more urban to rural environments were considered outsiders, even in cases where they shared a common ethnicity and lived in the local community where they taught. For Patricia, Dorothy, and Volene, experiences were more complex. While they possessed ethnic membership, they had not grown up in the area, and as such were not only perceived as outsiders, but they themselves had conflicting (or different) values, practices, and beliefs. The following excerpt from an interview between Dorothy and myself illustrates one way in which difference played itself out and the extent to which competing beliefs in addition to urban teacher status worked to produce experiences of co-presence:

> RESEARCHER: So what does it mean, because the place is quite rural [speaking about her place of birth]
> DOROTHY: Ja, but it's not as rural as here.
> RESEARCHER: So what is the difference when you grew up there, and coming into a pretty rural environment, would you say there were differences?
> DOROTHY: Ja, like in this place there is no water, pit toilets you see, all those things.

RESEARCHER: But in terms of the way people live their lives, and in terms of the way they believe things

DOROTHY: Ja, Ja, most people of this place believe in Sangomas. [They] believe in many things which in our place are not so very much important. But I've learned not to judge a person because of his belief. Because I'm a Christian, everybody must be a Christian ...

RESEARCHER: So how did your parents become these devoted Christians in a community that might not have been very devoted?

DOROTHY: I don't know, what can I say?

RESEARCHER: Did they sometimes think, maybe we should go to the Nyanga?

DOROTHY: No never, never, never. Never, never, never, never. Even our children like I told you I had a child before I got married, nothing. Even now as I'm getting divorced, people will tell you, go to this Nyanga. But I will tell them, it will never work for me because I will never believe the guy in the first place. Because you must, everything works with your belief ...

Vera and Kobie from Bloukoop and Paul from Joseph Rhodes claimed community membership by virtue of living or having grown up in the area, and not necessarily as a result of a common ethnicity. These teachers had insider status because, as they stated, they held similar values and knew the social practices of the community. Often, these teachers would use 'we' as the pronoun in discussing community practices and values, signifying their insider status. For some teachers, familiarity with the community provided a sense of comfort and security derived from shared values and meanings. Vera and Kobie from Bloukoop were particularly emphatic about sharing common values with learners and parents. Their descriptions suggested a close relationship between teachers and parents since, as they said, they attended the same churches, participated in the same social gatherings and shared an implicit belief in homogeneity regarding values and social practices.

In summary, emerging from the above is a picture that suggests self-monitoring irrespective of whether or not teachers were insiders or outsiders. Insider status translated into teachers recognizing the need for adherence to the rules, while outsiders self-monitored for fear of breaking the rules.

When one is perceived or when one perceives oneself as an insider or monitored has consequences for teaching something tacitly understood as being 'outside the practice'. For many of these teachers, as the next chapter will illustrate, possessing 'insider' knowledge produced varying enactments of teacher behaviour that did not always reveal their group membership. Conversely, those teachers who 'did not belong' felt under scrutiny and indeed, monitored their own behaviour, since they were conscious of what was at stake. Often, but not always, they adhered more rigidly to the official text.

Teachers, religion, and membership

Religion provided another important signifier of group membership and often served as the discursive space within and through which many in this cohort made sense of themselves. As one of many frames of reference from which respondents invoked a teacher identity, religion acted as a structured and structuring mechanism. Its regulatory properties, instantiated in respondents' significations of their membership in one or other religious affiliation, produced and reproduced particular identifications. All twenty respondents reported a religious association, with nineteen claiming Christian affiliations. Shahida, as already mentioned in the respondent profile earlier, was the only Muslim teacher. Respondents were differentiated by their orientation towards religion as opposed to their religious affiliation. Points of difference, therefore, were apparent in the pronouncements teachers made about the nature of their religious commitment rather than in the type of religion itself or associated denominations within a particular religion. Commitment to a particular religious orientation was evident in the way respondents identified themselves, which might include the way they dressed or spoke. The manner in which religion acted to produce and reproduce self regulation is discussed below in four categories: the fundamentalists, the conformist/traditionalists, the (un)conventionalists, and the nominalists. These analytical frameworks were useful as a way of identifying how in the performative context that is described in the next chapter, teachers concealed aspects of their identity through teacherly behaviours that were often removed from what they proposed as significant in their lives.

Dorothy, Pauline and Gugu were 'born again' or fundamentalist Christians. Teachers used particular speech and claimed to have undergone particular experiences, which identified them as belonging to a particular religious orientation. While Shahida practiced a different religion, her speech was nonetheless coded in much the same way as that of the fundamentalist Christians. The overriding claim made about themselves by these four was that of their new birth. It was also one expressed as life changing. Dorothy illustrated this well: "[I will] ... never forget it. It happened on the (she gives the date and place). There was a youth camp, I just went there because I wanted to see ... (place). But it has changed my whole life." Another common feature amongst the three 'born again' teachers was their experience of 'new birth' after a negative life experience. For example, after a brief period in which she 'went astray', Pauline offered the following explanation:

> PAULINE: Then I definitely *went back into the world* and it was also in that time that I rebelled, I just went very bad. Then after, in my third year, it was the end of my third year in college, I *got saved again.* I returned to *my walk* and I've been saved ever since. I will never ever trade, at the cost of not a thing, *will I trade my salvation.*
>
> RESEARCHER: Would you say that that was a significant moment in your life?
>
> PAULINE: Yes, very, very. I somehow believe God allowed the fall or the summer in my life so that when, I mean when I came back eight, nine years ago, ten years ago, I now can say I *will never ever go* that way again, because there is nothing in it. It's not worth it. Whereas now over the past nine, ten, years; I've actually got something to show. I've got nothing really to show for the time that I was not walking the path of righteousness.

Teachers making claims of rebirth, therefore, often described the moment of religious realisation as one of the most significant events in their lives. All three Christian female teachers gave elaborate descriptions of the day they 'dedicated' themselves to following a new religious orientation. Respondents often participated in some form of public ritual in which they denounced old ways in favour of new ways of being and knowing. These rites of passage signalled their membership. Coded speech, as that in italics above, was important as a marker of their identity. They often drew on this aspect of their identity when they invoked a subject position, as is evident in Shahida's narrative. She provided the following description of the pilgrimage she undertook, offering insight into the way she says it changed her outlook on life. She stated:

> When you stand on the plains of Arafat, it's an open field and you are at the mercy of your Lord. And you ask the Lord, [and say] 'please forgive [for] whatever I have done.' Whatever you have, maybe, lots of things that you were not happy about. Maybe you wanted to do more things and have a life full of pleasure, fulfillment and all that. Then you stand there and you ask your Lord, 'O Lord please, cleanse me body and soul.'... And I promise you that since I've been back from Mecca, everything has just gone very smooth for me, because you are like a baby when you come back. All your major sins and I mean you don't really go there with lots of sins, you know, but you do have the white lies that you tell, and you have lies that [you] also tell to gain or whatever, you know. But I think I've come a long way since, because it's just that.

The four teachers above suggested that their religious orientation influenced all the decisions they made in and out of school. It influenced their attitude towards learners as well as how they perceived their role as teachers. Pauline gave what was a common response amongst this group regarding conceptions of life purpose and its association with the role of the teacher. She stated:

> It's amazing the impact that it has because I've got to remember that these learners are here for a purpose and more so, I am here [for a purpose]. They're not there by chance. It's by design basically, that they are there and it's by design that I am there. And I have a particular function to fulfill in their lives, and I think that's why I like my subject because a lot of the time I teach them a lot of the things that you're not able to teach them in the biology lesson, or the geography lesson, values and standards and morals and those kinds of things, not that I would enforce mine upon them, but I often think that if teachers were more teaching us about life when I was at school, I think my life would have just turned out a tad differently.

The Conformists/Traditionalists

Religious identity was also evident amongst the six teachers (Zandile, Gwen, Kobie, Vera, Paul and Carol) who claimed to be conservative but not 'born again' Christians. For this group, membership was by virtue of family connection, having been born into traditional Christian families. In other words, many described being 'born into' or socialized into their respective religious practices from a young age. As with the group described earlier in this section, this cohort made pronouncements signifying their particular religious orientation. However, their claim to membership and insider status was different. Assertions associated with membership here stemmed from what they regarded as a long history of family membership in the group. Religious rules and resources that they as members drew on were embedded in a past integrally linked with family 'tradition', an association that made complex how they as individuals made sense of themselves outside the structure of family. What emerged, therefore, was a picture of a double structuring through religion and family, unlike the experience in the previous group where the religious trajectory seemed more personally/individually constituted. The role of family in shaping religious orientation was taken for granted and legitimated through respondents' pronouncements and enactments. Rules and practices included rituals to which respondents tacitly subscribed. Importantly, rituals were embodied as a way of being or becoming, with embodiment of such practices taken up and assumed as a natural and expected trajectory to follow. Gwen, one of four teachers from the middle-income cluster, described her experience in this way:

> [We were] taken to church every Sunday. We were at Catholic schools, the primary school especially. Once moving out from there, you would have to attend your Sunday school classes ... get confirmed and all that kind of thing. I was at a Catholic school high school as well. Yes, then as I say, [I was] involved as a youth leader in the church too.

Kobie too, described his family values as "very strong values ... very good examples (by parents) ... principled ... God-fearing. My father never showed anger, he didn't become angry. He never swore; I didn't ever hear my dad swear. He was hard working and took good care of his family." He went on to suggest that these were "absolutely" the values and practices to which he subscribed. In describing the interconnection between family values and his Christian values, he stated:

> Maybe, [it's] because I want to have a meaningful life and be of value. Also because I am also Christian I want to follow Christ's example. I know that it is a difficult thing to say, because you know, I mean, you must live up to that. But in such an honest conversation like this, I can tell you that this is what's expected of me to follow Christ's example. I am required to give a message, which is what my belief requires of me. [I cannot] just keep quiet about this message. I must play a role. Now I think teaching is a good place where I can be a good testament, a good example. I can be a good witness in teaching. I can influence childrens' lives in teaching.

In the section above, teachers foreground an assumed interrelationship between family history and religious patterns of being and becoming. They subscribed to family religious practices because they were expected to do so. Simultaneously, the practice becomes the structuring apparatus from which this cohort of teachers speaks. In other words, subscribing to such practices meant speaking from a particular position, making specific pronouncements and displaying particular sets of behaviours and practices. What emerged amongst this group of teachers, therefore, was that they all claimed to be 'strict' and 'disciplined' while at the same time 'loving children' and making sure that children were taught 'right and wrong.' All put forward that it was their *duty* to teach children (right and wrong). Duty in this instance was associated with Christian responsibility.

A distinctive characteristic amongst this group was the naturalized or assumed interconnection between religious association and their role as a model of good behaviour in and out of school. Gwen illustrated the point in the following excerpt:

> I've always been aware of the fact that I am a role model I suppose. As a young person, I was also quite involved in the church and the youth there as well, being the chairperson of a particular music group in the parish ... so I suppose I've always been aware of the fact that people look up to you. So, I've tried to live a morally correct life, I suppose one could say.

The relevance of the above and its association with understanding co-presence (and group membership), though, is the degree to which teaching seemed accepted as an extension of their life purpose; that is, to be a role model who influenced, shaped and actively sought to change children's behaviour. The upshot of this was conflation of religious commitment with their duties and responsibilities as a teacher, a stance that served as a regulatory framework from and through which teachers made sense of, not only who they were but also of what was expected of them in their role as teacher.

Interestingly too, this group of teachers made pronouncements such as, for example, "I grew up Catholic" in a way that assumed that I understood. Such declarations often signified accumulated religious capital that they perceived as symbolically significant. Such capital, though, included family positioning. Unlike the previous group of teachers whose religious orientation occurred as a result of individual choice, early socialization through family practices offered less choice in what was possible for this group. While respondents recognized the worth of membership in a 'privileged' group, they also seemed aware of the implications of such belonging. In other words, they understood what they needed to hold onto or give up in order to retain membership in two fields of practice: religion and family. Put differently, they needed to play by the rules of the game if they sought to retain membership of their respective families and faiths. Such positioning had implications for how this group operated in the classroom, as is evident from their classroom behaviour, described in Chapter 10.

The (Un)conventionalists

A small group of three teachers (Sipho, Mzi, and Jabulani) practised what I describe as Christianity and African Traditionalism. It is, however, important to state that the teachers themselves did not see these as distinct from one another. Jabulani and Sipho provided insight into how this group understood and practised religion. Jabulani said: "You see these two, the Christianity and the Amadloti (Ancestral worship), (pause) I believe that God is there and I believe that the Ancestral spirits are also there. So these two ... for some children they are taught that there are no Amadloti. There is the [holy] spirit only." She explained that she does not interpret them as differentiated in that, "Christianity, believing in God ... mmhh! I believe that long ago, Christianity was there. But for us Black people, we took the Christian belief together with our ancestral worship and made it one." Sipho too, provided important insight into how he understood religion and how he positioned himself within this constructed framework. He said:

> I used to tell my kids, my youngest is here at school that we've got different religion but they are all directed to the one person, the omniscient and omnipresent one, magnificent. Some call him Jehovah, some call him Allah and some call him Amadloti. And there are various ways ... there is a medium of passing our messages to God. So I believe that my mother and my ancestors are the ones who are passing all my prayers and guidance to the Almighty.

Jabulani explained that such positioning helped her understand learners and their experiences. She said:

So the way I believe helps me to understand the way the life of the children here, in (place); the way they interpret life. (pause) But if I had to say I am a Christian, I would not be able too, because sometimes, others come here having evidence that they have undergone the ritual. When you ask them why they have this evidence, they would say; 'We took part in the ancestral worship ceremony at home.' So if I came along with the Christianity, I would have, I would have discouraged this child. But because I grew up with both these beliefs, I am able to understand these children.

This group presents a commonly held beliefs concerning the distinction between these two religious universes. To this group, there was no contradiction in their practices since they viewed these as complementary rather than conflictual. Ease with living in 'two worlds' was encapsulated in the next description by Jabulani, a female teacher from Mpumalanga. In describing how she comforted a student on the death of her parents, she suggested that the little girl continue praying to her parents because they were watching over her. Our interaction below illustrates why she made the point and how it exemplifies her belief:

JABULANI: In between, we also believe in the "Ancestors". Ja! As that is the way the grandparents would also speak (pause). They do say ... perhaps, wherever you are, they are watching you. Even if they are dead, their spirit is in this room (home), watching you, you see. This is what I meant, that even though they are dead, they must not say, 'My mother is not here, the person you are living with is looking after you.' Your mother sees you, the one you loved, is it not? You are just like the other children. I wanted them not feel different to the other children.
RESEARCHER: And you, what do you believe, and how does it influence how you teach?
JABULANI: What do I believe?
RESEARCHER: Yes, would you also say, in similar circumstances, my mother is gone, but she is looking at me?
JABULANI: Yes, I believe in that (pause). Even as I am speaking like she is here and she is looking at me and is very pleased with what I am doing, I believe in that (pause).

Explanations relating to the complementarity of the two religious practices under discussion were common and even taken-for-granted among the other three respondents in this group. They took for granted that 'everyone did it' in their community. The ease with which teachers appeared to navigate their way within such discursive spaces is instructive. Jabulani provides an example in the excerpt below:

JABULANI: [In the past] ... we were speaking about those who have died and combined it all and made it all one. We did not separate it. But when the Western civilization came along, they took away our belief, and replaced it with the Western belief only. But if you can combine both of these beliefs, because life is no longer the way it was before, it would be right!
RESEARCHER: How do you combine the two, for yourself?
JABULANI: I go to church and I worship my Ancestors
RESEARCHER: How do you worship your Ancestors?
JABULANI: OK, if I have a problem, I go to church and pray. After that, I go there to my corner or to the gate, with an earthen pot of "African Beer" and do my ritual to my Ancestors. That is how things go well.
RESEARCHER: Do you think there are people in your community who do the same thing?
JABULANI: Yes. Many of them. (Pause) ... Many of them.

Sipho made the following observation in describing his mother's death: "... [S]o her departure did in a way make us to see the other side of life." In probing the meaning of the statement, this teacher offered the following explanation, "[M]mm ... our tradition, in our tradition I believe there is a guardian angel. If I can now raise some other incident where I escaped death I think I can write a bible-sized book." He went on to describe an incident in which, he proposes, his mother acted as a guardian angel that saved him from injury: "I felt she was with me there and I happened to survive, I don't know how."

This group stood out from the entire cohort in that, unlike the first two groups described in this section, they did not associate their role in school with some form of religious conviction. In other words, for this group, there was a distinct separation between their religious practices and beliefs, and their role as teachers. While they may have claimed to be role models in earlier discussions, such a position was not necessarily connected to their religious beliefs. Instead, being a role model was more closely related to social status and standing in the community rather than as a consequence of some religious orientation. This was different from the previous two groups, who claimed a more direct correlation between their religious beliefs and their role and duty as teachers. While the former groups also spoke of being role models in the community, such declarations were more closely aligned with their religious rather than professional identities.

The Nominalists

Patricia, Volene, Xola, Ester, Thandi, Lizzie, and Jenni did not explicitly foreground their religious orientation as did the groups discussed above. All except Xola in this group were from Mpumalanga. Nevertheless, all admitted to believing in God and understanding 'his hand' in shaping and 'guiding' their lives. Most of them went to church regularly. They participated in women's Christian groups and sang in choirs. Volene, Thandi, and Jenni, in particular, led school assemblies regularly and also led music and prayer sessions in teacher training workshops the researcher presented to a group in Mpumalanga. Xola, for instance, did not offer any explanation of his religious orientation. However, in talking about his HIV-status, he said that he understood it as God's will (to become infected). He says, "[If] it has to happen to a person and if God has chosen me to be that particular person then let it be."

In the main, this group exhibited the 'expected' behaviours of teachers and Christians. In other words, as teachers and 'Christians', they displayed the sets of norms and 'role model' behaviour that identified them as Christians even though they did not specify this. They took up the positions described above only when the occasion arose.

I bring this first section to a close by providing a diagram and a summary, below. What the diagram illustrates is the way in which the performative manifested to conceal aspects of the teachers' identity they had described in detail in this section.

Diagram 3: Early Influences and Subject Positions

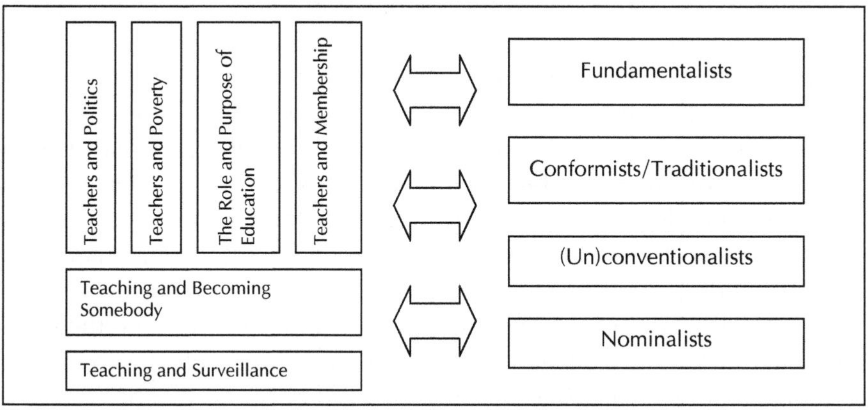

The potential for exercising agency was strongest where group membership included a convergence of religious beliefs or where teachers positioned themselves as 'nominal Christians'. Rather than act as a constraint, such positioning offered possibilities for teachers to navigate their way either between sets of beliefs, invoking one (over the other) when called upon to do so, or between subject positions, depending on the occasion. Interestingly, the former group did not necessarily interpret their actions as a deliberate denial of one belief system because, according to them, the systems were not separate. Neither did these groups consider their 'performances' as a form of masking. Instead, they associated foregrounding one practice or subject position over another (at any given moment) with appropriate behaviour, depending on the moment of instantiation. The upshot of this, as will be evident in the next section, is that often these teachers were more concerned with demonstrating teacherly behaviour (associated with being a role model in the community) them with teaching children the 'right' thing out of a sense of religious or moral duty. Thus teaching was more about performing teacher behaviour as opposed to what schools expected, namely, teaching to change behaviour.

Religious beliefs, however, did not always offer easy membership, and did not always co-exist in non-conflictual ways as the explanation above suggests. Holding fundamental and conformist religious values (irrespective of orientation) produced responses from teachers that often either masked or 'revealed' their 'true' identity. For teachers who reported conformist religious beliefs, flexibility in dealing with other ways of knowing and concomitant sets of beliefs and practices proved challenging. The rigid frame of reference in terms of which these teachers operated was unaccommodating to other ways of understanding the world, and led to specific forms of teacherly behaviour. So while all four groups produced particular teacher behaviours, these were different in their enactments, as the next chapter will illustrate. The fundamentalists and conformists not only displayed heightened awareness of their actions, but also a double awareness: an awareness of their awareness, a condition that often led to highly or exaggerated performative enactments. In such instances, some teachers were more concerned with always displaying particular sets of teacher behaviours that demonstrated their positions as either a 'good teacher', a role model whose duty it is to exhibit good behaviour, or a 'witness' of the religion, one who teaches out of a sense of duty to change students. Change in student sexual behaviour (as an expected outcome of learning) for this group was associated with moral change. Others, on the other hand, concealed their religious positions through exaggerated teacher enactments that often led to nonsensical interactions between teachers and learners which, as the next chapter will illustrate, had the unintended consequences of subverting the very discourse they were called upon to mediate. As Chapter 10 will illustrate, teaching the 'right thing' or concealing a 'true' identity sometimes stood in the way of teaching 'the expected' and thus framed the pedagogical discourse in very particular ways.

Giddens's (1984) theory of the duality of structure is helpful in understanding teachers and their response to what might be perceived as contradictory positions held in the classroom. While all groups exercised agency in the classroom, as the next chapter will illustrate, the achieved outcome yielded different results.

Experiences of co-presence and the panoptic of self also produced particular teacher behaviours that highlighted the performative nature of teaching. These were, as the final part in this section highlights, mainly influenced by constructions of what makes 'a teacher' and perceptions of what this group reported on as 'appropriate' teacher behaviour. Role models, mostly teachers, served as an important influence on teachers' constructions of 'a teacher' as well as in their perceptions of what constitutes a teacher's demeanour, dress code and behaviour. The next section therefore describes the interplay between early schooling experiences, perceived teacher conduct, and constructions of what makes a 'good' teacher. I then proceed with descriptions of the behaviours teachers privilege as those that make a 'good' teacher. I end this section with a discussion on how invocations of 'teacher' work to construct, while at the same time serve as the condition from which teacher subject positions are called up. The categories I use in the following include: role models and a 'good' teacher; disciplinarians or nurturers; teachers and deportment; and teachers and constructions of 'the teacher.'

Self-monitoring included adherence to a tacitly defined code of conduct (inside and outside the school/classroom) as well as to a particular dress and speech code. The following interaction between Paul and myself was instructive in highlighting what was a commonly held belief about teacher behaviour in and outside the classroom:

> PAUL: There are certain ways that you behave at home and at school ... you behave like that. If you're a teacher you must behave like a teacher, so what I bring from my (schooling experience) is that I believe that teaching must still be in the very, very formal phase if you are teaching in situations like these. Try to make it as formal as possible ...
> RESEARCHER: So you say when you're a teacher you must act like a teacher, what does that mean?
> PAUL: Well, not discussing, but if you look at the teacher corps, people think when it comes to, what can I call it, student excursions, then it's okay to have a beer while the kids are around, light a cigarette while they are around. Things like that and try to be friends, especially in situations. I'm referring to situations where we've got kids who belong to various gangs, and teachers try and be friends with them, and things like that.

Teachers' perceptions of how they ought to behave were regulated, too, by conceptions of who a teacher is and what a teacher does. Admiration (or a lack thereof) for teachers as role models also shaped teachers' conceptions, attitudes, and subsequent behaviour. Teachers, however, agreed on the following as the admirable characteristics their role models commonly displayed: deportment; knowledge and control of the content; good oration and meticulous attire (particularly possessing *good* dress sense). I use four categories as an analytical framework in this section: the influence of role models and the way they carried themselves (deportment); role models on teachers' constructions of a 'good' teacher; constructions and value in calling up 'the teacher', and the role of discipline and control in conceptions of teaching.

Teachers and deportment

Respondents reported that they admired how the teachers they identified as role model teachers 'carried themselves'. They confirmed that even today, teachers are 'expected' to carry themselves in a particular way because they are perceived as those members of the community who dress and converse well. This perception held true for at least ten teachers (two males and eight females). They described dress/attire/deportment as a characteristic feature that differentiated teachers from the rest of the community. Female teachers were especially likely to comment on teacher deportment. 'Deportment' devoted a way of being, comprising speech, dress and the way one carries oneself. Ester, a shy teacher from Mpumalanga, describing a teacher she admired suggested that "the way she dressed, the way she talked ... meant a lot for [her]." Mzi described two male teachers whom he admired in this way:

> There is a guy, who I can still remember. He was quite great in terms of dressing, and he made me to wish that if one day I can dress like that gentleman ... very nice. And another guy, by the name of Mr. [name]. By then I think I was doing Standard Six. You see there was this adolescent stage at the same time which makes one to familiarize himself with good things. But those were the guys, who were really my idols, in terms of dressing. Their code of conduct, so to put it, but they were also a source of inspiration to me.

Patricia, a black teacher from one of the 'new' schools in Mpumalanga, explained how her teacher cousin's demeanour and use of language intrigued her. It was her cousin's way of being that persuaded her to consider teaching as a career. She said:

> There was another ... a cousin of mine, who succeeded her Standard Ten and then went to the university. She was the first in the family to go there. Then I said, 'how could it be that she be the first and the last?' No, I had to follow suit ... Then she was a very encouraging courageous person. And what supported me and what actually helped me to put more courage in is that when she came there from the university she would say to us ... Do you know what a pedagogue is? You know pedagogue, you know education?' All these times when [she] asks what these terms are, what is pedagogue, you know, she would play with these nice words that we don't understand. And then I [would] say at home, one day I am going to know this pedagogue, even though I won't be able to go to the university, but I must make a plan to go to the college at least. Then the following year then I went to the college.

Teachers not only described how role models influenced their views on how teachers ought to carry themselves, but also on how they came to understand the power invested in 'the teacher', as the following section illustrates.

Teachers and constructions of 'the teacher'

Invoking 'the teacher' brought with it a historicity which, when instantiated in the pronouncements of some teachers, produced particular ways of being and knowing that sometimes revealed but more often concealed aspects of their identity. The next three descriptions illustrate the point. Gwen, the middle-class teacher who went to a private school and thereafter a prestigious historically white university, described her teacher role in the following way:

> [The children at my school] are capable if they want to; of speaking English properly. They don't speak English properly and I'm not here to perpetuate the slang or the playground language that they use. I'm here to guide them into a formal way of speaking and to help them get through matric and to get into a respectable position once they leave school ... [My role is to] empower the kids to be able to master English as best I can and to prepare them to deal with English in its various registers and contexts. There are times when I can relax and go into a different register. They're shocked when I speak Afrikaans or whatever, but one has to prepare them for the bigger picture, the bigger world.

Jenni, a nominal Christian who was the only black middle-class teacher, described her role in this way:

> To be a teacher, let me go back to the bible. The biblical teaching was one thing, which was done by God, in the Garden of Eden. God would come down to the Garden of Eden to teach Adam how to plant, how to take care of the garden. So teaching is, I think, a very good profession, whereby, it's only the people themselves, the teachers, who are supposed to behave well. And to be honest, and to teach the kids and to respect the community, respect themselves, and respect the kids, they need to be respected.

Lizzie, the only widow in the group who had not only gone against traditional practices and lived with her lover (rather than him paying lobola), but who also went back to school after having two children, described how her demeanour was often 'misleading' to students. She said:

> I think that the way I look, I am misleading my pupils, when I enter the class. My pupils think that I am educated, that I had a supportive family. When I say to them, 'you must study hard in order to be somebody tomorrow.' Those who don't have today, they look at me and think, Ah! And they say to themselves, *"She thinks we are like her, we are growing up in a situation where she grew up in."* They don't know the situation I grew up in! So I can sometimes realize that they are misled by my structure and by the way I dress and by the way I am driving a car.

She went on to say:

> Because if you look at us as teachers, we are not rich, we were not born rich, but we are self-made. We have made what we look like today. Not that we have inherited what we have today ... or that everything was just smooth for us, No! It was tough, just as it is today with you. We are here through hard work and determination.

Role models and a 'good' teacher

Perceptions and constructions of 'a teacher' and in fact, conceptions of what makes a *good* teacher were gendered amongst this cohort of teachers. While many held similar views of what teaching is and what teachers characteristically do, they were divided in the features and behaviours they foregrounded and privileged. Often the frame of reference in constructions of 'a teacher' was drawn from their own learning experience. Without exception, too, all named teachers as significant role models who sometimes encouraged them to consider teaching as a career of choice, but more importantly as those persons whose characteristics, sets of practices and behaviour they most admired and wanted to emulate. Admiration for teachers (as role models) and aspirations to become a teacher were, therefore, interconnected. The consequence for this study, though, is the extent to which experiences of schooling acted and continue to act as a lens from and through which teachers produce and reproduce constructions of 'the teacher.' Early learning experiences were disparate, often including strict and disciplined environments that, particularly amongst female teachers, tended to invoke negative recollections and images of the past. For them, as the following section highlights, a good teacher was one who displayed care and was nurturing. Male teachers on the other hand, admired strictness and what they construed as 'good' discipline.

Teacher as disciplinarian or nurturer

The most common recollections of schooling amongst this cohort of teachers were of spaces in which discipline and control took precedence. Teachers were strict and disciplined. Strictness was sometimes associated with good classroom discipline and control, while at other times it was perceived as evidencing a lack of emotions, with teachers displaying an uncaring demeanour. On other occasions control was linked to knowing one's subject content and holding principled and non-compromising beliefs about 'right and wrong'. Responses to this issue were gendered, as the descriptions below illustrate.

Most, but not all of the male teachers, admired teachers because they were either strict or restrained in their behaviour. It was often the principal who males most admired. In this regard, Kobie stated, "[m]aybe, the school principal ... he definitely had a great influence on my life. He stood for the right values that resonated with my values. And he lived them ..." Mzi, a black teacher from Mpumalanga, described a teacher he admired as follows:

> You know when he got to class; he had the confidence of knowing his matter, so to speak. So the thing was on his fingertips. So always, there was a time when I would think of dodging a period, I could dodge other periods but not his period because of the way in which he presents his lessons.

Teacher control was also associated with controlling one's emotions. Paul provided a rationale for why it was important to disguise (control) emotions and project a strict demeanour, especially when one taught in what he described as the 'township.' He linked past and present experiences, thus signifying his subject position and how he came to make meaning of his role and identity as a *strict* teacher. He stated:

> At high school also my principal definitely [talking about a role model]. They even knew how to run schools in those days. I am a believer in those ways. Discipline!

> We are too lenient today. I think we are just too lenient especially if we look at what happens in our township schools and we that grew up in the townships. There are times when you must not, and I say 90% of the time, you can't smile with these children even if you want to.

Strictness and control did not always produce constructions of a teacher identity as described above. Sometimes incidences of strictness and control produced negative learning experiences that led to different conceptions of teachers and teaching. Pauline provided insight into experiences that have caused her to think differently about her role as a teacher today. She said:

> A teacher at primary school, I remember I was in Sub B and since then I hated mathematics because I just couldn't get this sum. Then we had to know our 2x, 3x, right up to 12x tables. And she smacked me because I couldn't get to the answer quick enough. And since then I actually had a negative feeling and attitude towards mathematics.

She went on to explain how the above and following experiences below made her think differently about her own teaching. She said:

> Yes. Yes. I had a (subject) teacher who was terrible. She would just sit and the notes would be on the board and she never explained anything. And all we did was write down notes, answer the questions from our textbooks and that was in Standard Ten. That year, I often used to say that if ever I was a teacher, God forbid that I should ever be someone like this particular teacher. And I think a lot of it has to do with how she wasn't, is how I am today.

Her narrative also included recollections of teachers whom she found stimulating and who, she suggests, influenced her attitude and approach to teaching. She stated:

> At high school Standards Nine and Ten, there were two teachers, my history teacher, actually three, history teacher, mathematics teacher, and my biology teacher. Young teachers who were vibrant and made these things exciting and I think a lot of that influenced me in the way I am teaching today. You looked forward to getting to biology because Mr. (name of teacher) would definitely have something exciting or for history, it was just different. World War 2 wasn't World War like it was in the other years.

Her description echoes views commonly held amongst female teachers that suggest a different response (other than admiration) to strictness and discipline. Rather, they often described kindness, commitment, and nurturing as the attributes they most admired in teachers. Dorothy provided a description that captures both sentiments succinctly. She stated:

> There was this woman, she was teaching us. She was teaching us very nice; and you know during those days teachers were very harsh. So these other teachers, they were just punishing us ... calling us names ... doing all those things. But she was just kind, nice, a teacher really. Ja, and I wish if one day I can grow up and be the way she's doing it.

Commitment for female teachers was often linked to knowing and being able to explain subject content, unlike male teachers who associated subject knowledge with control and discipline. Gwen offered an example of the interconnection between commitment, subject knowledge, and nurturing that suggests a response somewhat different from the males' constructions of control and discipline. In describing some of the teachers she most remembers, she stated:

> The thing is that most of my teachers I still remember. I think they were committed teachers. They had their idiosyncrasies ... The maths teacher was an extremely good maths teacher. The Afrikaans teachers were also extremely good Afrikaans teachers, committed. I think the whole environment was quite a caring environment.

Lizzie provided a different perspective on nurturing, based on her experience as a student who returned to school after having two children. Describing the teachers she most admired, she says "... because I was older than all the other children in the class, they gave me support, they supported me, they did not discriminate against me that I was older than the others, instead they gave me support."

Diagram 4 below summarises Part 2 and illustrates the subject positions teachers took up in their descriptions in this section.

Diagram 4: Teachers, Perceptions of Teaching and Subject Positions

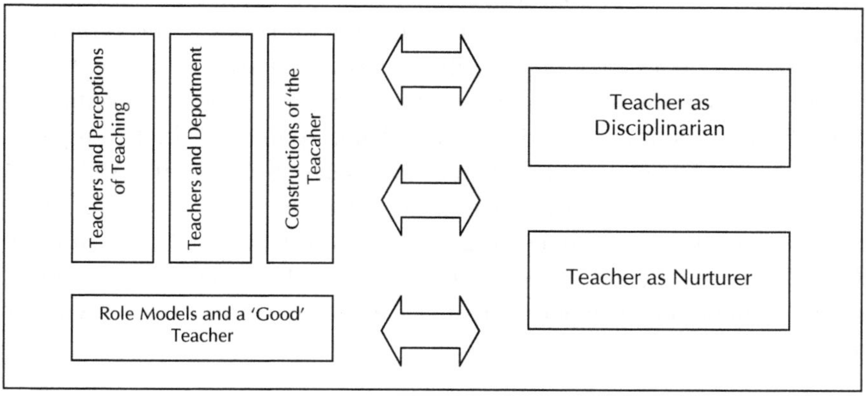

Understanding who a teacher is and what a teacher does was not always associated with individual roles and responsibilities. Rather, it was linked to the historicity of 'teacher', on one hand, and subject positioning, on the other hand. Althusser's (in Butler, 1997: 5) notions of interpellation are useful here in understanding constructions of 'a teacher'. Calling up 'teacher' produced a set of practices, or a series of performative behaviours whose historicity is neither clear nor linear. In other words, the respondents' constructions of a 'teacher' had a determinative history, but were only visible in what they proposed and in what they did, as will be illustrated in the next chapter. Teachers are [already] made through a history that understands teachers and teaching to be constitutive of a particular set of norms and practices. However, these norms and practices are only reproduced through iterative teacher enactments, which when reproduced are often rearticulated as emanating from the subject: as his or her own. Thus, while productions come from a place and have a history/past, teachers actively produce and as such act to remake 'the teacher.'

Butler's (1997) perspective on power is helpful in understanding how agents are produced while at the same time producing subject positions. Such an understanding takes as its premise the notion that the agent is constituted by, and constitutive of, power. In other words, teachers invoke subject positions and do so from a position that understands what 'teacher' means. But they *act* to produce and, as such, are not merely a production or a copy. They exercise power to produce through present pronouncements and enactments.

But who a teacher is and what a teacher does was also influenced by community expectations and experiences across a range of issues that included, but were not limited to, experiences and constructions of sexuality and the silences associated with sex; experiences of early pregnancy on the part of many females; obscurity in the use of language connected to body parts; feelings of inadequacy and unpreparedness in dealing with sexuality and HIV/AIDS; experiences and perceptions of HIV/AIDS, and conceptions and experiences of marriage. The final section in this chapter describes the experiences of teachers in respect of each of the above. As will become clearer in the discussion, taken together, these formed a complex network of experiences teachers drew on to make a teacher identity.

Teachers, sexuality, and HIV/AIDS

A whole range of issues associated with sexuality influenced teachers' conceptions of who they are and what they do. While I discuss these in separate categories below, they are all integrally linked and together produce a complex discursive site for the production of particular teacher identities. I begin the analysis with a description of teachers' experiences of sexuality and the associated silences in almost all the communities in this study. What was revealed was a strongly gendered discursive space in which the role of females was particularly precarious. This section includes commentary on the role of language in spaces where silence is the overriding response to discourses of sexuality and HIV/AIDS. The discussion is linked to Part III, where I described the influence of discourses of sexuality and disease on constructions, meanings and interpretations of HIV/AIDS. I highlight the consequences of the above for teachers and their work. In so doing, I describe teachers' perceptions of what parents expect from them as Lifeskills teachers as well as experiences of the pandemic in the communities in this study. This section ends with teachers' conceptions and experiences of marriage. Here I describe the identifications such conceptions produce and show how these were sometimes, but not always, linked to the religious orientations described earlier in this chapter. Importantly, though, I describe how marriage served as a site for specific and often conflictual subject positions by explaining teachers' experiences of condom use.

This section draws Chapter 10 to a close and brings together the dominant influences on teacher identity, and constructions and meanings associated with sexuality and HIV/AIDS. It serves as preparation for the next chapter, where the nexus between the two are examined through an analysis of teacher behaviour in some Lifeskills classrooms.

Teachers, sexuality, and silence

Irrespective of location, class, race, or gender, learning about sex or engaging in discussions on sexuality with parents and/or guardians was rare or non-existent among the teachers in this cohort. The silence associated with sex and sexuality in communities, as alluded to in the previous chapter, influenced the positions teachers took up and thus shaped their teaching of sexuality and HIV/AIDS, as the next chapter illustrates. For the most part, males and females experienced the effect of these silences differently. Males took it for granted that they knew how to relate sexually and that they did not have to be taught about it. All the female teachers, on the other hand, were acutely aware of the silences associated with sex. All but one of the fifteen reported having no discussion about sex with a parent. Carol, from the poor environment of Joseph Rhodes in the Western Cape, stated that she had discussions with her mother because they were "very close." She stated:

> When I was in Standard Two or Three, my friend in the class, her sister got pregnant and she was only in Standard Seven. For me this was something very new. I didn't know anything about pregnancies. Because I was the oldest girl in the family, I went home and I asked my mommy, 'Now why is she pregnant, what happened?' And she told me everything.

Carol's experience though, was atypical. For the rest of the females, silence was the norm. This being the case, in the main, no formal discussions were held on the topic, but some teachers reported being told not to play with boys or to stay away from boys once they began menstruating. For the most part though, these messages were obscure, as

Dorothy states, "[J]a, like they will never be specific, to be honest. They will just tell you, you must not even play with boys." Jenni, the only middle-class black teacher, supported this notion by describing what her parents said:

> Even talking about sex, telling their kids not to have sex ... it [was] not easy for them to do that. They just say, 'don't go around with boys'. They leave out: 'don't go around with boys and then what next'? And if the child asks them, they won't come up with an exact answer. I think it's the culture.

Jabulani, the black teacher from one of two deep rural primary schools, also provided an appropriate example. She had a child as a teenager and blamed this on the silences associated with sex in the community. She stated, "[A]s you know that they would not tell us where a child comes from. We will end seeing a person walking about with a huge stomach, but they would not explain where a child comes from." Similarly, in describing how she learnt about sex and sexuality, Pauline, one of two black secondary teachers who had relocated from a more urban environment to Mpumalanga stated, "When I started my periods I was given a book and told: read. But I was told to read and read I did. The other information that I got on sex and relationships and all that, came from friends. And very often, that wasn't the correct information." Subsequent discomfort in teaching sexuality, these teachers proposed, emanated from being poorly advised early on in life. Patricia put it this way:

> When we have to teach the kids it was not easy for me because you know we are not taught about it ourselves. And now here in front of them, I have to tell the children about themselves. So it was very much challenging for me to go out and look for information. And then give the correct information.

Descriptions such as the above were common, irrespective of the context in which the respondents grew up. The consequences this held for the group, though, were mixed. Some teachers grasped the implied meaning of 'don't play with boys' or 'stay away from boys' while for others, its meaning was opaque. A lack of understanding of their own sexual maturity and their sexed bodies contributed to teachers' describing their sexual development as shrouded in silence, coded language, and shame.

In general, the pattern was one in which the respondents' sources of information about sex and sexuality were siblings, friends, or through the experience of pregnancy. In some instances, older siblings were *ex-*

pected to convey information and educate younger siblings. Gugu, the female black teacher who grew up as the only girl in her family in the Eastern Cape and who became pregnant at 18, noted that such a practice was prevalent among the Xhosa group. According to her:

> Well, you know in our culture I grew up in a very ritual culture and tradition in Eastern Cape, whereby you don't just do anything. You have to, there is a generation gap [but] the gap within the generations is closed by the sisters, the brothers and the older ones. Like if I've got, if I'm the oldest at home, I'm the eldest at home, there are my sisters, the younger sisters at home. I am there to close that gap, that gap for the generations in this way. If I went, you know I went through the menstruation, I had to tell, I had to tell them [the younger ones], okay. Let's, [say] okay I'm already menstruating, when my sister, the younger sister, is getting to the menstruation, she doesn't know what to do [then you have to tell her].

Gugu went on to describe that she had no one to rely on to educate her sexually. Characteristically and in this case, as the 'older' sibling, her mother was expected to provide her with the necessary information. However, because of the generation gap, Gugu was not allowed to approach her mother concerning sexual matters. She stated:

> That's why I said it was difficult for me because there was no one to tell me what not to do. The only person that was my 'bigger sister', it was my mother. So because it was that [more traditional] time, the mothers they were not allowed [to discuss sex]. They were ashamed to tell us everything, [or advise us to] go for protection, [or to] go and do this, [or] don't do that. You were even afraid to say to your mother, 'mommy, I'm menstruating now.' Your mother [would] just see that you are menstruating now. Okay and she's afraid, what can I say to her? You know. You know it was very difficult for me because I was, there was no bigger sister for me to tell me, go for protection, don't do this, do that, so it was very difficult. That was why I said, I get this child, because there was no one to say to me this.

Her experience in this regard was not unique. Jabulani, a Swazi female, also described her experience with boys and subsequent pregnancy as the result of a lack of communication with older siblings who, she implied, were required to mentor her. She states, "I was not aware, I was not aware, as I was very young. I was only 15, turning 16 in December. I fell pregnant. And I was having a problem, as my eldest sisters did not talk to me about this. They even allowed me to go with boys." The assumption here was that older siblings were the sexual educators who needed not only to provide information, but also to act as mentors and guardians.

The lack of awareness and knowledge about sex, lack of mentorship and being uneducated in 'the custom' had consequences for five other black teachers. Lizzie, Thandi, Dorothy, and Patricia, all from poor communities in Mpumalanga and Zodwa, from the poor black community in the Western Cape, gave similar descriptions of their early experiences of sex and pregnancy.

While not all offered the same reasons for their condition (pregnancy), many described the subsequent shame associated with such an experience. Gugu gave a poignant example that was typical amongst this group of seven teachers. She tied a "stocking" over her stomach to conceal her pregnancy. She explained that, "[e]ach and every morning, I [tried] all my best to tie my stomach because, and the stomach was rising each and every day, as if it is trying to show me, you know (pause). And the uniform was trying to, [burst open] you know ..." She gestured what she meant as she described this incident.

She continued to explain the degree of embarrassment experienced in class. After refusing advances from her teacher, he humiliated her in front of her peers in a way that made her consider suicide. Gugu states, "I [thought that I] must just throw myself in one of those dams, there were big dams, they were constructed by the farmers. I said to myself, no, one day I should throw myself there."

While discourses on sex were silenced and obscured and even though teachers gave reasons that could have prevented these early experiences, pregnancy was normalised. None of the seven teachers questioned their condition since it did not appear uncharacteristic in the communities where many grew up. Lizzie described it as 'natural', something that happened during 'adolescence'. She says, "[A]s time went on, and adolescence caught up with me, I fell in love with another guy. We continued dating each other. I fell pregnant with my Standard 3, and had a baby!"

Even though the rest of the eight female teachers in this study did not experience early pregnancy they too obtained little or no explicit information from parents or guardians. For the most part, information was obtained either through experience or in resourceful ways.

Silence on the subject of sex seemed complicated by what was allowed and disallowed in the use (or lack) of sexual terminology, particularly, but not exclusively, amongst poor black communities. For all the black teachers, using explicit terminology to describe sexual organs in the vernacular was not 'allowed' since communities perceived it as vulgar or offensive. To them it had to do much more with 'culture' than with terminology. Ester, the divorced primary school teacher, stated:

> In the African community, if you use the terms for sexual organs it would imply that you are being vulgar. Because we know that you can use the words to speak nicely and yet you can use them to swear as well. Ja! So this could make the children lose respect.

Jenni corroborated this point. When asked why she experienced difficulty in talking about sex, after a long pause she said, "I think it is our culture. I think it is the culture." While she agreed that the difficulty was associated with cultural constraints, to her this should not preclude teachers from providing information that can change behaviour. She said that communities needed to reconsider such compromising positions. She stated, "[c]ulture is a barrier but we must at least try and forget about culture because people are dying. Culture or no culture, people are dying. We must talk to our kids. We must talk to these young ones."

While Vera and Kobie from the affluent but conservative Bloukoop community did not express similar sentiments about terminology, their actions in the classroom revealed a similar position in this regard, as I illustrate in the next chapter. In discussing how people contract the HI-virus, Kobie, for example, either overlooked or skimmed through sections on sex or said that learners already knew the information, implying that it did not need repeating. Vera, on the other hand, as becomes clearer in the next chapter, bounded classroom discourse in particular ways.

Carol and Paul, from the poor Afrikaans-speaking coloured community of Joseph Rhodes in the Western Cape, demonstrated similar patterns of behaviour to the teachers mentioned above. They too managed classroom discourse in ways that produced particular teacher identities and specific learner responses. Interestingly, all four teachers were characterised as conformist or traditional in their religious orientation in an earlier discussion.

Amongst some female teachers in secondary schools, though, and unlike the experience of teachers in the primary schools, the difficulty lay in the meanings rather than the terminology itself. For Thandi, Volene, Patricia, and Lizzie, all Swazi teachers from Mpumalanga, explaining the terms was difficult. All except Volene had been teenage mothers. They attributed the difficulty they experienced in explaining to their own discomfort, culture, and what I have previously described as a lack of mentorship and education earlier on in their lives. Thandi, who taught at Khonzani Senior Secondary, one of two 'new' secondary schools in Mpumalanga, said: "[I]t was also difficult because when you have to tell the children, how am I going to say it? You know? With our African culture there are things that we are not allowed to just say." She went on to describe how difficult it was to describe terms like masturbation. She said:

> Like you know, you tell a boy that masturbation so to say, what is it, what is masturbation? We are not you know, (their parents). [Our parents] did not talk about it. I knew nothing about that. I never knew that it existed. Here I have to stand in front of the class, and they [the children] come out with masturbation. [They ask] '... what is masturbation ma'am, because we have seen it somewhere?', and then I have to you know, go on [and explain the term]. It is just so difficult when they tell me it is something like this and you do this. So then how am I going to tell my kids? So really, it was difficult. Though I have the knowledge and the information, but it is difficult.

The experience of teaching sexuality for the two black male secondary school teachers, also from Mpumalanga, was much like that of the four teachers described earlier in this section. Unlike their female counterparts, these teachers put distance between teaching and their individual lived experiences. They managed sexuality in class as a topic in the curriculum that they were expected to mediate in their role as the 'teacher.' Their response to awkward questions or provocative statements in class was either with a joke or through disciplining the child for 'being rude', or – as with the four teachers above – through overlooking or skimming through sections on sex, or stating that learners already knew the information, which therefore did not need repeating.

On the other hand, Xola, the HIV-positive male teacher from the poor community of Gapeng in the Western Cape, responded differently in that he took it as 'his duty' or his 'calling' to teach sexuality and HIV/AIDS, as described earlier on in this chapter. He explained that he took every opportunity to educate learners about HIV/AIDS at Vuyani Primary School where he taught. This he did whenever he came across an unsupervised class or when called upon to do so. To him children must be told about prevention, but importantly, they must see him as a survivor rather than a victim of the HI-virus.

Cultural constraints, or difficulty in the use of sexual terminology and the meanings ascribed to sexual words, were not traceable in explicit ways amongst those teaching in the English-speaking environments of Gracious Park and Stanton. For the most part, Shahida from Macadamia Primary and Gwen and Pauline from Parktown Senior Secondary, all three from middle-class backgrounds, used explicit language and elaborated on their meanings voluntarily and sometimes even exaggeratedly as I will illustrate in the next chapter. Shahida suggested that she had little difficulty teaching sexuality because she "grab[bed] it by the horns. I'm just so straightforward. I say, today we are going to talk about sex."

Teachers in the poor black and coloured schools in both regions reported that using English to explain sexual terminology was not only acceptable, it was easy because they felt comfortable. So while language served to maintain linguistic hegemony during Apartheid, the experience in teaching sexuality and HIV/AIDS now was different. Especially amongst females, English offered some distance between the material and the 'self'. It also offered protection against communities who, as an earlier discussion showed, already marked them as outsiders. Ester, the shy divorced teacher from Siyabonga Primary School described it this way:

> When you use the English terminology, people understand that you have a goal for using it, unlike the times when you use the African terminology, it could cause a fight. Sometimes the children and even the adults when they get into an argument, they use the African vulgar terminology of the sexual organs to insult one another. But addressing them and using the English terminology for sexual organs is acceptable.

In summary, associations of silence and shame with discourses on sexuality were pervasive in all the communities in the study. The gendered nature of teachers' experiences was stark. For the most part, males were left to find out about sex without guidance from parents or guardians, while it was expected but not always practised that females would obtain information either from older siblings or older members of the family. For females the unintended consequences of silence regarding sex were harsh and included pregnancy and the non-disclosure of HIV-status for fear of stigmatisation. Many reported acute discomfort in teaching about sexuality. Silence and shame also held consequences for the ways in which the teachers in this study experienced, interpreted and responded to HIV/AIDS in the community, as the next section describes.

Silences in communities regarding sex extended to include silences regarding HIV/AIDS. Many reasons were put forward for this and experiences in the different communities differed. Teachers from the coloured communities of Stanton and Gracious Park and those from the white community of Bloukoop did not perceive HIV/AIDS as a serious threat to their respective communities, even in the face of a reported escalation in incidences of teenage pregnancy in Gracious Park. This group of teachers, as is shown in the final part of this section, offered marriage and their religious orientations as safe spaces for protection against infection. Thus, silence was associated with perceptions that their communities were safe and that they were protected from infection through marriage, perceptions that played themselves out in particular ways in the teacher behaviours I describe in the next chapter. Briefly, though, as with teacher enactments described in the previous section on sexuality, similar patterns of behaviour were traceable in teaching HIV/AIDS. Teachers also avoided or dismissed learner input, skimmed through sections of the work, or sequenced the lessons in a way that framed the discourse.

Unlike the group above, the majority of black teachers were in constant fear of infection, whether or not they were married. Fear of infection was associated with practices privileging males over females, as the last section in this chapter illustrates. Fear of the meanings associated with the pandemic and in some cases, fear of disclosure, resulted in practices of silence that more often than not compromised women's positions and their understanding of themselves.

Much like the discourses on disease described earlier in Part III, the meanings associated with HIV/AIDS among all the female black teachers were embedded in the dominant religious and moral discourses of punishment, silence, and shame. Ester gave what was a typical response regarding conceptions of HIV/AIDS in all these communities. She said, "It looks that if you have HIV you are punished." Lizzie described the shame associated with infection, in which she alluded to why people did not easily disclose their status:

> The shame, the way that AIDS was introduced, the way AIDS is transmitted, it was said that you get AIDS (HIV). It was said that AIDS (HIV) is transmitted mainly

> through sexual intercourse. So if I am HIV positive, it will take me time to disclose it ... Why ... because I will be ashamed! What the people will be saying. Are they going to say I am, I don't have a strong personality [in other words promiscuous] and that I just sleep anywhere.

Fear was also closely associated with constructions of the pandemic in the everyday. Popularly, teachers reported many perceptions about infection, prevention and cure. Examples included: men who are circumcised cannot catch HIV/AIDS; using a condom causes AIDS; HIV/AIDS is injected into 'black' people's water; HIV/AIDS is curable; one was bewitched if one became infected; and that if you slept with a virgin, you would be cured of the virus.

The way teachers positioned themselves and understood their roles was influenced too, by parent perceptions of what should and should not be taught, as well learners' "knowledgeability" (Giddens, 1984) on issues of sex and sexuality, issues described briefly in the next section.

Teachers, parent expectations, and HIV/AIDS

Female teachers in the study generally reported discomfort in teaching sexuality. The black teachers, for the most part, acknowledged the difficulty they encountered when their own values, influenced by tradition, differed from what they were required to teach. Additionally, their task was often made more arduous as their own cultural practices and religious beliefs precluded them from discussing certain issues. Teachers recognised the tension that existed between cultural practices and education. This, however, was made more difficult by perceptions parents held of teachers' roles and the content they deemed appropriate for children to learn. Many teachers agreed that parents often sent mixed messages about HIV/AIDS and whether or not it should be taught in schools. The prevailing perception, particularly among female teachers, was that parents expected them to teach the curriculum, but they often questioned the depth, nature, and appropriateness of the information. Teachers also indicated that many families were upset when their children were taught about HIV/AIDS and sexuality, when in particular 'cultures' and religions talking about such issues is prohibited. Many acknowledged how disabling at times cultural practices/beliefs/traditions were in an education system that required openness in this regard. Volene, the only HIV-positive female teacher in the group, encapsulates what was a common experience amongst black female teachers in Mpumalanga. She said:

> But nowadays you are looked at as an enemy because you don't teach their children what they think you are supposed to teach them, especially when it is coming to LO. You teach them about their sexuality, about their behaviour, their rights. So they [parents] look at you as somebody who is going to teach their children, [to] disrespect to them at the house, because they believe that these are things that children must not know at all. Especially when coming to the sexuality part.

Shahida, the Muslim teacher from Macadamia Primary School, stated that parents enquired about the appropriateness of the information she taught. Her response was instructive in that, rather than acknowledging the efficacy of the material, she said that it was mandatory and that the government expected her to teach the official curriculum. She said:

> [T]hey will come to the class and talk to me and ask me did I say those things. I say, I said those things [but] it's not what I am saying, it's what the government says, that we need to educate our children, it's not what I am saying. [I say that] if you feel that I shouldn't be teaching this to your child, then you have the right to take your child, but, how else, I'm not going to tell your child, if you're not going to tell your child, how is the child going to learn? I mean, there's going to be a child without any knowledge going into this world. He must pick up a little here, he must pick up a little there. So he must know the facts of life. Because when I grew up, I was told that babies were got on the mountains, you know.

Maintaining perspective on their role within a complex set of relations was not only complicated by silence regarding sex and mixed messages from parents, but also by the knowledge teachers had about learners. For the most part, secondary school teachers reported that they were aware of learners' sexual activities. They acknowledged that learners were not only sexually aware and/or active, but that their knowledge about sex and sexuality was sophisticated and well developed.

Notwithstanding the above, abstinence was the most common safe sex message learners received, irrespective of geographic location, race, gender, or religious orientation. Many more female teachers were unable or unwilling to propose the use of condoms as a precaution even in the face of their acknowledgement that learners were sexually active. Teachers' reluctance was partly associated with their own lack of experience in speaking about sexual issues in a public space, but more so, with what was perceived as a clash between cultural or religious beliefs and curriculum expectations. Teachers were the knowledge providers and yet at the same time, the moral gatekeepers; how these positions played themselves is described in the next chapter.

Interestingly, some fundamentalists and conformists in this cohort did not teach anything other than abstinence, since they said it compromised their religious beliefs. Kobie, the white male conformist from Boshendal Senior Secondary, stated that he did not experience any conflict between roles, either as a teacher or a Christian; neither was there any doubt about what he taught. For him, the only message was "abstain, abstain." Others felt that even though the information they were required to teach compromised their religious principles, they had an obligation to provide learners with options. Pauline, a fundamentalist who taught at Parktown Senior Secondary, made the following observation. "I do often voice my personal opinion in the lesson when I say that the best kind of contraception is 'No.' And I say if you really have to, if you really, really, have to, then use a condom. But the best form of contraception is 'No' because it's the contraception for your mind ... for your emotions ... for your body and for everything."

But this was not the whole story, as the next section illustrates. Silence about sex held serious consequences for teachers in their experiences of marriage, condom use and conceptions of 'culture'. Below, I briefly outline how conceptions and experiences of marriage acted as another layer of influence and thus a discursive space for the production of particular teacher identities.

Teachers, marriage, and HIV/AIDS

Conceptions and experiences of marriage or relationships influenced the ways in which this cohort understood and positioned themselves. Marital status was often portrayed as the norm from which other subject positions were read and interpreted and as such, an important marker of identity. It influenced responses to condom use and interpretations of 'culture'. I describe these experiences in two categories below: first I give descriptions of the meanings associated with marriage, and then I show how, interpretation of what is and is not allowed in 'cultures' shapes responses to condom use.

Teachers and marital status

I outlined the marital status of this cohort of teachers in the profile at the beginning of this chapter. Briefly, thirteen were married, four were single, two were divorced, and one teacher was widowed. This profile included a married couple, Carol and Paul, who taught at a poor coloured secondary school in the Western Cape.

Conceptions of and meanings attached to marriage differed. Marriage was often perceived as the rite of passage to adulthood and, for the most part, the 'expected' thing to do. These views were held by most of the women in the group. Pauline, the teacher who became 'born again' suggested that she did 'wild things before marriage' because she understood marriage as the signifier of change. She states, "I did everything that I was not supposed to do because my philosophy at the time was: enjoy it now while you can because once you're married you're not expected to do those kinds of things anymore." As such, and as a significant moment, it legitimated teachers' status either as adults or as responsible members of society. It acted as a signifier of adulthood and also legitimated their status as those who could speak about sexuality. However, while on the one hand marriage legitimated their status as Lifeskills teachers, it also acted as the site from and through which particular subject positions were invoked and produced.

I was struck by how the respondents opted to introduce themselves in the initial interview. After brief introductions, consistently and voluntarily, the majority of the married respondents reported being 'happily' married. There was also an indication from this cohort that marriage offered safety and security. Nine of the married teachers, including the couple, described their marriages as happy and secure. How this group defined 'happy' varied, as did the reasons. For some, happy was associated with financial security, while for others marriage offered companionship. For some, it was the *expected* experience: marriages should be happy. Kobie and Paul, from secondary schools in very different communities the Western Cape, stated that they were happily married because they had married their long-term girlfriends. In addition, Paul stated that his happy marriage was the result of his religious orientations. He and his partner had courted for ten years without a sexual relationship. This was possible, he said, because they were both Christians. He, therefore, could see no reason why children today could not abstain from sexual relations, since he and his wife did.

The remaining four within the cohort of married women, described marriage as difficult and challenging but, as Pauline said, 'worth it.' They gave various reasons for this. Thandi and Shahida stated that polygamy or the threat of polygamy was a challenge. Thandi, a Swazi teacher from Mpumalanga was currently in a polygamous marriage. She was the second of two wives. Mostly, this arrangement worked well because she was the favoured wife. She had also established a good relationship with the first wife whom she now considered a sister. It was comforting to her to have a husband who took care of her family of five children. However, she indicated how such an arrangement created anxiety. On the one hand, she took comfort in knowing where her husband spent his nights. On the other hand, she expressed concern about him "bringing home a new wife", the consequence of which would be a change in her role as the favoured wife. She also expressed anxiety about the increasing HIV-infection rates amongst women, described in detail earlier. She stated that while she was monogamous, she could not account for her husband or the first wife's sexual practices (before and during marriage). She was also unable to introduce the topic of condoms in her marriage since it would raise her husband's suspicions concerning her fidelity. She was eager to do so but was afraid of the consequences this would have and, as such, remained silent.

Shahida, the Muslim teacher, understood that her religious practice condoned polygamy. She too expressed fear and anxiety about the possibility of such an occurrence and the consequences this would hold for her. She stated:

> Yes, because I'm, that's for me, that's a concern. Because, we, the husband who can afford to marry another wife, he [doesn't] need the permission of his first wife. He can just go and just tell her that I am interested in this girl and then I'm going to marry her. And there's nothing that you can do. Well, if you love that man so much, you will share him with another woman. But my concern is you don't know this person from anywhere. You don't know how she goes about doing things, how clean she is, how she lives her life. Now the night when it is your turn, having sex

> with you, he sleeps with you right, because you are also his legal wife. Now next week he goes to that one, you don't know who she has slept with, you know.

Sometimes religion acted as a 'protector', as in the case of Paul, above. As a 'born again' Christian, Gugu's experience was that her religious orientation alienated her from her spouse. Her husband, she suggested, used her religious enthusiasm as the reason why 'he went out' as well as for his infidelity.

Dorothy, one of two divorced teachers in this study, highlighted how, as a born again Christian, she did not anticipate her husband's infidelity. She stated, "[b]ecause we are Christian. How could this happen to us?" Dorothy reported being ashamed of her 'divorced' status and was stigmatised as a divorced Christian woman.

The commitment of marriage did not always offer safety and security. Patricia from Buyisa Senior Secondary described her experience as wife to a husband who had fathered a child during their marriage. She expressed fear of HIV-infection. After a long explanation about her husband's infidelity, she stated, "[t]hough I am innocent, I've never done anything wrong, how could I get AIDS, you know, things like that, but it could be the other. But I wish I can, I can make a test."

Her descriptions implied, too, that male infidelity was 'normal' and even acceptable. She said "You know how it is with the men." The statement, however, also signified another meaning, one deeply embedded in constructions of gender and sexuality described in detail earlier on. She presupposed a common understanding about infidelity between herself and the researcher.

Male infidelity was not the only reason for divorce within this group. Ester, the shy female who had been a domestic worker for eighteen years, stated that her husband 'left' her because she pursued a career. She says, "[I went to] night school, until I get my matric. And then I went to Mzanzi College. That time my husband left me because I was going back to school, he left me with three kids." Like Dorothy, this teacher also understood the stigma attached to her status as a divorced woman. She did not remarry and was careful to have an impeccable profile. She stated, "[I]t is great that I have not had any scandals in my life, that I have been living nicely and not had anything to make me look bad."

Lizzie the widow's experience regarding marital status was instructive. She gave a detailed account of how married women generally responded to a widow in the community, namely, as one who took other women's husbands. Her status, she suggested, engendered suspicion and isolation, and sometimes even a loss of friendships. She stated that women (and men) associated widowed women with money.[42] It was, therefore, assumed that they did not need security but could, as she said, "give pleasure to the men."

The experiences of the single respondents in this study were disparate. Volene and Xola, I have already stated, were HIV-positive. Their status as single and HIV-positive elicited very different responses and experiences. Xola, as I indicated in an earlier discussion, disclosed his status to the staff of Vuyani Primary, his family, and the broader community. While he initially struggled to accept his status, and after a three-month coma followed by a prolonged recovery, he was perceived as a hero in his community. His new identification as an HIV-survivor, he said, gave him another chance in life. He says, "I don't celebrate birthdays. I say I am three years old now because it is three years since I was diagnosed." He added that no one asked how he was infected because, in his community, no one asked a man about his whereabouts.

Volene's experience was very different. First, she had not disclosed her status at the time of the fieldwork. Few people, other than her immediate family, a colleague and two other people (including myself as the researcher) knew. The reasons she gave for this included fear of stigma. Recognition that members of staff at Buyisa Senior Secondary had already diagnosed her, kept her silent. She said:

> I should think I was not yet ready. Especially the reaction of what happened last year. I took it lightly [gossip at school when she fell ill]. I thought to myself, I will not think about it because it's going to make me feel worse than I feel now. I remember when I was in hospital and then when somebody gets sick and they lose weight, and this is happening. You start to think about this obviously, and unfortunately it was in the staff room. One of the ladies, said, well it could be she is suffering from '*this*' [her emphasis]. You know, because she had come to see me in hospital, the whole staff came to see me.

Stigma was not only associated with misconceptions about transmission, like the constructions of disease described in earlier chapters in Part II, but also with promiscuity and lose morals.

42 The perception was that women received payouts from policies and pension funds after the death of their husbands.

Normalised conceptions of marriage as supposedly safe and secure discursive spaces did not include the way in which safety against disease was experienced. Often during interviews, discussions on relationships led to respondents' volunteering information about safe sex.

The silences associated with sex and sexuality reported on earlier extended to include silences around issues of sexual safety, but the reasons for these were many and various.

Twelve of the thirteen married teachers reported that discussion on safe sex was absent in their marriages. Patricia was the only married teacher who reported initiating discussion about safe sex in her marriage. In the following excerpt she described an experience that offers insight into what was common amongst women in these discursive spaces. She said:

> This issue of HIV/AIDS also affected me for one because you find that I'm married to a man and I take care of myself. I don't sleep around with other men, but only to find that my husband comes home late and being drunk sometimes. For that matter I don't have trust on him, because I don't know what he is doing when he is not at home till late. And when I ask him to practice [safe sex], he doesn't want to. He says it means I don't love him and I don't appreciate him. And if I say yes I don't trust you because I don't go with you at night, he fights me. I really don't feel safe when I'm with him in bed. We do unprotected sex, so this thing makes me to worry and I'm also scared to go and do HIV tests because I will feel it is the end of the world. Even if I ask him to go for HIV/AIDS test he says I don't trust him and I don't love him anymore. So I feel so frustrated I don't know what to do.

Knowing that her husband was not faithful to her, she broached the subject of his wearing condoms when he was not with her: "[w]e were talking about condomising, I said to him, please play safe. Make sure you are putting on a condom." Her husband's reaction to her suggestion was instructive. She said:

> It is very difficult, although I know I am unprotected, but then, he refuses to put it on, I don't know what's his problem. He refuses to put a condom on. He says, I can't put a condom on, you're my wife, you are not a girlfriend. You're my wife. Then I say if I am your wife [does that mean] you have to kill me. If you think you are HIV then [do you] also make me to have it.

The candidness in the conversation with her husband was telling. While she was subservient in many ways, she knew what was going on in their lives as a married couple.

The coloured and white teachers held the general view that they did not need to discuss safe sex. Kobie, Vera, Paul, and Carol were of the opinion that marriage was safe and by implication, it protected partners against infection. Vera and Kobie from the affluent Bloukoop community could not imagine the need for such discussions because they were 'Christians' and married. Vera, who was married to a religious leader, reported that it was not an issue that, as a community, they needed to discuss. As indicated in an earlier discussion, both respondents described their community as tight-knit, conservative, and God-fearing, and therefore under no threat of infection. The common response thus was silence.

Responses to safe sex in the rest of the group were mixed. Silences worked differently in the black communities and were produced from different spaces. On the one hand, silence regarding sexual safety was associated with silence about sex. But more importantly, silence about safe sex was embedded in acceptance of male infidelity as a normalised practice, just as not questioning men about their whereabouts, was accepted as normal.

There was also evidence that elements of traditional culture were extrapolated in a manner which, more often than not, compromised the position of women and put their lives at risk. Women were traditionally expected to play a subordinate role to men, and were valued as possessions. Examples of this, described earlier, are the practices of polygamy and lobola. The female black teachers acknowledged that their role in the household was to be subordinate to the man, regardless of their educational or career standing in the community. They all agreed that their roles were still very traditional: while at work they were the teacher, in the home they were silenced. This 'silencing of women' was a key element in the experience of female teachers across the two provinces, with women saying how they were taught to respect men and be silent. They pointed out that when they did speak out or retaliate, men contended they were 'disrespecting the culture.'

The story so far

This chapter has provided descriptions of the sources and resources that teachers draw on in constructing an identity. These sources were multiple and together created a complex set of practices that were often complementary but most commonly conflictual. The patterns that emerge are ones that illustrate how depictions of a discursive space that use the dominant categories of race, class, gender and location often obscure the complexity inherent in these spaces. Evident amongst these descriptions was how the dominant discourses of sexuality and disease detailed in Chapter 7 and their concomitant practices of silence, marginalisation and stigma, continued to be used to frame the HIV/AIDS discursive landscape. The result, as is evident in the descriptions above, was the production of particular teacher identities as well as particular teacher enactments exemplified in the next chapter. Importantly, too, this chapter has illustrated how, in different 'moments in time' teachers invoked different subject positions and, as I trace in Chapter 11, particular 'strips of behaviour' (Schechner, 1985). Rather than proposing a fixed teacher identity which is commonly the case in research on teachers (see Chapter 6), in this work teacher identity is understood as made up of a multiplicity of subject positions that teachers take up at a particular moment in time. Teacher identity is understood as a complex but deliberate 'performance' constituted in the moment, always (re)cognising what is at stake. This performance has its own almost existential – for the moment – character. It is here, as I shall suggest later, that much more work needs to be done to connect this seemingly discrete and autonomous moment with the teacher's sociological history.

And so we see that the influences teachers draw on have a historicity that only gets revealed when instantiated in teacher pronouncements or enactments. While in many instances there was evidence of how teachers were 'structured' by these discourses, the complexity of their subject positions suggested that they were more than the structures surrounding them. Rather than being produced by them, the discourses are the conditions that teachers rely on themselves to produce particular subject positions. In other words, these conditions provided moments of contingency in which the teachers spoke and acted either in compliance or resistance.

The early experiences recorded above, together with what was described in Chapter 9, were brought together to produce a picture of the complex discursive space from and through which these teachers take up positions. The next chapter traces their behaviour in the classroom, in such a way as to highlight its performative nature.

Four patterns of teacher 'being-ness', what I call 'teacherliness', emerged from the descriptions above and the behaviours I report on in the next chapter. At one level, these patterns of behaviour highlight the performative nature of 'being-ness' and, by implication teaching about sexuality and HIV/AIDS. While teachers concealed aspects of their identity when they produced particular teacher subject positions (as illustrated in the first two sections of this chapter), what emerged from the responses on sexuality and HIV/AIDS were patterns of 'being-ness' that were pronounced in their concealment and thus unrecognisable and irreconcilable with the teachers' own reflections on their experiences.

Importantly, the four patterns of 'teacherliness' exhibited by these teachers blurred the dominant inscriptions of race, class, gender, religion. Instead, what emerged were patterns of 'being-ness' that cut across these broad sociological frames at different moments in time, producing a picture that could not easily and neatly be stabilized into categories of religion, race, ethnicity, class or gender. Different moments in time invoked particular subject positions teachers took up, depending on what they understood to be at stake. Using broad sociological categories was, therefore, unhelpful in illuminating first, the complexity of this discursive space and second, the way in which performativity presented itself in this context.

At another level, therefore, these patterns of teacherliness acted as categories of concealment, obscuring what was actually happening in the lives and experiences of this cohort of teachers, particularly with regard to their experiences of sexuality and HIV/AIDS. While the evidence suggests that black female teachers' experiences were more challenging with respect to the nexus between their marital status and negotiations about their sexual health, the argument that their experience was different or amplified because of ethnic, racial or gender factors cannot be sustained. This was surprising, since these communities were embedded in a discursive space deeply inscribed by race, gender, and class.

Teacher behaviours were typically either exaggerated, framed, normalised, or bound discourses. As I stated above, these concealed what teachers put forward as significant markers of their identity. While I understood these as arbitrary and fluid, I present the data in the next chapter using the four as categories of description that typified the behaviour of the teachers. I was able to isolate these behaviour consistencies and reach conclusions on the basis of the extended observations I was able to make of the teachers.

The first two groups comprised teachers who complied with what was 'expected' of them through exhibiting behaviour that had the appearance of conformity either to prescribed norms and regulations or to the preferred pedagogical practices in national education policies. The last two groups, while maintaining an appearance of compliance, conformed to neither the 'expected' form nor the content of the curriculum, as the following discussion highlights.

The first group, the exaggerators, exhibited behaviour that had the appearance of adherence to prescribed or 'expected' pedagogical norms and regulations as stipulated in the national curriculum policies prescribed for the General Education and Training Band. In practice though, they modified and transformed the practices through their exaggerated teacherly behaviours. The *exaggerators* were those teachers who characteristically displayed behaviour that was animated with respect to the development of the pedagogical script in Lifeskills classrooms. Dorothy, Jabulani, Gugu, Ester, Shahida, Jenni, and Xola, all from primary schools, fell into this category of teachers. For the most part, these teachers exaggerated teacherly behaviour as well as overstated the content. Teacherly behaviour in this instance means the *process* or the *act* of teaching that teachers relied on in mediating the content. Exaggerating both aspects in the classroom had unintended consequences for not only what actually happened in the classroom but also the outcome of the lesson.

This group of teachers was concerned with being distinguished as those who complied with the 'expected' and met curriculum objectives through adherence to the prescribed content. Importantly though, they did so through the pedagogical approaches they privileged. Group-work was, therefore, common amongst this group. They often designated roles to learners and spent considerable amounts of time at the beginning of each lesson separating learners into groups and explaining each role. Ester, for example, spent as many as 15 minutes of a 35-minute lesson to group learners. Teachers were always well-prepared and had learner material readily available. They were always eager to teach and often inquired about their performance afterwards. They volunteered information about learners and regularly expressed concern about the emotional, physical, and academic needs of learners. These were teachers who were seen to be 'doing something' about improving the plight of learners at their respective schools.

Most of the teachers in this group used explicit terminology in mediating sexuality and HIV/AIDS. They often used repetition, rhetorical questions, and prolonged teacher/learner interactions as forms of mediation. The chalkboard was rarely used as a mediating tool. Rather, teachers used worksheets, charts, and textbooks and relied on the interactions they had with learners as the main form of mediation. *Exaggerators* were often perceived and also perceived themselves as 'good' teachers.

The second group, the *normalisers,* was much like the exaggerators in that they too displayed many of the characteristics outlined above. The teachers in this group were well-prepared and employed 'learner-centred' pedagogies in their class arrangements and styles of teaching. They adhered to the 'the expected' and (re)cognised it as their duty to follow the curriculum. Moreover, these teachers positioned themselves as counsellors or guides and were aware of teaching learners accurate information, first as a sense of 'moral' obligation, and second, because correct information was important for examination purposes. Regarding the former, Pauline stated, "[b]ecause I decided that many of my learners lack that kind of guidance, I don't want to say, [I give them] counselling, but more guidance." Unlike the exaggerators, though, these four teachers were more controlled in their teacherly behaviour and exhibited the performative through normalising the content in ways that reduced the impact of the message. While for the former group performative enactments included exaggeration of the content and the process, for Pauline, Thandi, Vera, and Nicolene, all from secondary schools, the teaching process was a relatively stable one. It was in normalising the content that the performative was exemplified.

Like the exaggerators, the *normalisers* were also perceived and perceived themselves as 'good' teachers, but for very different reasons. Unlike the former for whom 'good' meant 'performing' the sets of behaviours associated with teaching, in this instance, 'good' was interpreted as giving learners the 'right' information while maintaining the 'posture' of a teacher.

Normalisers raised questions that were either rhetorical or invited obvious text-based responses from the class. The upshot was that in these teachers' classes, learners were more controlled than was the case of classes of taught by the former group. While learners were given a voice, there was little room for deviation from the official text. When learners did ask questions or offer information that deviated from the expected, teachers referred them back to the text or provided a well-modulated response. In other instances, teachers discontinued the discussion by emphasising time on task or the insignificance of the point raised. Sometimes, but not commonly, teachers referred to the importance of the content for examination purposes, thus foreclosing further discussion on the topic.

Normalising the discourse was done in two ways: either through the use of the authoritative text or through modulation and task sequencing.

The third group of teachers, the *framers*, were those who structured their teaching around familiar practices that were underscored in the more conventional roles of schools, teaching, and teachers. Kobie, Carol, and Paul, all conservative Christian teachers from secondary schools in the Western Cape, were the group for whom teaching was about the performance of that which they believed constituted teaching and 'the teacher'. This group (re)cognised the authority invested in calling up 'the teacher' and were knowledgeable about its capital value. Thus, these teachers relied mostly but not exclusively on the authority that 'the teacher' invoked. They came across as knowing what is 'best' for learners and as a result, often ignored, skimmed through or paraphrased information. They presented themselves as the 'knowledge bearers' and 'knowledge producers', and regularly reminded children that they had the experience and understood the developmental phase [puberty] and context of their learners and, as such, knew what was important for children to learn. While they used the official text as the basis for producing the lesson, they regularly emphasized what they took for granted as important and directed learners to underline important text and ignore the rest.

The common response when learners interjected was to dismiss their comments, or to offer an explanation that included personal experience, or to propose that the issue be dealt with at a later stage.

Discipline was an important identification that marked their teacherliness. All three marked themselves as disciplinarians and said that they were known as such to parents, staff, or learners.

Lecture modes of mediation were common amongst this group. Teachers asked closed or rhetorical questions much of the time. More often than not, though, they did not wait for responses but volunteered the desired response. Learners were often passive during lessons and would respond either in chorus or in 'yes/no' tones.

In teaching sexuality and HIV/AIDS, many of these teachers used their authority in directive ways not only to pace lessons, but also to foreclose discussion. In this way they framed the content and the process of mediation. This group used the rhetoric of assessment, lesson pacing or their authority as primary resources to frame teaching.

The final group, the *binders*, were a group of teachers whose characteristics mirrored the framers in many ways. Sipho and Mzi fell within this category of teachers. Much like the group above, they were both very articulate and displayed teacherly behaviour in their deportment. Mzi, for example, identified himself as one who, "... [is] disciplined, honour[s] time, dedicated to [his] job ..." They too were disciplinarians and perceived themselves as 'knowledgeable'. Unlike the group above whose "knowledgeability" (Giddens, 1984) was embedded in the official as well as the everyday, this group was distinguished by their knowledge of the everyday. In other words, they relied more on what they knew about the community and their practices as well as the behaviour of adolescents in the region, than on the specific content they mediated. Their 'insider' status rather than being expert in the content authorised their positions as teachers, the consequence of which was an assumption that children knew the topics under discussion and their meanings, and, therefore, that these did not need elaboration or clarification.

A common response from teachers was either prolonged explanation that included personal experience, reprimanding learners for being trivial or facetious or trivialising the discussion. For example, in a discussion about ways of transmitting and preventing the spread of HIV/AIDS, Sipho from Hamba Senior Secondary used the text book to provide learners with the information on the ways of protection. He described two ways and after referring to his text book, realised that he had not mentioned monogamy as another form of protection. He asked children what the word 'monogamy' meant and got no response. He offered the following by way of explanation: "... it is the opposite of polygamy" and thereafter proceeded to give them an analogy of the Swazi king who practiced polygamy. Smilingly, he suggested that the class was still too young to understand, and that the children should not have many partners. The children on the other hand laughed, and one said "[b]ut Sir, the king is finishing all the wives." Sipho laughed in response and continued the lesson by asking, "Who is more – males or females?" The children (mostly boys) shouted out "the women." He laughed again and stated that there were more women because men had died as a result of protecting the country during war and protecting their homes from intruders. Important in this group was that their authority as teachers, unlike the framers, rested in their control of the process of mediation rather than in content knowledge and the mediation process.

This group perceived themselves as adhering to the requirements of the new curriculum as well as its pedagogical orientations. 'Group work', therefore, was the preferred pedagogical strategy, with teachers relying on learners as co-constructors of knowledge. While there was an appearance of this in the class arrangement, teachers held the floor for most of the time. Learners were often distracted and spoke to each other during lessons. Teachers were often not well-prepared, because, according to them, learners should offer the information. They had a general idea of the topic but did not have a definite plan beyond the information proposed in the textbook. Teachers also understood that learners, as co-constructors, were to be consulted, as Mzi said, "... you go to these learners first ...".

Unlike the *framers* whose authority lay in their knowing and thus framing the content, this group relied on the text book as not only their primary source of information but also the authoritative text. Teachers asked closed questions that required monosyllabic responses which children provided in chorus. This group, concerned more with *being* a teacher, like the *exaggerators* and *normalisers*, also perceived themselves as concerned for children's well being. Unlike these two groups, though, the *binders* were more concerned with appearances and role modelling because that was who teachers were and what teachers did.

The use of the chalkboard was common, even if it was to write down a word given by learners in response to a question. Teachers also used rhetorical questions and statements. They employed some form of discipline, albeit ineffectively, and tacit knowledge was used both as a mediatory tool as well was the main source of information.

Presented in Chapter 11 is the evidence for the assertions made above. Using observational and post observation interview data pertaining to two teachers in each category, I give a short description of the episode followed by an excerpt. This section does not include lengthy discussion since it sought to provide the evidence rather than an interpretation of the data, which follows in the final chapter.

Diagram 5, below, illustrates the multi-layered factors that influenced teachers' understanding, experiences and subsequent teaching. Importantly, the diagram highlights how in producing a subject position, teachers concealed aspects put forward as significant markers of their identities.

Diagram 5: Iterativity of Factors and Four Levels of Influence Shaping Teachers' Subjective Experiences and Patterns of Performativity

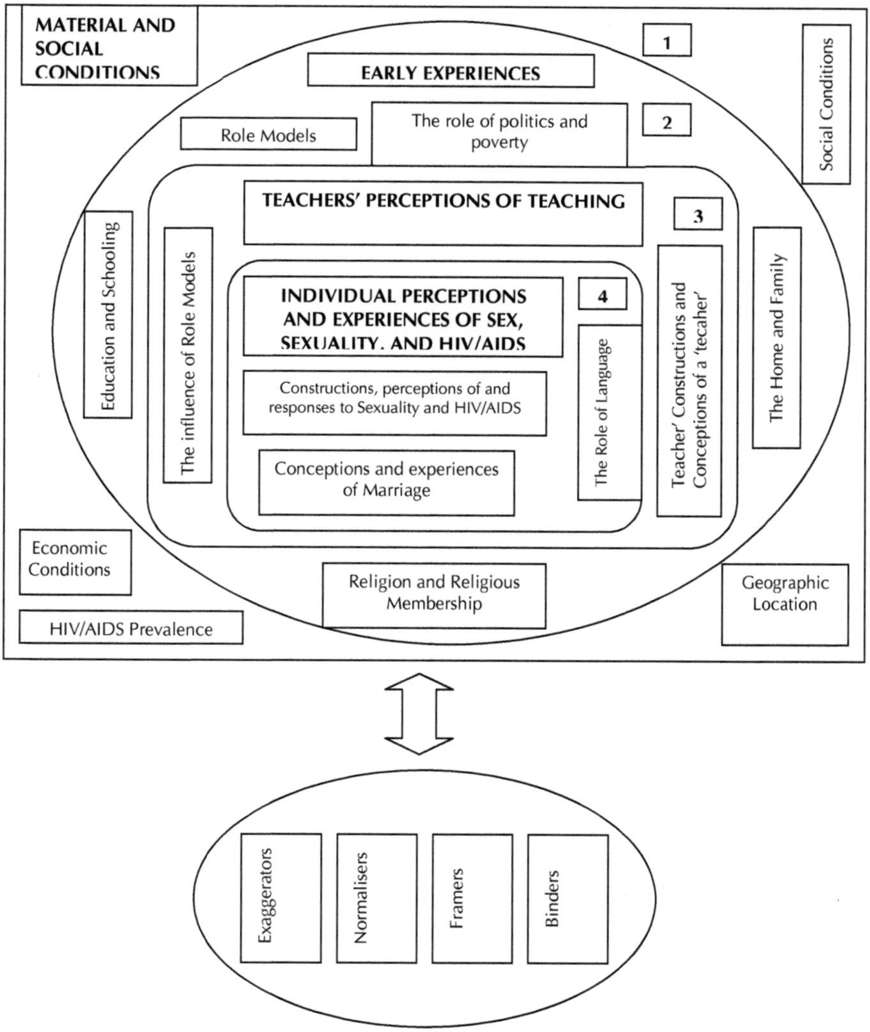

11 Subject positioning and teaching: understanding the performative teacher

The intention of this study was to investigate the nexus between teacher identity and classroom practice through examining factors shaping teachers understanding, experience and teaching sexuality and HIV/AIDS. The previous two chapters gave evidence of how the multiplicity and complexity of subject positioning foregrounds the performative nature of teacher identity and teaching. The four patterns of teacherly behaviour that emerged blurred the categories of race, class, gender, and religion. Importantly, the study and the identified teacherly patterns have highlighted the performative nature of identity and 'being-ness', and by implication teaching, particularly in the area of sexuality and HIV/AIDS. Teachers invoked positions in the moment, ever aware of the aberrant, the uninhabitable, in an attempt to come as close as possible to the 'ideal.' This in turn, necessitated them 'turning on themselves' through reiterative enactments (Butler, 1997).

Reiterative enactments or performances are repetitive actions which assume an 'act-like status' in the present (Butler, 1990). Teachers displayed sets of norms that were reified and ritualized, accumulated over time and taken for granted. Their historicity, however, was neither clear nor known and their production never clear or complete (Butler, 1990). An explanation of identity from such a perspective foregrounds the issues of temporality and spatial situatedness. One cannot assume, therefore, that such enactments arise out of a 'true' or 'fixed' identity, but rather, the reverse. What appears as a 'stable' identity is actually that which is structured through repetitive acts that attempt to come as close as possible to what is assumed as 'true' or 'real' or 'ideal'. However, as Butler (1999) says, enactments are themselves not stable, continuous or linear in their appearance. It is precisely because they are sometimes discontinuous that they reveal their arbitrariness and their constructed nature. Also, it cannot be taken for granted that acts will be produced in precisely the same way each time they are taken up.

The performative teacher

What follows below are episodes from the observational data of teacher behaviours in each of the four categories outlined at the end of Chapter 10. I selected illustrative data for two teachers in each category. Each category includes an episode of uninterrupted interaction between teachers and learners that exhibits the performative behaviour identified as characteristic of each teacher type.

The Exaggerators

The *exaggerators* included Dorothy, Jabulani, Gugu, Ester, Shahida, Jenni, and Xola. Using observational data from Shahida and Jenni, below, I illustrate how through their teacher enactments, the performative quality of teaching was exhibited. This group of teachers positioned themselves as facilitators and as meeting new curriculum expectations[43] in their practice as well as in the content of what they taught.

The *exaggerators* generally exhibited behaviour that was exaggerated both in its *process* as well as in *content*. They were not authoritative and invoked a process of teacherliness that was unfamiliar to them since, in the main, it was disembedded from the historicity teachers recognised as shaping their teacherly behaviour in Chapter 10. In other words, in their attempt to meet new pedagogical and curriculum requirements and to be *seen* to be meeting expectations, these teachers drew on resources that were in conflict with what they understood as 'the expected'. Expectations in the new curriculum required that they be facilitators rather than knowledge producers. They were also expected to adopt collaborative teaching strategies that included learners as co-constructors in knowledge production. Such expectations were at odds with what was stated

43 A discussion on these requirements is beyond the scope of this work. Briefly though, learner-centred pedagogical approaches are privileged in Outcomes-Based Education, particularly through the Revised Curriculum Statements of 2001. Concomitant practices within such frameworks assume learners as co-constructors in any pedagogical endeavour. This requires arranging learning in ways that encouraged participation and collaboration. Learners are assumed to be knowledge constructors and teachers are positioned as mediators or facilitators rather than knowledge bearers or producers.

as constituting a *good* teacher in Chapter 10, where most of the female teachers reported their role as nurturing and guiding learners. Guidance implied providing learners with the 'right' knowledge that would enable them to make the 'right' choices. Unfamiliarity with 'the expected' meant that teachers relied and drew on the familiar to make a teacher identity. The consequence of this lack of resources resulted in a masquerade of the familiar in dramatic ways. For the most part, their behaviour was animated and caricatured. They all 'grouped' learners and 'involved' them in lessons. They 'encouraged' learner participation and at one level, created the space for learners to offer information or opinions. At another level, the participation was restricted to monosyllabic responses through the rhetoric the teacher used and sometimes through prolonged explanations or repetitions, as I illustrate later on in this section.

Processes of mediation were characterised by repetition, rhetorical questioning, and prolonged teacher explanations and intermittent teacher/learner interaction. Teachers used analogies to simplify and get through the content. The consequences were often inconsistent interactions between teachers and learners that at times showed signs of coherence but, for the most part, went awry. Learners and teachers equally found it difficult to sustain the logic of the discussion or to come to logical conclusions on the process or the content, and as such, intended outcomes went unaccomplished with regard to both aspects. For the most part, the interactions were concealed

What follows below is an episode in which Shahida mediated a life skills lesson to a group of 40 Grade 6 learners at Macadamia Primary School, a middle-income but primarily working class community in the Western Cape. Briefly, she was the Muslim respondent who was fundamentalist in religious orientation. She adhered to a strict dress code that identified her as a Muslim who had gone on pilgrimage. The children sat in groups of four to six with desks facing each other. The lesson was aimed at teaching learners about changes from childhood to adulthood. In the interaction that follows this teacher used repetition, rhetorical statements or questions, closed questions and prolonged interactions to sustain the *process* of mediation. She used analogies either to ask questions about or to explain sexual concepts. She adhered to the structure of maintaining learner involvement.

The teacher introduced the lesson by giving children a picture with a boy lying in bed with a smile on his face. He had a book under his pillow. The class discussion began with the teacher asking learners what they see in the picture.

SHAHIDA: He is smiling! And what else?

CHILDREN: He is sleeping!

SHAHIDA: OK, He is sleeping! And what else?

CHILDREN: There is a book under his pillow!

SHAHIDA: There's a book under his pillow! OK, can you see we are moving now! We are moving, the picture is now moving! What is he seeing? More!

CHILDREN: He is hiding the book away from his parents!

SHAHIDA: He's hiding! What makes you say that? He's hiding! What makes you say that! "He's hiding the book away from his parents?" [She calls out a child's name]

KASHIEF: He's hiding things like that until his parents are fast asleep

SHAHIDA: OK! Things like what! Things like what!

CHILDREN: Naked people!

SHAHIDA: Naked people! Have you seen naked people already?

CHILDREN: Response: Yes Miss!

SHAHIDA: Is it the most natural thing to do? To see …!

CHILDREN: Mumbling around the classroom

SHAHIDA: Most natural! Do you see your own body? [She asks Thabiet]

THABIET: Yes!

SHAHIDA: All the time!

THABIET: Yes

SHAHIDA: All the time! Shannon!

CHILDREN: Yes!

SHAHIDA: How does that make you feel when you see you're naked all the time? Your body

SHANNON: Shy

SHAHIDA: Craig do you feel shy of your body? Do you say shy!

Same Child: I was thinking out loud! Miss

SHAHIDA: You were thinking out loud! OK. Shannon, we stick to Shannon! Remember your body is now, OK, we put another word also in it. Your body is now nude or naked; your body has no clothes on! Right! So, when is your body nude, when you don't have any clothes on? And you don't … when is it likely like that? Right!

SHANNON: When you take a shower!

SHAHIDA: When you take a shower, Yes! Adiela!

Child: When you bath

SHAHIDA: When you bath! When else? When you are getting undressed! Yes! Now we are going back to the picture! Remember now! We, he said now that the child is sleeping, his got a book under his pillow and his hiding it! Why do you think his hiding it? Because he said … what?

JOE: He may be daydreaming of the book!

SHAHIDA: He may be daydreaming of the book! Now, if you are daydreaming of the book! Are we going to talk just about now, about the picture! Where he is, he got the book under him or are we going to talk about the evidence! Where we must now be more specific, that we need to do the thing of the programme or what are we going to concentrate on? Colin!

COLIN: On the book!

SHAHIDA: Are we going to concentrate on the book! Now why do you want to concentrate on the book? Zabir! Come Zabir, quick! Remember it's your mind and how you feel, right! You are all children and you need to learn the facts of life! Right! You need to know what is happening with your body and you need to learn these things and you will only learn it with the life skills and if some adult person is going to inform you or tell you what to do. Yes, Colin!

COLIN: Or something else that is in the book!

SHAHIDA: Or some thing else that is in the book! Is it, can it only be an ugly book, where there are nude people or things like that?

CHILDREN: No!

SHAHIDA: It doesn't have to be, does it! The photo, the picture here, does ... it can do just that! Look at the picture, look at the picture and look again! We had one scene where she said it's a, he gave a meaning, right! Of a book that his hiding! How do we know that! How do we know that! Jack!

JACK: May be he's having a wet dream.

SHAHIDA: May be he's having a wet dream! Do you know what is a "wet dream"?

CHILDREN: mumbling

SHAHIDA: Jack! Explain to us what a wet means!

Child is silent

SHAHIDA: Do you know anything about a wet dream?

JACK: He's a big boy Miss!

SHAHIDA: OK, He's a big boy. Is that all? Is that a wet dream?

CHILDREN: ah! Ah!

SHAHIDA: Explain yourself! Because remember, I don't know what a wet dream is, now! Right! There are lots of children. Let's be honest now! And we ... I am asking you a question, do you know or do you not know what is a wet dream? If you know, you put your hand up and if you don't know you sit quietly and wait for the response. But I won't tell you the answer so easily. We can than think what you possibly think what a "wet dream" might be. OK, Elam?

ELAM: It is when you dream of having sex.

SHAHIDA: It is when you dream of having sex! You dream of having sex! Right! Remember we are children! Does that boy look like a child or does he look like a man? How do you feel?

CHILDREN: Like a child!

SHAHIDA: Like a child. More or less what age is he in?

CHILDREN: May be thirteen!

SHAHIDA: May be thirteen. Why do you think he is thirteen? Vernon? Come!

VERNON: He's still young.

SHAHIDA: He's still young! Now thirteen, is thirteen still young or old for you?

CHILDREN: Young!

SHAHIDA: OK, he's still young! Thirteen and he is having a wet dream. Jack explained what is a wet dream and Elam now said that he is dreaming that he is having sex. Can you explain to me now, one of you, if you know what is sex, and what does it mean to have sex? What does it mean to have sex!

CHILD: When a person gets intimate!

SHAHIDA: When a person gets intimate! What is intimate? What is intimate, being intimate with a person?

CHILD: When two people love each other! Miss!

SHAHIDA: When two people love one another! What kind of people? Can children! Young, as fourteen?

CHILDREN: No Miss!

SHAHIDA: Why not?

CHILD: He has his whole future ahead of him!

SHAHIDA: He's got his whole future ahead of him! Let's talk about that! Your future! Do you think he might engage in things that you are not supposed to? Shannon, David! How would that make you feel?

CHILDREN are silent

SHAHIDA: Tammy! How would that make you feel? How are you going to feel? You are not going to feel anything?

CHILDREN are silent

SHAHIDA: You are just going to not talk about it? So! Can you talk about it?

CHILDREN mumble

SHAHIDA: Don't you feel free to talk about it? OK, than we leave her! OK! All those who think they know what it is! Just by the feeling of the class, before I am going to tell you what it really is, I want the class to tell me what you think it might be! Not just Elam, and not just Colin! All the other children! Sherman, are you going to try to tell me? Tyron?

CHILDREN are silent

SHAHIDA: Come Tyron!

Children are silent

SHAHIDA: Are you still thinking about it? OK! Why don't you volunteer and tell me? So that we can all understand. When, what, they said, he said "a wet dream"! Jack! He doesn't know himself, but he said he knows what a wet dream is! Right! Sherman!

Sherman: When your sperm comes out of your private parts!

SHAHIDA: Sorry,

Sherman: When your sperm come out of your private parts!

SHAHIDA: When your sperm come out of your private parts! What does that mean? When does that happen?

CHILD is silent

SHAHIDA: Look you are going to tell me! Right! You must talk about this! You must, this is ... you know! You have to talk about it! If you don't understand you must ask questions! And if you are too shy, you must, you must talk about it! Right! OK! You have to talk about it because you are at this age whereby you need to learn all these things! Right! Because you don't get it in books to read about it! Right! Because it is feelings and experiences that you yourself, one day will, will ... understand what it is all about, right! OK! Jack, since you came out with it, you are going to tell us!

Evident in the above was how the teacher took up a particular set of behaviours. She relied on repetition, rhetorical statements or questions, closed questions and prolonged interactions to sustain the process of mediation and maintain a teacherly posture. There was an appearance of teacherliness in the sequencing: question/response; perceived 'learner involvement' and an impression of progress in the explanations of the content. As regards the latter, the teacher relied on the use of analogies to sustain and stabilise the discussion as in the case of 'wet and dry dreams' above. Another example in the use of analogies was in another section of the same lesson where the discussion evolved into one around erections, masturbation, and ejaculation. She asked learners what masturbation meant and a child responded "... skommel, Miss"[44]. Her response was:

> OK, but we are not going to repeat that. We are not going to be rude and not going to repeat that! Remember I told you Jack! Yes! We are going to just keep to the simple terms, masturbate! Right! They go into the toilet and they rub themselves and they will ejaculate! Stuff will come out, sperm will come out. EJACULATE! So we are now hereby where they dream, they can either masturbate and they will ejaculate. They will reach that pleasure. It is a pleasure that they will reach. Right! Now when you win in a game you get pleasure right! When you play a game on television or whatever one-day, a little game, you get pleasure out of it. Now those people when they do those things, they get pleasure when they ejaculate, when sperm come out of their private parts.

In the post observation interview, the teacher reported her aim as wanting to "involve" learners and "educate" them about their bodies because, as she said, "parents don't talk about this, if I don't who will." Performative behaviour was evident in the way Shahida was able to conceal significant markers of her identity, particularly those as a fundamentalist and as a woman who was concerned about the sexual consequences of polygamy for her life. Importantly, the above illustrates the way teachers exercise their agency in making the pedagogical script, consciously or not. The unintended consequences were exaggerated in the production of a script where teachers had few resources to draw on.

Jenni, a female black teacher who was married and whose intention it was to become a counsellor also taught a Grade 6 lesson at Yiso Primary School, a poor community in Mpumalanga. Learners, as was the case in the above, also sat in group formation. However, the episode

45 Skommel is a colloquial word meaning 'masturbate'.

below illustrates that as the lesson proceeded, the teacher took a dominant position. Jenni too displayed many of the teacher enactments described in Shahida's class in that she used rhetorical statements, repetition, question/response and supposed 'learner involvement'. While in her lesson on growth and development, she relied on repetition and question/response, unlike Shahida, her interaction with learners was abbreviated. She introduced the lesson by pre-empting the discussion with the following:

> JENNI: OK! As we have been talking about growing up, I want us now to come to the most important and the most sensitive part! OK!
>
> CHILDREN: Yes!
>
> JENNI: I say it is sensitive because some of you are going to be shy! Some of you will be shy! But please don't be shy! OK!
>
> CHILDREN: Yes!
>
> JENNI: Don't be shy! Don't be embarrassed! During this time, you will experience a lot of changes! That you are not even sure about! You don't know what is happening! What is happening in your body? Is it a mistake, or is it something that is supposed to happen. So! We will be dealing with that now! OK.

The lesson proceeded with her asking learners the function of each part of the body; from the brain to the function of the private parts. However, while she named every part of the body, she hesitated when she talked about the sexual organs and actually did not name them but rather said that we need them to survive. Her lesson progressed in the following way.

> JENNI: We've got these different parts of the body, which are very much important to us! Without your hand, there is no complete you, isn't it?
>
> CHILDREN: Response: Yes!
>
> JENNI: Without your brain! There is no complete you, isn't it?
>
> CHILDREN: Response: Yes!
>
> JENNI: Each and every part has got its' function, isn't it? So! Whatever, the body that you have, it's just natural, isn't it? OK!
>
> CHILDREN: Yes!
>
> JENNI: Natural that we have all the parts of the body! Having the brain, the ... the intestines, the lungs and did you see the functions of all this, how important are they?
>
> CHILDREN: Response: Yes!
>
> JENNI: Without the brain, would you be able to live?
>
> CHILDREN: Response: No!
>
> JENNI: Without the lungs, can you live?
>
> CHILDREN: Response: No!

JENNI: Without the stomach, can you live?

CHILDREN: Response: No!

JENNI: It's where the food is being digested, isn't it?

CHILDREN: Response: Yes!

JENNI: Without the intestines, can you live?

CHILDREN: Response: No!

JENNI: Without the ... the ... the private parts, can you live?

CHILDREN: Response: No!

JENNI: So! You see that the whole parts, they make a complete "us"! And how should we handle them? Carefully! OK! Isn't it?

CHILDREN: Response: Yes!

JENNI: It is very much natural and normal! And the composition of the body makes up a healthy you! It makes up a healthy you! It makes a healthy ... you, OK! It makes you be what kind of person? A healthy person! You understand?

CHILDREN: Yes!

Teachers in this group 'involved' learners and 'mediated' the prescribed content. They displayed appearances that masqueraded as 'the expected' in the performance but were far removed from it in practice. A common pattern of behaviour in dealing with the content was to either to normalise it through the use of analogies or present the body in its physical form. When a sexed body was introduced, teachers normalised it through associations with the 'normal.' Teachers supposedly followed the requirements of the new curriculum but had, as the episodes above illustrate, few resources to draw on to make the *new* teacher identity. Instead, the resources they relied on were ones that had a historicity that when called up, produced caricatured enactments of the familiar. These included different patterns of repetition, rhetorical statements or questions, prolonged explanations or drawn out interactions between learners and teachers, with the latter playing a dominant role in the discussions. The teacher enactments and their sets of practices, while familiar and recognisable, were conflictual with both the 'expected' teacher behaviour and the outcome of learning, the latter of which was ruptured and open to multiple possibilities. Teachers, though, as the post-observation interview revealed above, misrecognised their behaviour and assumed they were adhering to and meeting curriculum requirements. The consequences of such teacher enactments are discussed in more detail in the analysis in the next chapter.

The Normalisers

The *normalisers*, Pauline, Thandi, Vera and Nicolene, displayed teacherly behaviour that followed a prototype exhibiting well-modulated demeanours and control of the content through their own 'expert' knowledge of the topic, the sequence or assumed internal logic of the content. The performative was exhibited through modulation as well as through task or lesson sequencing, and through presenting the teacher as the expert but not the only knowledge producer. While the separation between content and process is arbitrary, it is useful in understanding the subtleties of teacher performativity. While the exaggerators relied on notions of co-construction as a means of knowledge production, this group of teachers used the authoritative text as the primary source to produce the pedagogical script in the classroom. They did this through showing little emotion or attachment to the content. The monotony in teachers' voices changed only when teachers disciplined learners or reprimanded them for comments they interpreted as 'facetious' or 'out of order.' The upshot was regulated and 'sequenced' lessons that had a form of coherence with an introduction and an end. For the most part, the interaction in class complied with the 'expected' with regard to content. Teachers in this group achieved the objective of 'having taught' well-prepared lessons. They 'involved' learners in the 'right' way, but more often than not, the impact of the intended message was minimised and reduced to an educational objective far removed from the intended. I use observational data from Pauline and Vera to illustrate the performative nature of these acts.

Vera, the white teacher from a predominantly Afrikaans-speaking environment, taught Grade 9 classes at Boshendal Senior Secondary, a school community she 'knew' very well. Her husband was a priest in a neighbouring community. Children always stood outside the class and waited to be invited in. She greeted them, told them where to sit and also directed them to take out their work books as well as the worksheets provided in a previous lesson. She directed some boys to take front seats; ones she told me in the post observation interview were sometimes disruptive in class. Learners were seated in pairs. She proceeded with the lesson as follows:

> VERA: OK. Let's turn back to the page that you have about HIV/AIDS. Now keep that page open and turn to today's work. Let's work on the TRUE or FALSE section

again so that we can see whether you have applied the information well. Right, lets look at the first statement: 'There is no cure for HIV/AIDS'. True or false?

CHILDREN: True.

VERA: Yes, true. Right. Remember what we said the last time. If a person uses anti-retrovirals then you can prolong your life. You can live healthily. But there is no medical cure that has been discovered by scientists yet that can take AIDS away. If you become infected one time, then you have it for the rest of your life ... Right ... Number 2; A person who contracts HIV becomes HIV-positive for the rest of his/her life. True or False?

CHILDREN: True

VERA: Yes, true

The relatively stable pattern of teacher behaviour Vera exhibited included question/response and learner responses mostly in the affirmative. Generally learners responded in chorus. She used the 'official' text as a tool for mediation. There was an assumption that the text held an internal logic and was thus presented as coherent, logical, sequenced. She also used the assumed coherence and authority of the text to produce the lesson. She was calm and showed very little emotion in dealing with a topic, despite assertions made in an earlier interview that discussion about sex, safe sex and HIV/AIDS was generally non-existent in the community. The same pattern was evident with another class when she mediated the same topic.

VERA: How does one contract HIV/AIDS?

CHILDREN: Sexual contact, blood

VERA: Blood, contaminated blood or blood transfusion, yes

CHILDREN: Dirty needles

VERA: Dirty needles. Someone else?

CHILDREN: Sex without a condom

VERA: Yes. Something else? Can someone think of another way? Right, the two important ways to remember of how someone gets HIV/AIDS is first through blood-write it down in your books. The first one is blood and then bodily fluids. Who can think and tell me of a typical body fluid that can make someone contract HIV/AIDS, not just blood but a body fluid.

CHILDREN: Sperm

VERA: yes, sperm hey. What else? Right so let's write that down. Let's number the work 1–5 and then we are going to write down the ways in which one gets HIV/AIDS. Right, the first one we said is through sexual contact and during sexual contact, body fluids are involved. We spoke about semen and also vaginal fluids, that's how a person can get HIV/AIDS through sexual contact. Right. Either the man's semen or the woman's vaginal fluids. Right, sexual contact. Has everyone written that down? ...

VERA: And the fourth one we said is contaminated needles. If you remember the article that we read last year about these two medical doctors that contracted HIV/AIDS. They both got it from contaminated needles. Right number 4 ... contaminated needles. That is also why we said drugs are dangerous. When you use drugs then you can also contract HIV/AIDS through contaminated needles.

VERA: And then number 5, when you can get HIV/AIDS from contaminated blood like when you get a blood transfusion. Contaminated blood or blood transfusion with contaminated blood ... right, does everyone have that?

At one level, her knowledge on the topic was such that learners did not question the accuracy of the information. At another level, control was evident in the *way* she presented the material. In drawing on the historicity of 'the teacher', this teacher positioned herself as calm, in control and an 'expert' in the topic. While she too proposed 'following curriculum requirements', unlike the previous group, she maintained control of the content through the use of the 'official' task and its inherent logical sequence. The result was the production of a script that appeared logical and successful in meeting the specified objectives, but was actually far removed from the intended outcome of possible behaviour change. Teacher agency and the performative were demonstrated in the way Vera concealed her conservatism with regard to issues of sexuality. Producing a position of teacher as 'expert' resulted in the teacher being able to distance herself and get through the content while maintaining a 'stable' teacher identity.

Pauline, a coloured teacher from Parktown Senior Secondary School in Gracious Park proceeded along much the same lines as the teacher above. As already stated in Chapter 10, she identified herself as 'born again', caring and accessible to learners when they needed to discuss any issue because, as she saw it, it was her duty or calling to guide learners. She had command of the content. She too used the content and the task sequence to produce a lesson that was consistently familiar and exhibited the 'taken-for-granted' sets of teacherly behaviour. She engaged in prolonged explanations and sometimes posed rhetorical questions that led to an expected or predetermined yes/no response. She asked for learners' opinions, but often provided the response. At other times, her questions were more open and received responses that she overrode with her 'expert' knowledge. She directed learners to underline the relevant content. While the class was arranged to facilitate group-work and while there was a sense of learner involvement, the teacher provided most of the input and for the most part, responded to her own questions. She sequenced the lesson, therefore, through the supposed 'internal coherence' inherent in the authoritative task as well as through her 'expert' knowledge, as the episode below demonstrates:

PAULINE: Now I put on your table a list for your own personal reading. What is the six steps or stages of AIDS and what I want you to do is just to look at that picture, and the headings there, can you spot the person with AIDS?

CHILDREN: No.

PAULINE: Does AIDS have a face?

CHILDREN: No.

PAULINE: So you unfortunately or Ja, unfortunately you cannot determine by looking at someone if they are ill, or that they have HIV or that they in fact have full blown AIDS. Okay, do you know the difference between HIV, being HIV positive and having AIDS full on? Anybody? Anybody have an idea? What is the difference between being HIV positive and having AIDS.

HANNA: If you have AIDS then you're at the final stages.

PAULINE: Your immune system gets affected. You have the HIV virus but it's not full blown. And is there a time period in which this virus can develop into AIDS?

CHILDREN in chorus: Ten years.

PAUL: Five years.

PAULINE: It depends on how you take care of yourself, and something like stress, which I think is very important, is that when you decide that you are HIV positive, then you actually take steps to take care of your body, to build up the immune system, and to look after yourself. Because that virus can lie dormant for a number of years, dependent on how long or how you care for yourself. Okay. Some people from between 5, 8, 10 to 15 years. A couple of years ago we actually had a speaker at the school, when we ran our AIDS programme for a week ... and every day we would actually have programmes and the final, well to finalize the week, we actually had a gentleman who came in and came to address the learners. He had AIDS. And the learners looked at him and said how can he have AIDS he doesn't look as if he has AIDS? And that is I think the scariest part about AIDS. If someone has the flu, you can hear, they cough their nose is congested, their voices are infected. AIDS isn't the same. It's a virus but it is very different to any of the other viruses that we know.

CHILDREN talk amongst themselves

PAULINE: We, we say that you have full blown AIDS, it means that your immune system is so, the white cells are so depleted that they can't build themselves up and you don't actually die of AIDS per se. You die of illnesses like the flu, TB, pneumonia, just the common cold, okay? So people often say that cancer is the worst, because you suffer, I often think and try and justify why people say that about cancer, because in my opinion, I think AIDS is far more stressful, far more painful, in more ways than one. Just like we are, if someone doesn't have a pleasant smell what is your reaction in the class?

CHILDREN talk amongst themselves

PAULINE: Now that is something that that person can actually get help for. Maybe, maybe the person has a problem at home, maybe the person just has a very strong body odour, we don't know. But our reaction pushes that person away. Okay, now if, look at some people investigating their armpits now.

Laughter by children.

PAULINE: Now unfortunately just the way that we are reared, we are all stigmatised in the sense that we, if someone was walking here and the person was deformed somewhat, lots of learners at Grassy Park High will probably laugh and joke about him. And like you say make gay about it. Why, did she walk into the back of a bus! Not thinking of how that person feels. Because the fact that that person is almost physically deformed, that already puts the person, or makes the person feel different to everyone else who is kind of normal. Why aren't you walking on all four your legs and that kind of thing? How much more then because of the risk of HIV, of being HIV, how much more then will we reject the person who is HIV positive.

CHILDREN talk amongst themselves.

PAULINE: If Tamsin comes tomorrow and says Miss, I've discovered that I'm HIV positive, and the class gets to know about it, will you still be Tamsin's friend?

PUPILS comment but they can't be heard because they do so at the same time.

PAULINE: Now how would you like to be treated if you were HIV positive?

GWEN: Normal Miss.

PAULINE: Normal, now what is normal?

GWEN: Like you were treated before everybody found out.

PAULINE: Okay, now I want to ask you another question, if you were tested and discovered you were HIV positive, will you choose to tell anybody or would you keep it a secret?

CHILDREN respond by discussing amongst themselves

PAULINE: Okay Keith said he would keep it quiet. Why?

KEITH: I'll be scared that I'll lose my friends.

PAULINE: Just taking the four ladies again [pointing to the three seated with Tamsin]. Tamsin did not tell anybody that she is HIV positive, but she will tell somebody who is very close to her because you are friends; those are the kinds of things that you share. Now there's nothing stopping the three girls from going to tell their mothers. Mom do you know, Tamsin is HIV positive. Will your mothers' treat her the same should she come to your house?

CHILDREN: No.

PAULINE: And knowing mothers, – are you okay, do you feel fine? And just that kind of thing. A lot of people are indifferent about the concept of HIV and AIDS. And that's why they act and react the way they do. Now that could be the response, the other response could be: 'Hello Tasman, how you? No she's not here, bye.' In fear of that that person might contact the virus as well. Does anybody know, yes Keith?

KEITH: Miss, would you ask the person how they got it if it was through a blood transfusion or …

PAULINE: Do you think that makes a difference about how you treat that person?

KEITH: No miss.

PAULINE: Okay, let's say me. I contracted AIDS because I was raped. Would that make you more sympathetic towards me than someone who is a prostitute maybe and contracted AIDS that way. Then you'll be more sorry for me who has HIV/AIDS

CHILDREN: Yes Miss

PAULINE: Because I was raped, in comparison to the lady I was describing.

CHILDREN discuss amongst themselves

PAULINE: Would you feel more sympathetic, we'll use Hanna as an example, if Hanna was sexually active with her first boyfriend and she discovered she contacted HIV from him, in comparison with the girl who would probably be called easy at school. Who would you have more sympathy for?

CHILDREN discuss amongst themselves

PAULINE: She didn't know that the boyfriend was a lying filthy dog and she loved him and he said they would marry, and all of that and now she ends up having HIV. Would you have more sympathy for her or the girl who is so called easy, even this girl has taken the necessary precautions and all the rest to make sure that she doesn't fall pregnant. So did the girl who is easy ask for AIDS or HIV?

CHILDREN discuss amongst themselves

PAULINE: Okay, can we actually, should we try and justify why we feel more sorry for the one and less sorry for the other. Shouldn't we feel sorry for whoever has contracted HIV no matter how they did? And just feel sorry for them and sympathize with them, and actually try and assist them in living, whether we know them or not, treat them equally. Because I don't think anybody asks, nobody stands there and says – fall upon me, I want HIV. Nobody in their right minds would ever do this because it is such a dreaded disease. You can't take cough mixture, you can't pop a pill and it disappears. It's once you have it you have it forever. Should we not then treat everybody as we would like to be treated?

CHILDREN: Yes Miss.

PAULINE: Remember that whole respect thing, it goes a step further now, respect even with a dreaded disease. Okay. If you'll just flip this page over, this one that you've got and with a highlighter in your right hand, if you don't have a highlighter, use your pencil. Now we have a few minutes before the end of the lesson, before it has been completed. I want you to highlight for me behavioural patterns that can lead to contracting the disease.

Sexual intercourse. Now you all know that by sexual intercourse you can contract HIV. You know what the risks are especially if you have more than one partner. The next one, blood to blood. And then you need to highlight those little arrows. This can happen when you share unsterilised needles to inject drugs, using unsterilised medical needles or being pricked by one accidentally. Sharing unsterilised cutting instruments in traditional practices such as scarification and circumcision. Are you following?

CHILDREN: Yes miss.

PAULINE: Using unsterilised needles to pierce your ears or tattoo your skin. And you often do that hey? And you write Lana and Muneeba forever. Don't go and get ideas now,

CHILDREN mumble

PAULINE: Okay, the next one, mother to baby. And there's a 39% risk if you the mother are HIV positive, that the baby will also be infected. Have you all heard of AZT? Then there's Niviropeen that they give to mothers only, if they are HIV positive. Can anybody tell me what is the motivation behind that? Why do they only give to the mothers who are HIV positive?

CHILDREN talk in their groups. Teacher does not wait for a response from learners.

PAULINE: If they do not give the mother the drug, there are babies who have contracted HIV while in the womb.

CHILDREN mumble in their groups.

PAULINE: I think when the baby is a few weeks it needs a mother's touch. And there is no guarantee that the mother is going to live long enough to rear that child. So I will strongly motivate to give pregnant mothers the drugs. Free of charge of course.

CHILDREN mumble in their groups

PAULINE: Behaviours you need not worry about. Sharing food, clothing, baths, toilets, cigarettes, classrooms or busses with someone who is infected. An infected person coughing or sneezing near you, TB spreads like this but not HIV. So these are the things you don't, these are the okay things. Getting infected body fluids like blood, semen, vaginal fluid, tears on to your skin will not cause you to become infected. Dry kissing, hugging, and caressing. What is dry kissing?

CHILDREN have a discussion but the teacher does not request a response. Instead, she continues ...

PAULINE: Wet, deep or French kissing, as long as you have no open sores or inflammation in or around your mouth. So if you're going to kiss someone dry mouth, you don't actually think about, do I have a sore? ... Sometimes you have a sore in your mouth but only when you eat something acidic, that burns in your mouth, then only you discover Oh but my mouth is sore.

PAULINE: The next one, masturbating yourself or your partner.[children snicker] Come on now you are far older than that. Come on now. Having a long term relationship like being married to someone who is uninfected and when both of you are faithful. Using condoms during sex, as long as they are used properly. Condoms should be used only once and they are used with a water-based lubricant. We'll come to that later ... Procedures which use needles or cutting instruments that have not been used before or they have been properly sterilised. Donating blood if properly sterilized equipment is used. Receiving a blood transfusion in South Africa today. Being bitten by a mosquito, or another insect. You are unlikely to become infected in this way as long as you don't have ... in your mouth, gums, etc. ... I do see you tomorrow. For homework tomorrow I want you to read the HIV antibody tests. Okay, and then we're going to have a very brief discussion about it.

In the post-observation interview, Pauline stated that she was obligated to discuss particular content, because it was 'the expected' thing to do; to follow the curriculum, even though she did not believe in what she said. The following was an episode from the post-observation interaction between the researcher and Pauline in response to the lesson above, particularly a question on masturbation:

> PAULINE: I am totally against it personally, I ... I ...
> RESEARCHER: Because?
> PAULINE: I just, I don't think of it as godly, it isn't. And I have actually gone to read, because I need too. My only sustenance is the Bible and I need to know the fact that it is in fact written in Bible. And, through asking, because I did not know exactly where to find it, I ended up reading a book on deliverance. And ...
> RESEARCHER: So it's in the Bible?
> PAULINE: Yes, masturbation, I can't tell you exactly where! But, just like I don't believe in safer sex, but I need to realize that there is a reality out... other sides to this. And this is exactly where I'm at with masturbation. Many years I've been exposed to it, whether it's through hearing, discussions, um! And its often joked about. But I need to put my personal feelings aside, because that is my opinion that is my beliefs. Well, it's the same the same kind of way which I handle the safer sex.

This group of teachers displayed sets of behaviours in which teachers appeared controlled and in control. They framed discussions through relying on the authority of the text. It was the text, too, that produced a particular set of behaviours. These often led to an outcome that for the most part appeared to be 'the expected', but was in practice far removed from it. In this group, the curriculum objective of producing the content to meet schooling rather than behaviour change requirements was evident. Framing the discourse in the above occurred even under circumstances when the discourse was ruptured and when the teacher hinted at opening the discussion. Pauline, for example, in continuing the lesson above on HIV/AIDS, developed a line of engagement that projected openness and frankness. However, rather than continue with the open discussion, what arose was a reversion or slip back to the content in a way that silenced what might have been a useful discussion outside of the 'expected', as the episode below illustrates:

> PAULINE: Let's say Moenira and Kurt are in a relationship (lots of laughter). Okay let's say Moenira and Kurt is a couple. Okay, let's say Dave and I are a couple. Okay, Dave are you listening, let's say Dave has the flu, I have the flu. Does that mean that we cannot kiss anymore because we both have flu?
> CHILDREN: No Miss!
> PAULINE: Is my flu going to get any worse if he kisses me?
> JOHN: Miss you obviously going to get more sicker because you actually have germs that he doesn't have.
> MARTHA: But flu is just the flu, you just have more flu.

RAFIEK: And AIDS isn't something that you can cure.

DAVE: Miss if the one partner is positive and the one is negative then you must abstain because there is a risk. But if both the partners [omitted by learner: are HIV-positive] then you can still use a condom.

PAULINE: I think Dave has got a very good point. And I did hear the point that a condom is not a hundred per cent. If I may just add to that, every contraceptive is not 100%. Whether it is an oral contraceptive or other contraceptives such as those you insert, it is not 100% safe. The point we, therefore, have to make is; if one is positive and the other one is also positive, and if they are happy together, they can probably have controlled protective sex. Okay, not saying now, okay they're both HIV positive so they might just as well have sex because they won't get it.

PAULINE: So you have to know that just as anybody out there is susceptible to contacting AIDS, so are you.

CHILDREN: Yes, Miss.

PAULINE: But a lot depends on the decisions that you make. If you take a wise decision, then obviously it means that you have thought through the consequences of everything. If you have taken an impulsive decision, then it means that you did not have time to think about the consequences of that decision. Now I put on your table a list for your own personal reading. What is the six steps or stages of AIDS and what I want you to do is just to look at that picture, and the headings there, can you spot the person with AIDS?

Pauline, like Vera, used her knowledge of the topic to maintain teacherly behaviour, in as much as the content served as the site of production of the 'appropriate' teacherly behaviour. But unlike Vera, Pauline was subversive in her performance. While she employed similar strategies to Vera, she allowed more learner participation and the insertion of a sexed body in the discourse. However, she subverted the very discourse she invoked by ignoring some comments or interpreting others as childish or facetious.

In contrast to the first group where teachers used analogies to 'get through' the content, these two teachers used their 'expert knowledge' to progress and invoke a 'stable' teacher identity. They relied on the 'internal logic' of the task or lesson to sequence and thus produce the lesson. Pauline's teacherliness illustrates another way in which teachers exercise agency in concealing aspects of their identity.

The Framers

The third group of teachers, Kobie, Carol and Paul, were the *framers.* The sets of behaviours this group displayed were invoked through the authority invested in 'the teacher', unlike the previous group, for whom emphasis lay primarily in the authority of the text. Their modes of mediation centred on their authority as the knowledge providers and the gatekeepers of what children should and should not know. While they maintained the façade of 'the official' by working from the text book and by 'complying' and working within the confines of the official curriculum, this group framed the discourse through ignoring the official text, skimming through 'unimportant' sections of the work or paraphrasing information. Children were rarely heard in these classes, other than giving monosyllabic responses. This group relied on the rhetoric of assessment, task pacing, or their authority as primary resources to frame the discourse. The result was learning information to fulfil a pre-established curriculum objective, either through completing a set of tasks, portfolio, or as preparation for the examination. Unlike the previous group, who used their knowledge of the topic to produce teacherly behaviour, the teachers in this group relied on the authority 'teacher' invoked to produce teacherly behaviour. I use observational data from Kobie and Paul to demonstrate the performatve nature of these teachers' behaviour.

Kobie, the white male teacher from Boshendal Senior Secondary, taught a Grade 9 class. Like Vera, he is from Bloukoop, the Afrikaans community that rarely spoke about HIV/AIDS because, as indicated in an earlier discussion, they did not perceive the community as vulnerable. Kobie invoked 'teacherliness' in a way that positioned him as the authoritative voice. By so doing, he (the knower), was able to constrain the discussion. He made decisions regarding what was 'correct' and appropriate for learners to learn and what they were to ignore. He not only controlled the process of mediation through the 'teacher' authority but also the content of the lesson, unlike the group above, whose control was much more in the process than in the content. The following three episodes from different lessons illustrate the point. In the first episode he states:

> The next important paragraph is about managing people ... that's important ... The rest of the stuff on that page is nonsense ... don't tell your parents that I am saying that the book is nonsense. I teach Grades 12 and I know what is required of you in

the exam so that is why I know what you have to concentrate on in the book and what you will need to pay attention to for matric.

The episode above demonstrates how the teacher used his authority to privilege bits of information and direct learners to ignore pieces of information he deemed irrelevant. He did not only rely on his authority as 'a teacher' but its historicity, evident in his calling up his knowledge of the 'matriculation' requirements.

While he used the sequence of the task to produce the content, in the following episode the teacher positioned himself rather than the text as authoritative and in this way was again able to privilege certain knowledge and ignore 'unimportant' text. In addition, he used his tacit knowledge of the learners to frame the discussion, as the following episode illustrates:

KOBIE: At the top of the question it says 'Read the information below and complete'. You are going to complete that part at home. I am just going to help you with the question about what is AIDS. I want to make sure that you give the correct definition of the term because I know that you people names it all kinds of different things. So, who can tell me what AIDS is?

CHILDREN: Acquired Immune Deficiency Syndrome

KOBIE: Right, Acquired Immune Deficiency Syndrome. Write it with the question. Now I want to quickly go over the questions with you, not because you have already answered it but so that I know you are on the right track. Has everybody written down the answer ... Acquired Immune Deficiency Syndrome

CHILDREN: Yes

KOBIE: Okay, now the second question. I don't want you to answer it now; I am going to give you the answers where it is necessary ... not for every question.

KOBIE: What is the cause of HIV/AIDS? We have already mentioned this, right? So it is not necessary to discuss it again, sexually transmitted diseases and all that stuff, you know it.

At one level, he too relied on the authority of the text, but unlike the group of teachers in the second category who rarely deviated from it, Kobie inserted himself as more authoritative. The upshot was that he was not only able to shape the discourse, but also present it as 'official' and by so doing remain detached from the content:

KOBIE: Okay, let's go further. The following paragraph ... The last part of that paragraph, let's read through it

KOBIE: The fact that the spread of HIV/AIDS can also be due to sexual behavior, is altogether denied and actually ignored. Right, in other words what is the cause of HIV/AIDS?

CHILDREN: Sexual Contact

KOBIE: Sexual contact. Is that the only cause of AIDS?
CHILDREN: Injection needles
KOBIE: Injection needles, what else?
KOBIE: Drug abuse, hey ... with injection needles
CHILDREN: A mother can transmit it to her newborn baby
KOBIE: A mother can transmit it to her newborn baby. 100%. Right now let's go on.

Kobie also used assessment as a way of privileging information and thus not only produced the lesson through his authoritative position, but also through that which he stated as important for the examination. While he relied on the official text, what he privileged produced something other than the 'expected', as was the case with the previous group. He discussed the 'facts' that needed to be known for the examination and encouraged learners to write these down for assessment purposes. In the following episode Kobie states:

> KOBIE: Look here, this short paragraph that I have just given to you. It is, paste it in your books. It was actually meant for your portfolios. I wanted to ... but I was scared you will lose it. I want you to reproduce it. In other words you are going to repeat it in your own words and then put it in your portfolios. I am going to enter the marks in my book because you have already given yourselves a mark for this. I trust that the mark you have given to yourself is the same as in your portfolio.

On another accession he said, "Mark the definitions because that is all you need to know for the exams" and then went on to say "You are already writing a test next week. Well this means that we have to go faster with our work. I am not preparing the exam paper but that does not mean I don't know what's happening." The teacher in this instance combined the task sequence with authoritative performances that secured his teacherliness, thus positioning himself in a way that made it difficult for learners to question his authority or the authority of the text.

In the post-observation interview Kobie insisted that the aim of his lesson was to provide one message only: abstinence. In response to a question about the aim of his lesson, he said "one message only ... so there is nothing else that is acceptable ... it is either right or wrong, either day or night. Day or night." When asked to explain what he meant by that analogy, he said:

> When you are in the dark, then it is night and when you are in the light, it is day. You can't be in-between ... God stands for 'right' He does not stand in the middle for indecision. He is willing to forgive you when you go wrong and because I live

> righteously and understand the consequences of my actions, here and at home. Because … I stand for particular values. I can't be otherwise, it would be hypocritical. What I teach learners and what I teach my children at home has to be consistent, exactly the same.

This teacher was thus able to produce a 'stable' teacher identity through leaving out what he considered unimportant or irrelevant.

Paul, the coloured teacher from Redhill Senior Secondary, exhibited similar teacherly behaviour in that he too produced teacherliness through invoking the authority of 'the teacher'. Like Kobie, he relied on his knowledge of the community as well as aspects of the 'official curriculum' to produce the strips of teacher behaviour. However, rather than tell learners to ignore pieces of information, he offered personal experience as a way of authenticating the knowledge. While he used the taken-for-granted internal logic of the official lesson, and thus relied on its sequence, he foregrounded his teacher authority rather than the content to produce enactments that offered a stable teacher identity.

In a discussion about myths regarding HIV/AIDS, Paul used the text, task sequencing, as well as his authority as 'the knower' to produce the lesson. However, his deeply held beliefs and constructions of who a teacher is and what a teacher does not only found expression in the teacherly enactments but also consciously framed what he did and did not allow in the classroom. In a post-lesson interview, he suggested the following when asked how he had made decisions about the pedagogical approach he elected to use. He stated:

> Ja. I will say my training consists of, I believe that in the Teacher's Training College, they very much put emphasis on the didactics of the teaching. So the methods, how to get the teacher involved, other than concentrating on what is it you give to them. So, I think because of that throughout my three years of teacher's training, I enjoyed that and I think that is where I learned to get involved with the pupils.

Recognition of his teacherly role rather than emphasis on the content is also evident in the strips of behaviour below:

> PAUL: Good, I want at least one more fact about HIV Grades 8 and 9. (Grade 8 teacher was absent so the classes were combined that day). You quite correctly have said blood transfusion, you have sexual contact, you have said breastfeeding, blood contact … sleeping with children … this is a myth and it is going around. And psychologists and social workers tried to address the myths when this disease first became known in our country. We noticed that babies were raped and what is

happening now what is being talked about, people are trying everything because they know that the disease has fatal consequences. Because they know that once you are ill, there is no cure. As soon as the virus enters your body, then you are finished. That is why they, this, that's why they believe that you will be cured if you rape a baby. *Lets write it down* ... She says there is, you can research it a little more, she says when a mother is pregnant and she is infected with the HI-virus, they can predict that the child will more than likely not be infected. (Children have a discussion about the statement). Good, oh we haven't come here yet ... sexual contact

Discussion amongst learners

PAUL: Mark says sex without a condom. Let's look again at the myths again as well as the facts. Sex without a condom, I will put it with prevention to protect yourself against picking up the virus. We are going to discuss prevention some time later.

CHILDREN have a discussion amongst themselves.

PAUL: blood contact. Let's write it down like this, it is a fact ... Another one ... another myth? You get, I know people who shun family members who have been infected with this virus. Because they believe that you cannot live with someone who is infected because they will transmit the disease ... Now I am going to put up this chart ... Let's look at the ways of prevention against the virus. Incidentally, I found this chart in 'Die Burger' [A daily newspaper in the Western Cape, South Africa]. Come let's, before we look at the chart, do you see the difference between myths and true facts regarding this deadly disease. Do you understand what is a myth and what is a fact? Now well, I agree wholeheartedly with you, here are a few facts and we will examine them later. I am also going to add a whole lot more facts, only when we get there though. Let's look at the 'facts' column – through blood transfusion from a person who is already infected, that's one. Two – if a mother who is infected breastfeeds her child...the virus can be transferred to the child. Three-sexual contact, right? and sleeping around. You sleep here today and there tomorrow. In other words, to sleep around can result in you contracting the virus. And then we say through blood contact ... Facts, think now about more facts.

In presenting the lesson, the teacher first positioned himself as 'the knower' who provided information. Moreover, his teacher-like behaviour made it possible for him to produce the content in a detached manner evident, for example, in the way he numbered the facts as well as in the way he selected what was or was not important to record in learner books. In addition, positioning himself as the knower worked to produce another element of teacherliness: the teacher as the decision-maker. This position enabled him to make choices concerning not only the process of engagement but also what did and did not get discussed during the lesson. In the episode above, the teacher provided long explanations about issues which, while related to the topic, were not necessarily integral to understanding ways of transmission. When a virulent form of transmission was introduced (sexual contact), he suggested that it would be discussed at another time. His positioning foreclosed the discussion even during moments when information was introduced that could potentially expand the argument to include learners' own experiences. In continuing the discussion on HIV/AIDS, and while he made use of information concerning the social environment of learners he knew so well, rather than perceiving it as an opportunity to engage learners, the teacher maintained the discourse within the realm of the official, as the next episode illustrates:

> PAUL: Lift up your hands, those of you, with all the sickness going around, who says it is worth going to the yard to sit and have a beer, a drink and that for sex. Show by lifting your hand that you think it is worth it, who says it is worth it?
>
> No child lifts a hand
>
> PAUL: Who of you think it is not worth it? 100% of the class! Why do you specifically say it is not worth it?
>
> PAUL: Come, name one person who is not afraid of death. Do you know the facts? Grade 8 and Grade 9? Do you know the facts?
>
> CHILDREN: Yes Sir!
>
> PAUL: So what are you going to do? What do you stand for" What is a priority for you? Do you want to get control of *this* disease?
>
> CHILDREN mumble
>
> PAUL: You say" Sir, the best is to abstain from sex
>
> CHILDREN mumble
>
> PAUL: You are going to sign a pledge and hold up and then when you come to Grade 12, I want to see to how many of you I can give a form again!
>
> PAUL: See what is on this page. It says: I have good plans for my future, I value love, and that is why I will wait. [He repeats this sentence]
>
> PAUL: What do these wonderful words mean to us? What are they saying? [He repeats this sentence three times]. The words actually mean, to me they mean: 'You know the facts about this deadly virus, so why would you expose yourself? Should I take a chance or should I not' ... The boys say ...
>
> CHILDREN mumble
>
> PAUL: Let's go on, time is against us. We will learn about the specific facts later. I think that you are now all aware of the virus. So to talk about the facts, that will be another lesson. There are many people in our community who are walking around with the virus. Many times you come to me and say, 'Sir, there is an 'uncle' who has AIDS ... The disease is here, but treat the person as part of the community. You know the facts, you know the facts ... carry these over to those who don't know. People with the disease need empathy. Good, lovely ... be helpful. Now give each one a page.

Paul and Kobie both produced lessons using their authority as 'the teacher.' As such, they were able to privilege some knowledge over others. They both used their knowledge of the community to produce a particular discourse in the classroom. However, the difference lay in the way they used such tacit knowledge. While Kobie used tacit knowledge of the community to ignore, overlook or 'block off' information, Paul used it to reinforce the 'uninhabitable' and supposedly ensure learners understood the consequences of their actions. These teacher behaviours were produced through teachers taking up positions as the authoritative and as 'the knower'. Instructive in the above was the extent to which these two teachers understood and recognised the positions they held. For them, performing teacherly behaviour and being acknowledged as 'the authority' was important. The content was presented as the 'truth'; bound by their conceptions of 'truth'. Unlike in the case of the previous group, for whom providing knowledge was a duty, the expected thing to do, for this group emphasis lay in the practised teacherly behaviour, with them positioning themselves as the gate-keeper against 'untruth', irrelevant information and the 'uninhabitable.'

The Binders

The final group, the *binders*, much like the exaggerators, displayed masqueraded behaviour but they invoked teacherliness through the authority invested in 'the teacher'. However, unlike the group above, the binders' patterns of behaviour were invoked through calling up the historicity of 'teacher' rather than the authoritative 'teacher.' In other words, calling on the historicity of 'the teacher' and emulating this in the present was evident in these teachers' enactments. They called up the 'official' in appearance but did not always comply in following the content or the process of mediation. Put differently, they followed a learner-centred pedagogy in the group formation but did not adhere to the practice. The results were lessons that appeared to have the form and traces of content but in practice were ends in themselves. Sipho and Mzi are the two teachers used to illustrate teacher enactments in this category.

These teachers regularly used tacit knowledge as a source of information and, importantly, as a form of mediation. While the previous group used tacit knowledge to frame the content as well as the process of mediation, this group used tacit knowledge to mediate. The teaching strategies this group relied on were by and large opaque. Traces of recognition lay in teachers calling on the specified official text verbatim and writing words or sentences on the chalkboard. Often what was written did not cohere since words or sentences were written in isolation. The 'official text' was taken as authoritative and was used verbatim and as such, teachers did not prepare. Unlike the group of teachers in the category above, who concentrated on the 'facts' rather than the actual wording, the two teachers in this group relied on the actual wording even in instances when learners understood the concepts and suggested comparable responses and sometimes insight into the topic.

Mzi was the black male teacher from Vuyani Senior Secondary, the only deep rural school in the Mpumalanga group. He taught a Grade 9 class in the area where he grew up. His lesson was on love and relationships. In the episode that follows, he introduced the lesson by giving it a title and writing the word 'love' on the chalkboard:

> MZI: Our lesson today is about love. [Teacher writes the word 'Love' on the board].
> MZI: Now class very good question. What is love? [The question is repeated by the teacher]
> MZI: You can speak in any language you prefer – in your mother tongue.
> [The children are silent]
> MZI: How can you define it?
> Bafana: It's a natural bonding
> MZI: "Love is an intense feeling for a person or things" [verbatim from the text. The sentence is written on the board.]
> MZI: What are the reasons that teenagers fall in love?
> [The teacher asks learners to discuss this question in groups and he walks around observing them 'work.' He suggests that one child write down the responses and another report to the class.]
> MZI: I want one response from each group
> CHILDREN's responses
> Group 1: Reason is to share love together
> Group 2: Girls want money from the boy
> Group 3: Recruitment – they are forced by friends – one has been enticed by their friends
> Group 4: Because of the adolescent stage
> MZI: What is the adolescent stage? It is a stage that controls your mind, when most of the changes occur in your body, when you don't know whether you are a boy or a man.
> MZI: The reasons are fine and maybe because of the environments or circumstances therefore these facts are relevant, but let me give you *the* reasons why people fall in love: [from the text-book]
> 1. For company
> 2. Share happy moments with ... right?

3. Sharing problems – maybe you have been raped-then you have a close friend to share the problem
4. Care- caring for each other ... right?
5. People fall in love for fun ... pure fun.

While learners provided important signals about individual experiences, thus offering opportunities for a potentially important and relevant (critical for the learners) discussion, the teacher foreclosed it by briefly acknowledging the points and continuing to introduce the official text verbatim from a sheet, containing information far removed from these learners' reality. The following was Mzi's response regarding the procedure he followed in the lesson. What he intended was far removed from what he actually achieved:

> Ja ..., I say that one has to do with the experience I have acquired in teaching. You know there are lessons which become, which are boring to the learners and there are lessons which make them to be willing to communicate or to speak in whatever way. So for this one because I know that I am dealing with adolescents, when once you come up ... with the topic of love, everyone would want to have an input on whatever you are saying. That is why I said that my best way of getting information from them is to pose a problem and in that way I know immediately how much information they have with regard to the subject ... Ja. I would say to some of them it is a reality. To some of them it is things that they hear from their sisters or whatever and they discuss. So my purpose is to make them not to do the wrong things. So you see when dealing with such people in that age group, you must be very careful, because you might develop an interest on that very same bad thing to that learner. Some actually, from their homes, they have it where a mother encourages a young girl to fall in love so that the girl can bring bread to the family, you see.

As opposed to those teachers in the previous group who seemed to use assessment processes, the content or the task sequence to develop the lesson, teachers in this group used the act of teaching in and for itself to 'get through' the lesson. Put differently, teachers understood the process they engaged in as 'what teachers do'. What emerged, therefore, was a noticeable and consistent set of practices which produced content as an end in itself. Producing teacherly behaviour became the aim rather than mediating content. Put differently, for this pair, emphasis lay on *that* they were 'teaching' rather than on *what* they were teaching; in other words producing the practice rather than providing information, content or knowledge for use by learners.

Sipho was the single black male teacher from Hamba Senior Secondary, the school with some of the worst matriculation results in Mpumalanga. The class he was due to teach for the observation session had 'disappeared'. He went to other Grade 9 classes that were unattended and made up a class to teach. A colleague harassed him on a few occasions, asking why he was working. He responded in isiSwati that he had a guest for whom he was teaching. The lesson follows below:

> SIPHO: Our lesson today will be about a common disease … HIV/AIDS. (Teacher writes the words HIV/AIDS on the board)
> SIPHO: What is it going to be about?
> CHILDREN: HIV/AIDS
> SIPHO: What does HIV stands for?
> CHILDREN: Human – Immune – deficiency Virus
> SIPHO: What does AIDS stands for?
> CHILDREN: Acquired Immune Deficiency Syndrome
> SIPHO: A virus is a sort of disease and once it enters the body, it kills the white cells. The body has two cell types-white and red. This immune virus-they are protective cells. You can see when you have a sore – sometimes you don't need to go to the doctor because your white cells can protect your body. Your body can heal itself. Most people who are HIV are prone to getting TB – what is TB?
> CHILDREN: tuberculosis
> SIPHO: Where are the people found who have TB?
> CHILDREN: At SANTA
> SIPHO: People who have HIV – they can do whatever we can do
> SIPHO: When someone has AIDS we must treat them compassionately: to be compassionate means to love someone.
> SIPHO: How does a person get AIDS?
> MAX: [in isiSwati]: when you are naughty doing rude things
> XOLANI: When you have unprotected sex
> SIPHO: When people engage in unprotected sex, if you sleep with someone who is HIV and you have unprotected sex, you can get infected. Bodily fluids, when you touch someone else's blood. How else can you get HIV?
> [The CHILDREN giggle and remain silent]
> SIPHO: Paging through the book says "There are certain myths-certain things people believe that may or my not be true. Before we talk about myths, let's talk about how someone can detect AIDS – so you don't get HIV
> CHILDREN: Abstain and then they repeat this in isiSwati [leave all forms of naughtiness and doing rude things]
> SIPHO: You can have sex but use a condom and when you work with blood, you should wear protective gloves.

Sipho, referring to his text book, realised that he had not mentioned monogamy as another form of protection. He proceeded in the following way:

SIPHO: you can protect yourself through monogamy. What is monogamy?
No response from children
SIPHO: It is the opposite of polygamy. King Sobuza is a polygamist because he has many wives. But you are still young ... you should not have many partners.
BEN: But Sir, the king is finishing all the wives
[Sipho laughs in response and continues the lesson by asking]
SIPHO: Who is more: males or females?
The CHILDREN (mostly boys) shout out, 'the women'
[He laughs again and states that women are more because men died as a result of protecting the country during war and protecting their homes from intruders]
SIPHO: There is another way in which we can get HIV – through drugs ... like dagga, heroin. When you use drugs and someone shares a needle with you, you can get the virus.
SIPHO: Any questions?
CONRAD: They say condoms are not 100% safe.
SIPHO: It is true that the condom is not safe because it can tear. [he and the boys laugh] So if it tears then you can get infected.
LINDI: But there *is* a way, through abstaining
SIPHO: When you go to heaven God will ask you what you did with your asset [private parts]. How are you going to respond?
TOM: I will use my penis to go to toilet.
SIPHO and the CHILDREN laugh and he ends the lesson [unceremoniously, as I wrote in my journal].

While there was an appearance of coherence in the content, what was produced neither cohered nor met the intended outcome processually or as regards the content. In the post-observation interview and in response to a question about the analogy he used, Sipho replied:

> I wanted to show them that when someone is having so many wives it becomes a problem because you cannot be able to satisfy all of them. I remember last week, I read in the newspapers. There was a second wife and she killed her husband because he could not satisfy her. So she said that the first wife was taking everything out of her husband, so when he comes to her, he comes very tired and he could not sexually satisfy her. So many things are going through my mind ... wife of a soldier, who was a soldier sent to the forefront of the battle, so that he can have the wife. Ja, so I just wanted to show them that.

What the two excerpts above foreground is how these two teachers understood that procedurally the following was a requirement in the pedagogical endeavour: introducing the topic and writing it on the chalkboard, asking an introductory question, allowing for some responses and then producing the official version as closure. Mzi supported this assertion in the post-observation interview, when he stated there was a particular way to mediate. He said, "Yes, actually, the *best* approach is to pose a question and then give them time to think about it, then you get their response. They respond differently. From their responses you take whatever, but then you give them the correct things to follow."

In summary, teaching about sexuality and HIV/AIDS invokes different subject positions, and these often threaten what teachers put forward as the 'ideal.' The specificity of this HIV hermeneutic space forces those living and working in these spaces to rethink notions of love, proximity, relationships, and trust. In the case of these teachers, it forced them to confront the 'aberrant other' in the public space of the classroom. It brought a physical and sexed body into the sacred arena of the school and classroom, a discursive space usually reserved for mindful, rational bodies. The upshot of this was the production of performative behaviours that had consequences for their teacher identities as well as the outcome of learning.

As I outlined in Chapter 10, teachers speak and act within a discursive space that is charged with conflictual messages. The messages they put forward and the actions they set in motion in their classrooms, therefore, are not neutral, as the results above suggest. They are not mere implementers of, in this case, a pre-scripted uncontested Lifeskills curriculum whose aim is to ensure learners are taught safe and safer sex messages, the outcome of which would be informed decision-making with regard to sexual choices. The attempt to maintain the ideal while at the same time mediate about sexuality and HIV/AIDS cannot be a more threatening space for the 'self'. The result, therefore, was first, the production of a set of performative behaviours that often concealed the most threatened aspects of themselves, and second, a modification and transformation of the prescribed pedagogical script, which changed the intended outcome of the lesson.

The consequences of these performative behaviours resulted in teachers not always complying with their own or prescribed sets of outcomes, as I briefly summarise in the next and final chapter of this work.

Part V
Unintended consequences of 'performing' teaching

Introduction

The study of contexts is intrinsic to any analysis of social action. And any commentary on contexts implies an examination of the human interaction that constitutes the strips of behaviour people call up within a particular space and time. It involves examining ways in which people understand themselves as members of different groups, each with their own rules and regulatory practices. It requires examining words and actions in their presented form, 'in the moment' of instantiation with all the gestures, facial expressions, and feelings that accompany them. It also requires an awareness of the reflexive nature of identity construction (Giddens, 1984).

The study that forms the basis of this book was aimed at examining the factors shaping teachers' understanding, experiences and teaching of sexuality and HIV/AIDS. It began with questions about who the teachers were and what it was about themselves that they brought into the classroom. I put forward the argument that individual and collective influences and experiences serve as mediatory resources teachers draw on to produce and reproduce knowledge and teacherly enactments in the classroom. Such an argument challenges constructions of, on the one hand, teachers as mere *deliverers* of an uncontested, sanitised and agreed upon body of content and, on the other hand, schools as stable or neutral environments where safe sex messages are effortlessly delivered by a complying teacher to a relatively passive audience of learners.

The fundamental question, therefore, was about the relationship between what teachers bring into the classroom of themselves and what happens when they invoke the body in its physical and sexual form, a body usually absent in the public arena of the classroom and the sacred discursive space of schools.

The results suggest that the influences on teachers' lives are multiple and complex. What teachers bring into the classroom of themselves, particularly as it relates to sexuality and HIV/AIDS, is not only complex, but also mediated in discursive spaces outside the school that make teachers rethink and confront their own constructions of love, proximity, and trust in their relationships. This discursive space is extremely threatening to the ideologies these teachers hold about the 'self'. The influences teachers bring into the classroom that serve as the discursive space from which they speak, are a threatened, unstable and contestable hermeneutic space riven by contradictory messages. Their attempt, therefore, to present a 'stable' teacher identity concealing their own vulnerabilities became the condition from which this group invoked subject positions and, in so doing, exhibited the performative nature of teaching.

Part V thus brings the book to a close, through a brief analysis of the value of applying notions of performativity in understanding teachers' work in Lifeskills classrooms. Through analysing what actually happened in the observed classroom, this section offers some insight into the unintended consequences of teachers' performative behaviour and the implications this holds for teaching about sexuality and HIV/AIDS. In discussing the unintended consequences in the identified teacher performances, I suggest that they, more often than not, leave the outcome of teaching and learning open to multiple and contradictory interpretations rather than what was 'intended.' I do this by analysing first, the content of sexuality and HIV/AIDS classroom discourse and second, the unintended consequences resulting from the four types of teacherly behaviour portrayed in Chapter 11. While the final outcome of teaching is never guaranteed, these teacherly behaviours, I argue, have consequences for what is proposed as the outcome of teaching sexuality and HIV/AIDS in schools, namely a change in sexual behaviour.

This chapter concludes with some commentary on the policy, teacher training and curriculum implications such an investigation holds, and in so doing raises questions rather than provides answers.

12 Teacher performativity and classroom discourse

In the introductory section of this book I put forward the argument that teaching sexuality and HIV/AIDS disrupts the practice in schools in particular ways. I proposed that, in the main, schools privilege 'mindful bodies' with the chief goal being that of ensuring the academic success of learners. By and large, the functioning of schools depends on the absence of a physical body and its sexed form, that is, its disappearance in a system of education that is most often presented as rational and academic. For the most part, curriculum material is presented as possessing an internal logic and as that which, when presented, follows a rational linear pattern. The goals of teaching about sexuality and HIV/AIDS, however, are different. They are put forward with the view to ensuring that the outcome leads to learners making informed decisions about their sexual practices; goals that invoke a body in its physical and sexual form. As a consequence, teaching about sexuality and HIV/AIDS also invokes aspects of teachers' identities that are riven by contradictions. Teaching about sexuality and HIV/AIDS forces teachers to confront aspects of their identities in ways that animate the complexity of their lives and the discursive spaces in and through which they make meaning of their individual and collective identities. The upshot of this, as the evidence in Chapter 10 illustrates, is a disruption in constructions of schools as appropriate spaces for the mediation of safe sex messages and presents classrooms as discursive spaces where neither the mediation process nor the learning outcome can be guaranteed or taken for granted.

Performativity and biologised, (dis)membered bodies

The insertion of sexuality and HIV/AIDS into the curriculum, involving the calling up of discourses of sexuality and disease in the public space of the classroom, had the potential to disrupt and as such render the pedagogic space and relationship open to negotiation and reconstruction. However, teachers' attempts to 'teach' or 'mediate' about sexuality and HIV/AIDS, more often than not, resulted in their presenting a biologised (dis)membered physical body. In their attempt to maintain 'stable' teacher identities, most teachers produced the content in a sanitised, 'official' form. The consequence of this was twofold. First, such an orientation highlighted the authority invested in the dominant discourses of sexuality and disease described in Part III and foregrounded the extent to which teachers relied on these to produce a pedagogical script. Teachers normalised the content in a way that often neutralised the impact of the message, even in instances when a body in its sexual form was invoked. The upshot of this was that, while the content had the potential to destabilize classroom discourse as well as temporarily rupture a stable teacher identity, through invoking particular teacherly behaviours teachers were able to reframe the discourse and by so doing insert their authority as the mediators of *particular* messages rather than 'the expected.'

However, and this is the second point, reframing the discourse resulted in a reintroduction and thus, reproduction of the very thing which teachers' teacherliness intended to conceal – the physical, sexualised body. In other words, in instances when inscribed notions of what constitutes a teacher identity were temporarily troubled or ruptured by learners and not as a deliberate act by the teacher, these were reinstituted and reproduced by the teacher through their teacherly behaviour. The power to invoke rested with teachers and was made visible through the patterns of behaviour they brought into play. These distinguishable patterns of behaviour were invoked through the possibility of the 'uninhabitable' or 'aberrant other' (Butler, 1997). In other words, the physical and sexualised body was only revealed in its absence. Thus, inscriptions by teachers through their enactments produced iterative processes that in turn reproduced the content in particular ways. It could also be said that the content was the condition through which particular iterative behaviours were invoked. The consequence of this for teaching about sexuality and HIV/AIDS, therefore, was reinforcement rather than a disruption of the dominant discourses of silence and shame that were described in detail in Chapter 10. While no unitary meaning can be associated with 'constraint', in this instance discourses on sexuality and disease were constraining and manifested through the production of the silences experienced in and outside the classroom.

Performativity and normalised discourses

Giddens (1984) suggests that the unintended consequences and conditions of actions have to be interpreted within the flow of intention rather than according to the reasons people give for their actions. All the teachers normalised the discourse in the classroom, but in different ways and with varying unintended consequences. Normalized here refers to the *way* in which teachers discussed issues of sexuality and HIV/AIDS. While the outcome of teaching is never complete, what was evident through observing classrooms was that particular teacher behaviour produced particular sets of perceived outcomes.

The *exaggerators* used different ways to normalise 'the private'. Sometimes they highlighted 'its' naturalness and sameness. In this instance, biological or physical bodies were presented as unmarked. None of the social meanings that mark bodies as raced, classed, gendered and sexed bodies were invoked. Calling on the naturalness of a physical body, therefore, obscured the complexity of meanings inscribed on a social body.

In normalising the discourse, the *exaggerators* also disrupted their own constructions of 'the teacher' and were often not able to sustain the process or the knowledge produced in a 'stable' way. Instances of teachers 'turning back' on themselves were evident when they objectified, itemised or 'dismembered' the body, or in their use of analogies to elicit information about sexual acts. The latter was often produced in ways that reduced or subverted the associated sexual meaning. Teachers normalised the private in ways that enabled them to, albeit temporarily, maintain a 'stable identity' and, in so doing, conceal aspects of their troubling identities. Their actions resulted in a rupture in the process and the intended outcome of teaching and learning. Instead, they established a discursive space in which multiple meanings could be attributed to the content as well as the 'invoked' teacher identity. Interestingly and conversely, these teachers were also the most adventurous in their behaviour. While normalising the discourse concealed aspects of their identity, the importance of their exercising agency to invoke a sexed body in the classroom cannot be underestimated. As I stated in Chapter 10, and as those who were attempting to adhere to the new curriculum requirements, these teachers had few resources to draw on to make a new teacher identity. This notwithstanding, they invoked the sexual body, being fully aware of what was at stake.

The *normalisers,* on the other hand, called upon a 'mindful' body as well as the authority of the text to produce a 'stable' teacher identity. Adherence to the 'official' text reduced the discourse about sexuality and HIV/AIDS to information that rational and logical minds process with the purpose of fulfilling the outcome of schooling: namely, passing an examination. In so doing, this group normalised the discourse as an outcome of schooling. In other words, applying the 'inherent' logic of the text and presenting it as coherent, itemized and sequenced, resulted in teachers' producing the 'official' content with the unintended consequence of its being perceived as information for the examination only. Its intended value and utility, namely, as providing information that would lead to learners' making informed sexual choices, were subverted and minimised through the performative strips of behaviour exhibited by teachers (Schechner, 1985).

The assumption that tasks or the content possessed an inherent logic also resulted in teachers being able to distance themselves from the content. Exercising their agency as 'the experts' who presented information in a logical way offered a glimpse of how these teachers 'turn back' on themselves in ways that concealed aspects of their identity, for example as conservative or fundamental Christians who actually did not believe in some of the aspects of the curriculum they were required to teach. These teachers drew on what was familiar in their past to produce, relatively intact, their established teacher identity and a conventional kind of learning outcome. The performative behaviours teachers produced reinforced the use of information as an outcome of schooling rather than something that had utility beyond the examinations or beyond the classroom. Performative teaching in this regard offered fewer possibilities than did the teaching of the previous group for the insertion of a more nuanced discourse on sexuality and HIV/AIDS. Importantly, too, these sets of behaviours foreclosed rather than ruptured classroom discourse, even though the opportunity to do the latter arose. The exercise of agency by teachers here reinstated their authority as producers of the mainly 'official' or 'expected' message.

The *framers,* in relying on the authority of 'the teacher' to invoke an 'ideal' teacher identity, also normalised the discourse through calling on the official discourse of schooling. However, unlike in the case of the normalisers, classroom discourse in this instance was framed through the use of the authority invested in calling up 'the teacher'. Normalisation here operated on two levels. First, teachers presented themselves and their sets of behaviours as normal. In other words, it was the duty of teachers to frame and demarcate what was or was not important and what was to be privileged in the classroom. Secondly and similarly to the previous group, teachers normalised the content through reference to its importance for assessment purposes. The consequence of these sets of behaviours was classrooms in which learners, for the most part, listened and 'agreed.' It was clear in teachers' behaviours that their power rested in the authoritative. For example, they defined 'difficult' words and explained them in a way devoid of the everyday or more complex social meanings attached to them. These words were often packaged in a way that created a separation between the 'official' and their everyday meaning, a process often embedded in discourses on assessment. The upshot of this was that teachers were able to disregard the social meaning and the more complex issues associated with the content and 'get on' with the task of 'teaching'. Any potential to rupture and expand the discussion outside 'the expected' or privileged bits of knowledge was, therefore, not possible.

The *binders* normalised the discourse through invoking tacit knowledge and through relying on the historicity of 'the teacher'. As males, they recognised and were aware of what was at stake and thus either trivialised the content or bound it through producing certain rules and regulations. They invoked particular patterns of teacherly behaviour that had the appearance of the familiar but were in actuality far removed from these. While there was an attempt to adhere to the requirements of the new curriculum through applying collaborative pedagogical processes, these were a masquerade for something else. The familiar manifested itself through teachers' following a process whereby they introduced the lesson with a question, 'encouraged' discussion amongst learners, obtained responses but ignored these and offered learners instead the 'correct' book definition on the board. Learners offered ample opportunity for the insertion of a physical and sexualized body into the discourse in these classes. But teachers subverted this in favour of a discourse that positioned them as knowledgeable. The outcome of this was the production of a relatively stable teacher position, 'the knowledgeable one', with the outcome of learning entrenching rather than subverting the dominant discourses of masculinity and sexuality operating in these deeply gendered discursive spaces (as outlined in Chapter 10).

The beginning: the researcher and the performative

Situating teachers as the locus of inquiry in this study brought four issues together that this work examined: (a) descriptions, constructions and interpretations of the pandemic; (b) understanding the disease beyond its effect on an individual, biologized body; (c) researching the social construction and material effects of the pandemic; and (d) examining the type of empirical questions researchers asked, particularly as they related to education in general and to teachers and their work in particular. In positioning teachers as the embodiment of structures and, as such, carriers *and* mediators, there was an attempt to expand current epistemological paradigms to include frameworks that insert more hermeneutic ways of understanding HIV/AIDS discourse and its articulation in classrooms. This was done through examining the nexus between teacher identity and classroom practice, on the premise that teachers operate within complex situated contexts that not merely produce them but to which they contribute. Second, such a focus on teachers offered the possibility of redefining schools as charged environments where structures and agents operate in complex ways to produce particular subject positions.

This study analysed ways in which Lifeskills classrooms serve as a discursive space for the production of particular teacher identities. It demonstrated how in the complex interplay between mediator and mediated, teachers not only act to produce but also are produced through iterative acts of teacherly behaviour (Butler, 1990). The evidence suggests that while this field of practice is regulated by deeply gendered, raced and classed apparatuses that often act as constraints, teachers take up positions, make choices and act to produce subject positions that are contingent. Their teacher identities are not formed through an adherence to a single or dominant signifier such as race, ethnicity, religion, class or gender. In other words, they do not call up the teacher through a singular or dominant marker of their identity. Rather they choose and take up positions, always conscious of what is at stake. As the teachers in this study demonstrated, what they choose to foreground in the moment of instantiation is more often than not, not the whole story. It is in the performative that they concealed aspects of their identity, which in the narratives, they had proposed as either important or troubling.

I advance the argument that these performative enactments are transformative. They are therefore never complete and thus cannot be reified. The corollary to this, and to make an epistemological argument, one cannot use reductionist, scientific, rational orientations to understand what happens in the complex space of a Lifeskills classroom where the public and private collide and animate the fragility of teacher identities. In the same vein, one cannot make simplistic associations between knowledge and practice or between knowledge and learning outcome. As this work demonstrated, Lifeskills classrooms are a discursive site for the production of troubling rather than stable teacher identities, leaving the message open and the messenger free to take up the position that is best suited for 'the moment.' Assuming that schools are the best repositories for the mediation of safe and safer sex messages, and that the mediated knowledge will potentially lead to a change in sexual behaviour, therefore, is simplistic. Bryant *et al.* put it succinctly when they state that classrooms are 'practiced' spaces where a host of intersecting discourses compete, "a site in which diverse beings come together in order to engage and negotiate knowledge, systems of understanding, and ways of being, seeing, knowing, and doing" (2005: 3). This negotiation is not random but performative.

Implications of teachers teaching about sexuality and HIV/AIDS

While they are not conclusive, it is important nevertheless briefly to describe the implications this work has for initial teacher training as well as for ongoing professional development.

Curriculum requirements notwithstanding, teachers bring themselves to the classroom, and learning outcomes, however these are measured, are hugely influenced by this. First, therefore, training teachers to teach about sexuality and HIV/AIDS requires an on-going dialogue about how such content invokes aspects of teachers' identities that they are usually not required to call up in the public space of the classroom. Often, as this study showed, teachers can conceal these aspects in ways that have unintentional consequences for the process and outcome of mediation. Encouraging this dialogue is important if teachers are to consider the outcomes of teaching about sexuality and HIV/AIDS as reaching beyond fulfilling externally driven outcomes, and towards changing learners' sexual behaviour or, at the very least, decisions they make about their sexual practices.

Second, and related to the above, addressing the issue of HIV/AIDS within South Africa where certain cultural practices, religious traditions, and socio-political realities exist, is highly sensitive. It thus becomes important to assist those who teach such sensitive subjects to develop their own levels of comfort around these topics and become sensitized about what they might be doing (perhaps due to lack of awareness, personal discomfort, or a host of reasons already articulated in this work) that is inhibiting their learners' opportunities to develop into critical thinkers pertaining to issues of sexuality and engage in healthy sexual behavior. Important, too, would be providing learners with a forum where they can more openly discuss sexual behaviour and sexual choices without being quickly 'shut-down', or re-focused in another direction, or given the 'official' answers, or in some way having their exploration of these issues 'foreclosed'. Indeed, this would seem an essential step in addressing the HIV/AIDS pandemic in South Africa.

Thoughts to ponder

This work is not complete and, therefore I do not offer a conclusion or a set of conclusive (or decisive) recommendations. Rather, I offer points to ponder.

The teacher research analysed in Part IV pointed to the use of teacher history and teacher subject positioning to understand how teachers can produce better learning outcomes in the classroom. I ended that section by proposing the use of an alternative epistemological orientation that I later applied in this work. Such a stance accounted for teachers as active agents who are not only constituted by, but who also contribute to making 'the teacher' and teaching. Such an orientation, as this work demonstrated, offered the possibility of bringing together interrelated issues that have not received attention in research in the way this work has proposed, namely, examining the intricacy in the relationship between structure and agency as it plays out in teachers' work on sexuality and HIV/AIDS.

The application of this alternative epistemology in this study emphasized two broad issues that I propose as points for further investigation. The first relates to how teacher agency is regularly depicted in teacher research, namely, as the ability to *change* teacher behaviour to produce 'expected' learning outcomes. The questions that arise from this work relate to what happens when the outcomes are open to multiple interpretations. What are the messages children actually hear? How do they make meaning of the intended and unintended messages?

At another level, teacher agency in this study was also translated as the ability teachers have to produce or reproduce outcomes that challenge racial, gendered or classed identities. But what happens when the application of these categories does not serve to reveal what actually happens in schools and classrooms? As was the case in this study, it would have been easy to use the deeply gendered, ethnic, racial and classed profile of these teachers to frame the analysis, particularly given their political and social history. However, such an approach would have obscured the complexity of their lives and the discursive spaces where they make meaning of their lives. This notwithstanding, it was surprising that these constructs did not manifest as more significant than others. This points to the second issue that like this work illuminates, namely, questions about the use of broad sociological constructs to explain identity and difference. At one level, like the sociologists I used to frame this work, I too invoked these constructs to take up a position. At another level, it was through rupturing them that another side of the story was revealed. One can, therefore, not ignore their utility, but finding the points of rupture as this work did, sheds light on another part of the story even though it, too, is not complete. The questions that arise, therefore, are both conceptual and epistemological. How can we claim to know what actually happens in classrooms when and if we subscribe, first, to dominant epistemological orientations, and second, to regularly invoked sociological constructs?

Appendices

Appendix A: Employment Status

Table 6a: Employment Status: Western Cape

	Bloukoop	Gapeng	Gracious Heights	Joseph Rhodes	Stanton
Employed	28 802	18 834	10 165	6 589	7 833
Unemployed	9 490	19 789	1 260	3 051	1 167
Not economically active	16 455	17 995	4 723	6 247	5 023

Table 6b: Employment Status: Mpumalanga

	Nyalunga	Mapagama	Elangeni	Thokoza
Employed	2 618	2 258	2 347	1 648
Unemployed	2 632	1 850	1 940	1 283
Not economically active	4 166	3 667	2 886	1 231

Appendix B: Highest Level of Education

Table 7a: Highest Level of Education: Western Cape

	Bloukoop	Gapeng	Gracious Heights	Joseph Rhodes	Stanton
No schooling	5 402	6 330	919	1 298	699
Grade 7/Standard 5	4 609	5 339	1 162	2 354	1 230
Grade 9/std 7/form 2	4 908	6 142	1 755	2 606	1 711
Grade 12/std/form 5/matric	16 103	12 285	5 422	2 872	4 360
Bachelor's Degree	776	451	128	29	185
Honour's Degree	369	81	37	8	62
Higher Degree (master's or Doctorate)	291	76	31	–	43

Table 7b: Highest Level of Education: Mpumalanga

	Nyalunga	Mapagama	Elangeni	Thokoza
No schooling	3 007	2 059	1 781	1 124
Grade 7/Standard 5	1 267	983	874	437
Grade 9/std 7/form 2	937	750	724	372
Grade 12/std/form 5/matric	1 431	1 573	1 343	706
Bachelor's Degree	10	13	10	–
Honour's Degree	6	5	8	
Higher Degree (master's or Doctorate)	–	3	–	–

Appendix C: Annual Household Income

Table 8a: Annual Household Income: Western Cape

	Bloukoop	Gapeng	Gracious Heights	Joseph Rhodes	Stanton
No income	3 200	4 348	244	347	184
R1 – R4 800	587	955	53	89	58
R4 801 – R 9 600	1 407	282	138	465	319
R9 601 – R19 200	2 599	3 959	279	813	458
R19 201 – R38 400	2 897	3 751	648	1 324	911
R38 401 – R76 800	3 569	2 310	1 613	1 268	1 446
R76 801 – R153 600	4 141	906	2 045	475	1 150
R153 601 – R307 200	2 906	209	758	83	462
R307 201 – R614 400	557	49	116	17	65
R614 401 – R1 228 800	95	14	41	26	13
R1 228 801 – R2 457 600	73	30	18	19	11
R2 457 601 and more	28	19	5	6	9

Table 8b: Annual Household Income: Mpumalanga

	Nyalunga	Mapagama	Elangeni	Thokoza
No income	575	385	214	391
R1 – R4 800	568	370	285	126
R4 801 – R 9 600	973	670	667	316
R9 601 – R19 200	907	728	735	437
R19 201 – R38 400	47	476	481	343
R38 401 – R76 800	143	175	166	133
R76 801 – R153 600	46	42	40	19
R153 601 – R307 200	7	7	10	4
R307 201 – R614 400	4	6	–	–
R614 401 – R1 228 800	–	–	–	–
R1 228 801 – R2 457 600	–	4	–	–
R2 457 601 and more	–	–	3	–

Appendix D: Occupation by Geography

Table 9a: Occupation by Geography: Western Cape

	Bloukoop	Gapeng	Gracious Heights	Joseph Rhodes	Stanton
Legislators, Senior officials & managers	2 196	364	629	164	484
Professionals	267	614	698	119	540
Technicians and associate professor	3 751	1 318	1 716	41	1 111
Clerks	4 713	1 939	2 372	1 074	1 589
Service workers, shop & market sales	2 750	2 381	1 063	646	874
Skilled agricultural and fishery workers	247	10	27	25	34
Craft and related trade workers	3 071	1 612	1 247	1 073	1 223
Plant and machine operators	1 481	1 296	663	1 240	540
Elementary occupations	6 059	6 216	659	1 255	901
Not economically active	25 945	37 784	5 983	9 298	6 190

Table 9b: Occupation by Geography: Mpumalanga

	Nyalunga	Mapagama	Elangeni	Thokoza
Legislators, Senior officials & managers	48	39	68	11
Professionals	51	73	59	23
Technicians and associate professor	146	136	166	47
Clerks	182	172	174	109
Service workers, shop & market sales	284	279	282	138
Skilled agricultural and fishery workers	38	35	19	21
Craft and related trade workers	544	430	489	294
Plant and machine operators	231	270	250	222
Elementary occupations	1 040	702	811	611
Not economically active	6 798	5 517	4 826	2 513

Appendix E: Type of Housing Unit

Table 10a: Type of Housing Unit: Western Cape

	Bloukoop	Gapeng	Gracious Heights	Joseph Rhodes	Stanton
House or brick on separate structure	11 239	8 017	5 595	3 613	3 980
Traditional structure or hut	625	268	44	99	76
Flat in block of flats	1 720	606	10	3	353
Town/cluster/semi-detached house	856	320	60	441	139
House/flat in backward	342	419	122	121	322
Informal dwelling/shack in backyard	1 923	1 103	16	576	99
Informal dwelling/shack not in backyard	5 000	6 119	33	12	33
Room/flat not in backyard	120	195	33	31	47
Caravan or tent	75	113	6	3	13

Table 10b: Type of Housing Unit: Mpumalanga

	Nyalunga	Mapagama	Elangeni	Thokoza
House or brick on separate structure	3 179	2 162	2 357	1 140
Traditional structure/dwelling or hut	249	252	104	102
Flat in block of flats	88	60	5	4
Town/cluster/semi-detached house	12	12	3	3
House/flat/room in backward	12	22	26	40
Informal dwelling/shack in backyard	35	28	25	74
Informal dwelling/shack not in backyard	53	103	102	308
Room/flatlet not in backyard	20	144	170	70
Caravan or tent	–	5	–	–

Appendix F: Toilet facilities

Table 11a: Toilet Facilities: Western Cape

	Bloukoop	Gapeng	Gracious Heights	Joseph Rhodes	Stanton
Flush Toilet (connected to sewage)	18 618	12 128	5 857	4 618	4 962
Flush Toilet (with septic tank)	733	276	12	115	11
Chemical Toilet	25	52		4	4
Pit Latrine with ventilation	43	61	4	3	
Pit Latrine without ventilation	26	174	18	14	4
Bucket latrine	874	5677	5	102	23
None	1 745	667	62	83	86

Table 11b: Toilet Facilities: Mpumalanga

	Nyalunga	Mapagama	Elangeni	Thokoza
Flush Toilet (connected to sewage)	48	145	56	1 050
Flush Toilet (with septic tank)	34	54	28	53
Chemical Toilet	131	11	7	–
Pit Latrine with ventilation	602	235	118	–
Pit Latrine without ventilation	2 525	2 189	2 423	189
Bucket latrine	20	33	16	202
None	313	195	155	256

Appendix G: Main Water Supply

Table 12a: Main Water Supply: Western Cape

	Bloukoop	Gapeng	Gracious Heights	Joseph Rhodes	Stanton
Piped water inside dwelling	13 197	8 544	5 620	3 811	4 650
Piped water inside yard	4 332	3 281	132	847	155
Piped water on community stand	2 271	3 217	65	30	84
Piped water on community stand	1 832	3 672	129	214	172
Borehole	16	–	–	4	–
Dam/pool/stagnant water	9	–	3	–	5
River/stream	–	3	–	–	–
Water Vendor	7	8	–	–	5

Table 12b: Main Water Supply: Mpumalanga

	Nyalunga	Mapagama	Elangeni	Thokoza
Piped water inside dwelling	108	88	98	16
Piped water inside yard	190	1 456	2 168	1 073
Piped water on community stand: dis	619	497	261	175
Piped water on community stand: dis	734	593	227	366
Borehole	3	11	–	–
Dam/pool/stagnant water	–	29	–	–
River/Stream	8	32	–	–
Water Vendor	–	3	–	7

Appendix H: Energy Source of Cooking and Lighting

Table 13a: Energy Source for Cooking: Western Cape

	Bloukoop	Gapeng	Gracious Heights	Joseph Rhodes	Stanton
Electricity	15 775	11 574	5 876	4 760	4 887
Gas	498	384	42	107	151
Paraffin	5 523	6 641	4	42	18
Wood	72	72	28	8	17
Coal	69	110	3	3	6
Animal Dung	55	133	–	7	4
Solar	31	71	3	7	–

Table 13b: Energy Source for Cooking: Mpumalanga

	Nyalunga	Mapagama	Elangeni	Thokoza
Electricity	1 551	1 563	1 705	403
Gas	85	43	75	31
Paraffin	1 151	729	885	487
Wood	830	493	113	61
Coal	28	8	13	747
Animal Dung	5	11	7	11
Solar	10	3	–	3

Table 14a: Energy Source for Lighting: Western Cape

	Bloukoop	Gapeng	Gracious Heights	Joseph Rhodes	Stanton
Electricity					
Gas					
Paraffin					
Wood					
Coal					
Animal Dung					
Solar					

Table 14b: Energy Source for Lighting: Mpumlanga

	Nyalunga	Mapagama	Elangeni	Thokoza
Electricity	2 458	2 020	2 128	1 274
Gas	3	7	10	3
Paraffin	442	214	202	98
Candles	753	604	458	368
Solar	3	8	–	3
Other	15	10	3	5

Appendix I: Mode of Travel to School or Work

Table 15a: Mode of Transport: Western Cape

	Bloukoop	Gapeng	Gracious Heights	Joseph Rhodes	Stanton
Not applicable	31 374	38 373	6 859	11 614	7 757
On foot	14 805	16 727	2 483	5 212	2 803
By bicycle	459	221	69	212	87
By motorcycle	300	102	35	39	32
By car as a driver	12 045	1 052	3 769	1 066	2 920
By car as a passenger	9 190	2 824	4 041	1 444	2 869
By minibus/taxi	4 499	5 983	2 967	1 728	2 101
By bus	848	3 424	3 045	585	525
By train	4 158	11 220	397	1 803	985
Other	324	356	284	83	79

Table 15b: Mode of Transport: Mpumalanga

	Nyalunga	Mapagama	Elangeni	Thokoza
Not applicable	8 022	5 924	537	2 992
On foot	5 955	5 078	4 522	2 140
By bicycle	16	24	7	41
By motorcycle	8	20	7	5
By car as a driver	143	151	117	106
By car as a passenger	98	137	52	274
By minibus/taxi	466	340	437	679
By bus	1 785	1 179	1 556	140
By train	15	12	15	4
Other	25	11	3	12

List of References

Acker, S. 1989. Ed. *Teachers, gender and careers.* Lewes: Falmer Press.

Aggleton, P., Davies, P. & Hart, G. 1989. *Social representations, social practices.* New York: Falmer Press.

Aggleton, P., Davies, P. & Hart, G. 1993. *AIDS: facing the second decade.* New York: Falmer Press.

Akoulouze, R., Rugalema, G. & Khanye, V. 2001. *Taking stock of promising approaches in HIV/AIDS and education in sub-Saharan Africa: what works, why and how.* [Online]. Available: http://www.adea.org/ [2003, February 20].

Aleman, G. 2005. Constructing gay performances: regulating gay youth in a „gay friendly" high school. In *Performance theories in education: power, pedagogy and the politics of identity.* Edited by B.K. Alexander, G.L. Andersen & B.P. Gallegos. New Jersey: Lawrence Erlbaum Associates. 149–171.

Alexander, B.K., Andersen, G.L. & Gallegos, B.P. Eds. 2005. *Performance theories in education: power, pedagogy and the politics of identity.* New Jersey: Lawrence Erlbaum Associates.

Althusser, L. 1971. *Lenin and philosophy and other essays.* Translated from the French by Brewster, B. London: New Left Books.

Andersen, N. Å. 2003. *Discursive analytical strategies: understanding Foucault, Koselleck, Laclau, Luhmann.* Bristol, UK: Policy Press.

Babbie, E., Mouton, J., Payze, C., Vorster, J., Boshoff, N. & Prozesky, H. 2001. *The practice of social research.* Oxford: Oxford University Press.

Bailey, P. 2002. Parasexuality and glamour: the victorian barmaid as cultural prototype. In *Sexualities in history: a reader.* Edited by K.M. Phillips & B. Reay. New York: Routledge. 222–246.

Ball, S.J. & Goodson, I.F. Eds. 1985. *Teachers' lives and careers.* London: The Falmer Press.

Ballenger, C. Ed. 2004. *Regarding children's words: teacher research on language and literacy: Brookline teacher researcher seminar.* New York: Teachers College Press.

Barbour, R.S. & Huby, G. Eds. 1998. *Meddling with mythology AIDS and the social construction of knowledge.* London: Routledge.

Barnett, T. & Whiteside, A. 2002. *AIDS in the twenty-first century: disease and globalization.* Basingstoke, Hants.: Palgrave Macmillan.

Baxen, J. & Breidlid, A. 2004. Researching HIV/AIDS and education in sub-Saharan Africa: examining the gaps and challenges. *Journal of education* 34: 9–29.

Baxen, J. & Gilmour, D. 2001. *GTZ/PEI-WCED. Baseline survey on some schools in the Western Cape.* Cape Town: GTZ.

Baxen, J. 2005. What questions? HIV/AIDS educational research: beyond more of the same to asking different epistemological questions. *UWC papers in education* 3: 58–63.

Bennel, P. 2003. *Telling it how it is? The UNAIDS 2003 update on the aids epidemic in sub-Saharan Africa.* Mimeo. (Unpublished).

Benyon, J. 1985. Institutional change and career histories in a comprehensive school. In *Teachers' lives and careers.* Edited by S.J. Ball & I.F. Goodson. London: Falmer Press. 1–26.

Birke, L. 1999. *Feminism and the biological body.* New Brunswick: Rutgers University Press.

Bhaktin, M.M. & Voloshinov, V.N. 1986. *Marxism and the philosophy of language.* Cambridge, MA: Harvard University Press.

Bloom, B.S. 1968. *Learning to master.* ERIC Document Reproduction Service No. ED 053419.

Bloom, B.S. 1976. *Human characteristics and school learning.* New York: McGraw-Hill.

Bloomberg, C. 1993. *The effectiveness of life skills project enhancing self-concept and self-empowerment.* Psychology Honours Research Project. Cape Town: University of Cape Town. (Unpublished).

Blumenberg, H. 1983. *The legitimacy of the modern age.* Cambridge, MA: MIT Press. (Original work published in 1966).

Bondi, L., Avis, H., Bankey, R., Bingley, A., Davidson, J., Duffy, R. et al. 2002. *Subjectivities, knowledges, and feminist geographies: the subjects and ethics of social research.* Lanham: Rowman & Littlefield Publishers.

Bourdieu, P. 1977. *Outline of a theory of practice.* Cambridge: Cambridge University Press.

Bourdieu, P. 1984. *Distinction: a social critique of the judgment of taste.* Translated from the French by Nice, R. Cambridge, MA: Harvard University Press.

Bourdieu, P. 1986. The forms of capital. In *Handbook of theory and research for the sociology of education.* Edited by J.G. Richardson. New York: Greenwood.

Bourdieu, P. 1990. *The logic of practice.* Translated from the French by Nice, R. Stanford: Stanford University Press.

Bourdieu, P. 1991. *Language and symbolic power.* Translated from the French by Raymond, G. & Adamson, M. Cambridge, MA: Harvard University Press.

Bourdieu, P. & Coleman, J.S. Eds. 1991. *Social theory for a changing society.* Boulder: Westview Press & New York: Russell Sage Foundation.

Bourdieu, P. 1992. *The logic of practice.* Cambridge: Polity Press. (Original work published in 1980).

Bourdieu, P. 2000. *Pascalian meditations.* Translated from the French by Nice, R. Cambridge: Polity Press.

Bourdieu, P. & Wacquant, L.J.D. 1992. *An invitation to reflexive sociology.* Chicago: University of Chicago Press.

Buczekiewicz, M. & Carnegie, R. 2001. The Ugandan life skills initiative. *Health education* 101(1): 15–21.

Butler, J. 2004. *The Judith Butler reader.* Edited by Sara Salih with Judith Butler. Malden, MA.: Blackwell Publishing.

Burger, E. Ed. 2003. *South African yearbook 2003/04.* Pretoria: Government Communications.

Butler, J. 1997. *The psychic life of power: theories of subjection.* California: Stanford University Press.

Butler, J. 1993. *Bodies that matter: on the discursive limits of "sex"*. New York: Routledge.
Butler, J. 1990. *Gender trouble: feminism and subversion of identity*. New York: Routledge.
Butt, R., Raymond, D., McCue, G. & Yamagishi, L. 1992. Collaborative autobiography and the teacher's voice. In *Studying teachers' lives*. Edited by I. Goodson. London: Routledge. 51–98.
Calhoun, C., LiPuma, E. & Postone, M. Eds. 1993. *Bourdieu: critical perspectives*. Chicago: Polity Press.
Campbell, C., Foulis, C.A., Mainane, S. & Sibiya, Z. 2005. The impact of social environments on the effectiveness of youth HIV prevention: a South African case study. *AIDS care*. 17(4): 471–478.
Carr, W. & Kemmis, S. 1986. *Becoming critical*. Lewes: Falmer Press.
Carr, W. 1989. *Quality in teaching: arguments for a reflective profession*. Lewes: Falmer Press.
Carrim, N. 2003. Teacher identity: tension between roles. In *Changing patterns of teacher education in South Africa: policy, practice and prospects*. Edited by K. Lewin, M. Samuel & Y. Sayed. Sandton: Heinemann. 306–322.
Carson, T.R. & Sumara, D.J. Eds. 1997. *Action research as a living practice*. New York: Peter Lang.
Cassell, P. Ed.1993. *The Giddens reader*. California: Stanford University Press.
Cheal, D. 2005. *Dimensions of social theory*. Basingstoke, New York: Palgrave Macmillan.
Christie, P. 1986. *The right to learn*. Johannesburg: Sached/Ravan Press.
Cicourel, A.V. 1993. Aspects of structural and processual theories of knowledge. In *Bourdieu: critical perspectives*. Edited by C. Calboun, E. Lipuma & M. Postone. Cambridge: Polity Press. 89–115.
Cohen, L., Manion, L. & Morrison. K. 2000. *Research methods in education*. 5th ed. London: Routledge/Falmer.
Cohen, D. 2002. HIV and education in sub-Saharan Africa: responding to the impact. *Perspectives in education* 20(2): 13–23.
Con Davis, R. & Schleifer, R. 1994. *Contemporary literary criticism: literary and cultural studies*. New York: Longman.
Coombe, C. 2000. *Managing the impact of HIV/AIDS on the education sector*. [Online]. Available: http://www.harare.unesco.org/hivaids/webfiles/Electronic%20Versions/Coombe%20Impact%20South%20Africa.doc [2006, August 14].
Creswell, J. W. 1994. *Research design: qualitative & quantitative approaches*. Thousand Oaks: Sage Publications.
Crewe, M. 2002. Reflections on the South African HIV/AIDS epidemic. *Society in transition* 33(3): 446–454.
Daniel Tatum, B. 1997. *"Why are all the black kids sitting together in the cafeteria" and other conversations about race*. New York: Basic Books.
Davenport, T.R.H. & Saunders, C. 2000. *South Africa: A modern history*. Basingstoke, Hampshire: Macmillan.
Delanty, G. 1999. *Social theory in a changing world: concepts of modernity*. Cambridge: Polity Press.
Denzin, N.K. & Lincoln, Y.S. Eds. 1994. *Handbook of qualitative research*. Thousand Oaks, California: Sage Publications.

Denzin, N.K. & Lincoln, Y.S. 1998a. *Collecting and interpreting qualitative materials.* London: Sage Publications.

Denzin, N.K. & Lincoln, Y.S. Eds. 1998b. *The landscape of qualitative research: theories and issues.* Thousand Oaks, California: Sage Publications.

Department of Education. 2002. *Revised national curriculum statement grades R-9 (schools): Tirisano.* Pretoria. [Online]. Available: http://www.education.gov.za [2006, August 10].

Department of Health. 2003. *Summary report: national HIV and syphilis antenatal sero-prevalence survey: 2002.* Pretoria: Department of Health.

Dodd, N. 1999. *Social theory and modernity.* Cambridge: Polity Press.

Dorrington, R.E., Bradshaw, D. & Budlender, D. 2002. *HIV/AIDS profile in the provinces of South Africa-indicators for 2002.* Cape Town: Centre for Actuarial Research, Medical Research Council and the Actuarial Society of South Africa.

Dubose Brunner, D. 1994. *Inquiry and reflection: framing narrative practice in education.* Albany: State University of New York Press.

Durkheim, E. 2001. *The elementary forms of religious life.* Translated from the French by Cosman, C. Oxford: Oxford University Press.

Durkheim. E. 1952. *Suicide: a study in sociology.* Translated from the French by Spaulding, J.A. & Simpson, G. New York: Free Press.

Eagleton, M. Ed. 2003. *A concise companion to feminist theory.* Oxford: Blackwell Publishing.

Epstein, D. & Johnson, R. 1998. *Schooling sexualities.* Buckingham: Open University Press.

Edelsky, C. Ed. 1999. *Making justice our project.* Urbana, Illinois: National Council of Teachers of English.

Eisner, E.W. 1985. *The art of educational evaluation: a personal view.* Lewes: Falmer Press.

Eisner, E.W. 1993. Forms of understanding and the future of educational research. *Educational researcher* 22(7): 5–11.

Eisner, E.W. 1995. What artistically crafted research can help us understand about schools. *Educational theory* 45(1): 1–6.

Fishman, S.M. & McCarthy, L. Eds. 2000. *Unplayed tapes: a personal history of collaborative teacher research.* Illinois: National Council of Teachers of English.

Foucault, M. 1976. *The archaeology of knowledge.* Translated from the French by Sheridan Smith, A.M. New York: Harper & Row.

Foucault, M. 1978. *The history of sexuality: an introduction. Vol. 1.* New York: Random House.

Foucault, M. 1989a. *The order of things: an archaeology of the human sciences.* London: Tavistock/Routledge.

Foucault, M. 1989b. *The birth of the clinic: an archaeology of medical perception.* London: Routledge.

Fraenkel, J.R. & Wallen, N.E. 1993. *How to design and evaluate research in education.* Boston: McGraw-Hill.

Gallant, M. & Maticka-Tyndale, E. 2003. School-based HIV prevention programmes for African youth. *Social science & medicine.* 58(7): 1337–1351.

Gallegos, B.P. 2005. Performing school in the shadow of imperialism: a hybrid (Coyote) interpretation. In *Performance theories in education: power, pedagogy and the politics of identity*. Edited by B.K. Alexander, G.L. Anderson & B.P. Gallegos. New Jersey: Lawrence Erlbaum Associates. 107–126.

Giddens, A. 1982. *Profiles and critiques in social theory*. Berkeley: University of California Press.

Giddens, A. 1984. *The constitution of society: outline of the theory of structuration*. Berkeley: University of California Press.

Giddens, A. 1987. *Social theory and modern sociology*. California: Stanford University Press.

Giddens, A. 1990. *Consequences of modernity*. Cambridge: Polity Press.

Giddens, A. 1991. *Modernity and self identity*. Cambridge: Polity Press.

Goffman, E. 1959. *The presentation of self in everyday life*. New York: Doubleday Anchor Books.

Goffman, E. 1973. *The presentation of self in everyday life*. Woodstock, NY: Overlook Press.

Goodman, D.J. 2000. *Promoting diversity and social justice: educating people from privileged groups*. Thousand Oaks, California: Sage Publications.

Goodson, I.F. 1991. Sponsoring the teacher's voice. *Cambridge journal of education* 21(1): 35–45.

Goodson, I. F. 1992. *Studying teachers' lives*. London: Routledge.

Green, L. 1998. *Narratives of cognitive development: some South African primary teachers stories*. PhD Thesis: University of Exeter. (Unpublished).

Halfpenny, P. 1979. The analysis of qualitative data. *Sociological review* 27: 799–823.

Hall, S. 1990. Cultural identity and diaspora. In *Identity: community, culture, difference*. Edited by J. Rutherford. London: Lawrence & Wishart. 222–237.

Hall, S. & du Gay, P. Eds. 1996. *Questions of cultural identity*. London: Sage Publishers.

Hammersley, M. & Atkinson, P. 1995. *Ethnography: principles in practice*. 2nd ed. London: Tavistock.

Hammersley, M. Ed. 1999. *Researching school experience: ethnographic studies of teaching and learning*. London: Falmer Press.

Hargreaves, A. 1994. *Changing teachers, changing times*. London: Cassell.

Harrison, A., Xaba, N., Kunene, P. & Ntuli, N. 2001. Understanding young women's risk for HIV/AIDS: adolescent sexuality and vulnerability in rural KwaZulu/Natal. *Society in transition* 32(1): 69–78.

Hartell, C.G. 2005. HIV/AIDS in South Africa: A review of sexual behaviour among adolescents. *Adolescence* 40(157): 171–181.

Hartman, H.J. & Glasgow, N.A. 2002. *Tips for the science teacher: research-based strategies to help students learn*. Thousand Oaks: Corwin Press.

Hartshorne, K.B. 1992. *Crisis and challenge: black education 1910–1990*. Cape Town: Oxford University Press.

Hechter, M. & Horne, C. 2003. *Theories of social order: a reader*. California: Stanford University Press.

Hekman, S. Ed. 1996. *Feminist interpretations of Michel Foucault*. Pennsylvania: The Pennsylvania State University Press.

Hetherington, K. 1998. *Expressions of identity: space, performance and politics.* London: Sage Publications.
Hopson, B. & Scally, M. 1981. *Lifeskills teaching.* London: McGraw-Hill.
Irvine, J.M. 2003. The sociologist as voyeur: social theory and sexuality research, 1910–1978. *Qualitative sociology* 26(4): 429–456.
Jagodzinski, J. Ed. 2002. *Pedagogical desire: authority, seduction, transference, and the question of ethics.* Connecticut: Bergin & Garvey.
Jansen, J. Ed. 1991. *Knowledge and power in South Africa.* Braamfontein: Skotaville.
Johnson, S. 2000. The impact of AIDS on the education sector in South Africa. *Presentation to the IIEP meeting on the impact of HIV/AIDS on education.* 27–29 September 2000. Paris.
Kaaya, S.G., Mukoma, W., Flisher, A.J. & Klepp, K.I. 2002. School-based sexual health initiatives in sub-Saharan Africa: a review. *Social dynamics* 28: 64–88.
Kalipeni, E., Craddock, S., Oppeng, J.R. & Ghosh, J. 2004. *HIV and AIDS in Africa: beyond epidemiology.* Victoria: Blackwell Publishing.
Kelly, M.J. 2000. *Planning in the context of HIV/AIDS.* UNESCO, Paris: International Institute for Educational Planning.
Kelly, K. & Parker, W. 2000. *Communities of practice: contextual mediators of youth response to HIV/AIDS. Beyond awareness campaign report.* Pretoria: Department of Health.
Kelly, K. 2000. *Communicating for action: a contextual evaluation of youth responses to HIV/AIDS. Sentinel site monitoring and evaluation project report.* Pretoria: Department of Health.
Kelly, M. 2002. Preventing HIV transmission through education. *Perspectives in education* 20(2): 1–12.
Kimmel, M.S. & Plante, R.F. Eds. 2004. *Sexualities: identities, behaviours and society.* New York: Oxford University Press.
Krais, B. Ed. 1991. *The craft of sociology: epistemological preliminaries.* Translated from the French by Nice, R. New York: Walter de Gruyter.
Lacquer, T. 1990. *Making sex: body and gender from the Greeks to Freud.* Cambridge, MA: Harvard University Press.
LeClerc-Madlala, S. 2001a. Demonising women in the era of AIDS: on the relationship between cultural constructions of both HIV/AIDS and femininity. *Society in transition* 32(1): 38–46.
LeClerc-Madlala, S. 2001b. Virginity-testing: managing sexuality in a maturing HIV/AIDS epidemic. *Medical anthropology quarterly* 15(4): 533–552.
LeClerc-Madlala, S. 2002. *Youth, HIV/AIDS and the importance of sexual culture and context.* Centre for Social Science Research: Aids and Society Research Unit. UCT. [Online]. Available: http://web.uct.ac.za/depts/cssr/papers/wp9.pdf [2003, August 1].
Levine, S. & Ross, F. 2002. *Perceptions of and attitudes to HIV/ AIDS among young adults at the University of Cape Town.* Aids and Society Research Unit, Centre for Social Science Research. UCT. [Online]. Available: http://web.uct.ac.za/depts/cssr/papers/wp14.pdf [2003, August 1].
Lewin, K., Samuel, M. & Sayed, Y. Eds. 2003. *Changing patterns of teacher education in South Africa: policy, practice and prospects.* Sandton: Heinemann.

Lieblich, A., Tuval-Mashiach, R. & Zilber, T. 1998. *Narrative research: reading, analysis and interpretation.* London: Sage Publications.
Lyotard, J. 1984. The postmodern condition: a report on knowledge. Translated by Bennington, G. & Massouri, B. Minneapolis: University of Minneapolis Press. Quoted by B.K. Alexander, G.L. Anderson & B.P. Gallegos. Eds. 2005. *Performance theories in education: power, pedagogy and the politics of identity.* New Jersey: Lawrence Erlbaum Associates. 2.
Mackey, S. 1993. Emotion and cognition in arts education. *Curriculum studies* 1(2): 245–256.
MacKinnon, C.A. 1982. Feminism, Marxism, method, and the State: an agenda for theory. In *Feminist theory: a critique of ideology.* Edited by N.O. Keohane, M.Z. Rosaldo & B.C. Gelpi. Chicago: Chicago University Press. 1–30.
Maykut, P. & Morehouse, R. 1994. *Beginning qualitative research.* London: Falmer Press.
McCafferty, R. 2003. *HIV/AIDS, cultural values and media.* A paper prepared for the project, 'Schooling, Cultural Values and HIV/AIDS. Mimeo. (Unpublished).
McCormick, T.M. 1994. *Creating the non-sexist classroom: a multicultural approach.* New York: Teachers College Press.
McDowell, L. & Sharp, J. Eds. 1997. *Space, gender and knowledge.* Feminist readings. London: Arnold.
McElrath, K. Ed. 2002. *HIV and AIDS a global overview.* Connecticut: Greenwood Press.
McLaren, P. 2005. Forward. In *Performance theories in education: power, pedagogy and the politics of identity.* Edited by B.K. Alexander, G.L. Anderson & B.P. Gallegos. New Jersey: Lawrence Erlbaum Associates. xv–xix.
McLaren, P. 1991. Decentering culture: postmodernism, resistance and critical pedagogy. In *Current perspectives on the culture of schools.* Edited by N. Wyner. Brookline, MA: Brookline Books. 231–257.
McLean Donaldson, K.B. 1996. *Through students' eyes: combating racism in United States schools.* Westport, Connecticut: Praeger.
McNay, L. 1992. *Foucault and feminism: power, gender and the self.* Cambridge: Polity Press.
Meyers, E. & O'Connell Rust, F. Eds. 2003. *Taking action with teacher research.* Portsmouth: Heinemann.
Mirembe, R. 2002. AIDS and democratic education in Uganda. *Comparative education* 38(3): 291–303.
Mishler, E.G. 1990. Validation in inquiry-guided research: the role of exemplars in narrative studies. *Harvard educational review* 60: 415–441.
Moi, T. 2005. *Sex, gender and the body: the student edition of what is a woman*? New York: Oxford University Press.
Morrison, A. & McIntyre, D. 1969. *Teachers and teaching.* Baltimore: Penguin Books.
Morrison, A. & McIntyre, D. 1971. *Schools and socialization.* Harmondsworth: Penguin.
Mouton, J. 1996. *Understanding social research.* Pretoria: J.L. van Schaik.
Neito, S. 1994. Lessons from students on creating a chance to dream. *Harvard educational review* 64(4): 392–426.
Neuman, W. 2000. *Social research methods: qualitative and quantitative approaches.* 4th ed. Boston: Allyn and Bacon.
Nietzsche, F. 1966. *Beyond Good and Evil.* Translated by Kaufmann, W. New York: Vintage.

Nkomo, M.1990. *Pedagogy of domination.* Trenton: Africa World Press.

Nye, R.A. Ed. 1999. *Sexuality.* Oxford: Oxford University Press.

Parker, R. & Gagnon, J.H. Eds. 1995. *Conceiving sexualities: approaches to sex research in a postmodern world.* New York: Routledge.

Peltzer, K. 2000. Knowledge and attitudes about HIV/AIDS of a sample of school teachers in South Africa. *Psychological reports* 87: 1065–1066.

Peltzer, K. & Promtussananon, S. 2003. HIV/AIDS education in South Africa: teacher knowledge about HIV/AIDS: teacher attitude about and control of HIV/AIDS education. *Social behaviour and personality* 31(4): 349–356.

Phillips, K.M. & Reay, B. Eds. 2002. *Sexualities in history: a reader.* New York: Routledge.

Pinar, W.F. 1994. *Autobiography, politics and sexuality: essays in curriculum theory 1972–1992.* New York: Peter Lang.

Pollock, D. 1998. Introduction: making history go. In *Exceptional spaces: essays in performance and history.* Edited by D. Pollock. Chapel Hill: University of North Carolina Press. 1–48.

Porter, W.J. 1999. ¡Si Se Piede! teaching for transformation. In *Making justice our project.* Edited by C. Edelsky. Urbana, Illinois: National Council of Teachers of English. 77–95.

Postone, M., LiPuma, E. & Calhoun, C. 1993. Introduction: Bourdieu and social theory. In *Bourdieu: critical perspectives.* Edited by C. Calhoun, E. LiPuma & M. Postone. Chicago: Polity Press. 1–13.

Provincial Administration of the Western Cape. 2004a. *Antenatal workload by district: booking April 2002–March 2003.* Cape Town: Metropole Region Department of Health. (Unpublished).

Provincial Administration of the Western Cape. 2004b. *Metro prevention of mother to child treatment (HIV) report, quarter.* Metropole Region Department of Health. (Unpublished).

Provincial Administration of the Western Cape. 2004c. *HIV-counselling and testing: Nyanga monthly district report, January–March, 2004.* Nyanga Region Department of Health. (Unpublished).

Provincial Administration of the Western Cape. 2004d. *Monthly District Reports, October 2002 to March 2004.* Metropole Region Department of Health. (Unpublished).

Provincial Administration of the Western Cape. 2004e. *Monthly district report: Grassy Park Civic, April 2002–April 2004.* Grassy Park Civic Department of Health. (Unpublished).

Rivers, K. & Aggleton, P. 1999. *Adolescent sexuality, gender and the HIV epidemic. HIV and development programme.* UNDP. [Online] Available: http://www.undp.org/hiv/publications/gender/adolesce.htm. [2003, January 17].

Rubin, G. 1975. 'The traffic of women: notes on the "political economy" of sex'. In *Toward an anthology of women.* Edited by R. R. Reiter. New York: Monthly Review Press. 157–210.

Rubin, H.J. & Rubin, R.S. 1995. *Qualitative interviewing: the art of hearing data.* Thousand Oaks, CA: Sage Publications.

Rummel, M.K. & Quintero, E.P. 1997. *Teachers' reading/teachers' lives.* Albany: State University of New York.

Rutherford, J. Ed. 1990. *Identity: community, culture, difference.* London: Lawrence & Wishart.

Sach, J. 2003. *The activist teaching profession.* Milton Keynes: Open University Press.

Scarth, F. 2004. *The other within: ethics, politics, and the body of Simone de Beavoir.* Lanham: Rowman & Littlefield Publishers.

Schatzki, T.R. & Natter, W. Eds. 1996. *The social and political body.* New York: The Guilford Press.

Schechner, R. 1985. *Between theatre and anthropology.* Philadelphia: University of Pennsylvania Press.

Scorgie, F. 2002. Virginity testing and the politics of sexual responsibility: implications for AIDS intervention. *African studies* 61(1): 55–75.

Scott, J.C. 1990. *Domination and the arts of resistance: hidden transcripts.* New Haven, CT: Yale University Press.

Shisana, O. & Sibiya, L. 2002. *South African national HIV prevalence, behavioural risks and mass media household survey 2002.* Cape Town: Human Science Research Council.

Shulman, L.S. 1986. 'Those who understand: the knowledge growth of teachers'. *Educational researcher* 15 (2): 4–16.

Sikes, P., Measor, L. & Woods, P. 1987. *Teacher careers: crisis and continuities.* Lewes: Falmer Press.

Silva, E.B. 2005. Gender, home and family in cultural capital. *The British journal of sociology* 56 (1): 83–103.

Simbayi, L.C., Skinner, D., Letlape, L. & Zuma, K. 2005. *Workplace policies in public Education: a review focusing on HIV/AIDS.* Cape Town: Human Science Research Council.

Simon, B. 1988. 'Why no pedagogy in England?' In *Frameworks for teaching.* Edited by R. Dale, R. Fergusson & A. Robinson. London: Hodder and Stoughton. 336–350.

Singhal, A. & Rogers, E.M. 2003. *Combating AIDS: communication strategies in action.* New Delhi: Sage Publications.

Sliedrecht, S. 1996. *Life skills for adolescence: evaluative research on the quest programme.* Master's Dissertation. Cape Town: University of Cape Town. (Unpublished).

Small, N. 1988. 'AIDS and social policy'. *Critical social policy* 21: 9–29.

Sontag, S. 1990a. *AIDS and its metaphors.* London: Penguin.

Sontag, S. 1990b. *Illness a metaphor and AIDS and its metaphors.* New York: Anchor Books.

Stadler, J. 2001. *Looking at loveLife the first year: summaries of monitoring and evaluation.* loveLife. [Online]. Available: http://www.kff.org/docs/sections/safrica/firstyear_report.pdf. 50 pages [2003, January 13].

Stenhouse, L. 1975. *An introduction to curriculum research and development.* London: Heinemann.

Stenhouse, L. 1985. *Research as a basis for teaching.* London: Heinemann.

Stephens, D. 2002. *Asking the way: researching culture, education and development. Mimeo.* (Unpublished).

Stockdill, B.C. 2003. *Activism against AIDS: at the intersections of sexuality, race, gender and class.* Boulder: Lynne Rienner Publishers.

Swartz, D.L. & Zolberg, V.L. Eds. 2004. *After Bourdieu: influence, critique, elaboration.* Dordrecht: Kluwer Academic Publishers.
Thomas, D. Ed. 1995. *Teachers' stories.* Philadelphia: Open University Press.
Thompson, L.M. 2006. *A history of South Africa.* Johannesburg: Jonathan Ball.
Tom, A. 1984. *Teaching as a moral craft.* New York: Longman.
Tripp, D. 1993. *Critical incidents in teaching: developing professional judgement.* London: Routledge.
Ulack, R. & Skinner, W.F. Eds. 1991. *AIDS and the social sciences: common threads.* Lexington: The University Press of Kentucky.
UNAIDS 2006. *Report on the global AIDS epidemic. Executive summary.* A UNAIDS 10th Anniversary special edition. [Online]. Available: http://data.unaids.org/pub/Global Report/2006/2006_GR-ExecutiveSummary_en.pdf [2006, August 14].
Webb, J., Schirato, T. & Danaher, G. 2002. *Understanding Bourdieu.* London: Sage Publications.
Weedon, C. 1987. *Feminist practice & poststructuralist theory.* New York: Basil Blackwell.
Weeks, J. 1986. *Sexualities.* London: Routledge.
Weeks, J. 1989. AIDS: the intellectual agenda. In *AIDS: social representations social practices.* Edited by P. Aggleton, G. Hart & P. Davies. New York: The Falmer Press. 1–20.
Weeks, J. 2002. Sexuality and history revisited. In *Sexualities in history: a reader.* Edited by K.M. Phillips & B. Reay. New York: Routledge. 27–41.
Weeks, J. & Holland, J. Eds. 1996. *Sexual cultures: communities, values and intimacy.* New York: St. Martin's Press.
Weeks, J. 1998. The „homosexual role" after 30 years: an appreciation of the work of Mary McIntosh. *Sexualities* 1: 131–152.
West, C. & Zimmerman, D. 1987. Doing gender. *Gender and society* 1: 125–151.
Willan, S. 2000. Will HIV/AIDS undermine democracy in South Africa. *AIDS analysis Africa* 11(1): 14.
Wolpe, H. 1988. Class concepts, class struggle and racism. In *Theories of race and ethnic relation.* Edited by J. Rex & D. Mason. Cambridge: Cambridge University Press. 110–130
Wood, K. & Jewkes, R. 1998. *'Love is a dangerous thing': micro-dynamics of violence in sexual relationships of young people in Umtata.* Medical Research Council. [Online]. Available: http://www.mrc.ac.za/researchreports/finallove.pdf [2003, January 17].
Wood, K., Maepa, J. & Jewkes, R. 1997. *Adolescent sex and contraceptive experiences: perspectives of teenagers and clinic nurses in the Northern Province.* Medical Research Council. [Online]. Available: http://www.mrc.ac.za/researchreports/contra.pdf [2003, January 17].
Woods, P. 1996. *Researching the art of teaching: ethnography for educational use.* London: Routledge.
World Bank 2000. *Exploring the implications of the HIV/AIDS epidemic for educational planning in selected African countries: the demographic question.* ACTafrica, AIDS Campaign Team for Africa, World Bank, March 2000.
Wyner, N. Ed. 1991. *Current perspectives on the culture of schools.* Brookline, MA: Brookline Books.
Zeni, J. 2001. *Ethical issues in practitioner research.* New York: Teachers College Press.

Index

Please note: Page numbers in *italics* refer to Tables and Figures.

abstinence 252–3
adult literacy rate 155
advocacy groups and civil society 130
Afrikaans-speaking environment 278–80
age 123
  appropriateness 30
  differentiated infection rates 161
agency 286
  centrality of 112
  exercise of 306
  see also under structure
agents, knowledgeability of 70–1
Althusser 50, 77, 79, 241
  see also language
analysis, units of 39, 51
anecdotal evidence 39
Apartheid history 154
  separate development 157–8
assessment process 289, 295
attachment 81
attire of teacher 234
attitudes 48
authority 265
autonomy, pursuit of 126
behaviour 261
  in and outside classroom 234
  patterns of 86, 261–2, 304
  repetitive forms of 75
  sets of 285
beliefs 48
biographical research 105
biographies 29
biological constructions 124
black teachers 114–15, 250
  female 259
  male 296–7
body
  biologically sexed 67
  constructions of 67
Bourdieu 18, 48, 49, 55–65
  see also practice, theory of 18
Butler 19, 48, 50, 77, 79–88, 111, 241
  see also performativity, theory of
capital 48, 57–8, 59, 153
  struggle for power 60–1
case study approach 29
chalkboard, use of 266
choices 79, 95–6
class 30–1, 123, 308
  divides 115
  inequalities 97–8
  relations 120
classroom 303
  discourse 110
closed or rhetorical questions 264–5
code
  of conduct 234
  dress and speech 234
  of ethics 40
cognitive ability 101
coloured community 247
coloured teachers 259, 280–5
commercial sex workers 133
communities
  categories 162
  economic disparities 163–4
  housing 164
  race 166
  unemployment and neglect 164–5
community
  expectations 242
  and membership 220–3

community
  teachers and HIV/AIDS 250–1
competition 56, 57
conceptual network 39
condoms 252–3, 258
conflictual messages 298
conformists 253
conformity 262
conscious 73–4
consequences, unintended 305
constructions of 'the teacher' 236
content or task sequence 295
control
  of content 234
  relations 73
  and strictness 238–9
co-presence 233
  and framing 48, 50, 72–3
corporeal body 124
corporeality 87
crisis of representation moment 97
cultural capital 59–60
cultural constraints 249
cultural fields 48, 55–6
cultural influence 47
cultural practices 17–18
  beliefs and traditions 252
culture 247, 248
  interpretations 253–4
curriculum and teacher's work 47
data 39–40
  collection process 35
  presentation 38
demographic identities 167–70
demographic profiles 161
  learner population 168
dependency 81
deportment 235–6, 234
differentiation categories 114–15
discipline 234, 264
disciplinarian, teacher as 238–42
disclosure
  fear of 250
  of HIV status 42
  reasons for actions 52
discourse 80
  analysis 38, 38
  health and medico-legal 130
  unequal relations of power 75
discriminatory practices 135
discursive conflict 80
discursive fields 80–1
discursive space 298, 303
disease and illness
  knowledge and perceptions 137
  meanings and interpretations 126
  medico-legal conceptions 134–5
documentary analysis 35
dominant discourses 21
  limitations 131–2
dominant structures 65
domination 19, 61–2, 77
economic capital 59, 162–7
economic divides 115
economic landscape 154–8
education 59, 98
  as class status 209–10
  and schooling 192
  research 139–45
  taken-for-granted activity 205–6
  way of becoming 206–9
Eisner 101
empirical data 22
enabling environment 107
enactment, pattern of 87
epistemological frameworks 22
epistemological orientations 21, 131–2
  teaching and teachers' lives 94–9
ethical considerations 40
ethnicity 30–1, 308
ethnographic research methodologies 96–7
experience 29
explanation, modes of 51
family 120, 192
female teachers 114–15, 197, 250, 251
  commitment 240
  deportment 235
  early learning experiences 237–8
  gendered discursive space 242–3

feminist orientations 21
feminist theory 19, 50, 77, 107–9
field(s) 48, 153
  in society 56–7
  notes 36, 37
flow of intention 305
force relations 80
formal school settings 14
frames of reference 18
framing 73
Foucault 19, 50, 77, 80, 123–4
  see also power and discourse
functionalists 53
fundamentalists 253
game, rules of 67–8
gender 30–1, 82–3, 120, 122–3, 137, 308
  and membership 219–20
  and sexuality 124
  pedagogical norms 262
geographic identities 167–70
geographic location 154–8, 162–7
Giddens 18, 48, 49–50, 51–2, 54, 69–78, 126–7, 233
  see also co-presence and framing; structuration, theory of 18–19
Goffman 18, 48, 49–50, 72
  see also presentation of self 18
Goodson 29
  see life history
government policies and plans 135–6, 138–9
group-work 262–3, 266
habitus, notion of 19, 48, 49, 63–4, 66, 153
  of the agent 61
health and economics 138
healthcare, access to 135
hermeneutic space of HIV/AIDS 29
hermeneutic theorists 53–4
heterosexuality 122
heterosexual relationships 135
historicity of 'teacher' 236, 241, 260
historical discourses on disease 118
HIV
  prevention 139–40
  transmission 14
HIV/AIDS 242–3
  constructions of 22, 48
  content and form discourses 15
  implications of discourse 125–8
  modes of contraction and transmission 14
  prevalence in Sub-Saharan Africa 13
  prevention 14
  research 21
  and sexuality 21
  understanding, experience and teaching 20, 242
homosexuality 122
human conduct, active reflexive character 54
identification 19, 77
  sexual 124–5
identity 81, 93, 236, 308
  and classroom behaviour 150–1
  construction 48, 191
  history of 120–1
  nature of 47
  and practice 77
  in relation to power 49
  social and cultural influences 194–5
  stable 269, 290
  true or fixed 269
identity positions
  non-singularity in constructions 82
  in social practice 20
ideology 79
„I", formation of the 84
'*illusio*' 63
individual 29
  choices 135
  and collective identities 136
  lives and experiences 51
  and state relationships 120
indulgence and consumerism 128
information
  collection 35
  managing of 38–40
  privileging of 289
  source of 293–4
informed choices 14

informed consent 40
intention 305
intentionality (medium) 75
interaction, focussed 73
interdependency of social systems 70
interpellation 79–80
interpretations 95
interpretivist orientations 102–10
interviews 17, 35, 37
  ethical issues 40
  semi-structured 35
  transcribed 38
intravenous drug users 133
knowledge 59, 103
  of content 234
  lack of 142
  tacit 293–4, 307
knowledgeability 251
Lacan 19, 50, 77, 79
  see also language
language 41–2, 79, 192
  body parts 242
  meanings attached to 62
  in subject formation 19, 50, 77
  Western Province *169*
lecture modes of mediation 264–5
Life Orientation 14, 197
Lifeskills 30
  classrooms 22, 116, 142, 308
  curriculum 298
  observation of lessons 36
  teachers 17–18, 254
life
  history 29–30, 105
  stories 29–30
  of teachers 30, 93, 301–2
literature 16, 21
  dominant discourses 20
  on HIV/AIDS 119, 144–5
Lyotard 111
males and females 122
male infidelity 256
male teachers 114–15, 238, 307
marginalisation 135
marginalised members of community 133
marital status 253–7
marriage 120
  conceptions and experiences 192, 242
  or relationships 253–4
  teachers and HIV/AIDS 253–7
masculinity and sexuality 307
material and social conditions 149
mediation process 16, 50, 271, 293–4
mediators, roles as 42
medical science 127
membership and teachers 218–19
memory
  traces 49, 194
  understanding of 74
men, roles of 120
mentors and guardians 245
mentorship, lack of 246
mission and vision 37
modernist constructions of HIV/AIDS 118
modernist framework 52–3, 103
modernity 126–7
modern moment 97
modification 76
monogamy 265–6
moral discourses 250
moral judgements 125–6
moral obligation 263
Muslim teacher 255–6
narratives 105, 308
  collective 191
  individual teachers 38
National HIV and Syphilis Antenatal Sero-prevalence Survey 159
naturalist constructions of body 124
networks 58–9
Nietzsche 62
non-linear forms of abstraction 101
normative script 76
norms 85
  and practices 241
nurturer, teacher as 238–42
object 39
oration 234
orientations towards disease 125–8

outcome of lesson 298
parent expectations 251–3
participant observation 35, 36
participation by teachers 32–3
    voluntary 32
patriarchal discourses 122
pedagogical norms, adherence to 262
perception 74
    and subject position *241*
    teachers and teaching 234
performance
    repetitive action 84–5
    of teachers 18
    theory 110–11
performative teachers 270
    binders 265, 266, 293–8, 307
    exaggerators 262, 263, 266, 270–7, 305
    framers 264, 266, 287–93, 306–7
    normalisers 263–4, 266, 278–86, 306
performativity
    biologised, (dis)membered bodies 303–4
    normalised discourses 305–7
    notion of 111–12
    patterns of *267*
    theory of 19, 50, 77, 79–88
personal dimensions of teaching 95
personal history and teaching practices 107
personal meaning making 102
policies 37
political discourses and HIV/AIDS 118
politics 199
    role of 192
    in South Africa 128–30
    and teachers 199–201
politicians and civil society 129–30
polygamy 255–6, 265
positionality, researcher 41–3
positioning 18, 50, 77
    and classroom practice 19
    meanings of 72
    modes of 74
positivist constructions 100–1
positivist orientations 99–102
postmodernist
    framework 52–3, 103
perspective 35
poverty 192
    and teachers 201–4
power 50, 66–7, 75, 80, 241
    conceptions of 19
    and discourse 19, 50, 77
    relations 48, 56
    reproductions of 49
power/knowledge relationships 80
practical consciousness 70–1
practice, theory of 18, 48, 55, 64–5
    limitations in 66–8
practices of silence 250
pregnancy 244–6
presentation of self 18
prevention programmes 14
private spaces 41
productive constraint, effect of 48
projection studies 137
protection from harm 40
punishment, silence and shame 250–1
purposive sampling technique 31–2
psychoanalysis 19, 50, 77
qualitative data 38
qualitative mode of inquiry 29
qualitative research 96–7
race 30–1, 308
    geographic location 166
    relations 120
reason, epistemological basis of 52
reconstructions 94–5
reflexivity 71
reiterative enactments 84–5
relationships 58–9
religion 192, 308
    born again Christian 256
    conformists/traditionalists 225–8
    fundamentalists 224–5
    nominalists 231–3
    subject positions *231*
    teachers and membership 223
    (un)conventionalists 228–30
religious beliefs 253

religious discourses 250
religious ideologies 120
reproductions of power and agency 107–8
researcher
  and performative 308–10
  role of 42
resignification 19, 77
resistance 19, 77
resource(s)
  access to 59
  material 36
respondents' profile 195–8
restored behaviour 85–7
Revised National Curriculum 14, 142–3
right to privacy 40
risk 127
role modelling 217–18
role models 192, 234, 235
  and 'good' teacher 237–42
routine 74–5
routinisation in practices 71
rural environment 158, 244
safe sex
  messages 17, 252
  responses to 259
  teachers and HIV/AIDS 258–9
schools 142
  selection of 31–2
science
  and education 101
  and medicine 122
  and religion 122
self 47
  concept of 73, 74
  and identity 96
  panoptic of 233
  productions of 49
self-discipline 128
self-improvement 128
self-interest 61–2
  and freedom 128
self-management 128
self-monitoring 222, 234
separatist policies in South Africa 114
sex 82–3
  community and silence 244, 250–1
  concepts of 120
  construction of gender 67
  drive 121–2
  education programmes 142
  lack of awareness and knowledge 246
  sources of information 244–5
sexology, terms of 122
sexual behaviour
  constraints 122
  decision making and choices 137
  prohibitions 120
sexual development 244–5
sexual deviance 122
sexual differences 122–3
sexual freedom 122
sexuality 14, 48
  definition 121
  discourses 15, 22, 118–25, 249
  historical perspective 120–1
  and HIV/AIDS 91–2, 115–16, 242–3
  implications of teaching 309–10
  multiplicity of 123
  orientations towards 119–25
  silence and shame 242–9
  understanding, experience and teaching 20
sexually transmitted infections 14
sexual terminology 246–7, 249
simple random sampling 32
sites 30–1
  schools 31–2
  teachers 32–3
social action 47, 52, 119
  and activity 51
  constituted nature of 18
  constructions of 48
social activity, complexity of 54
social and material conditions 149
  provinces, communities and schools 153–8
social capital 59, 162–7
social class 97

social classifications 30–1
social cluster of schools *162*
social evolution 51
social identities of teachers 150, *151*
social influence 47
social interaction 71–2, 74–5
social interactionism 104
socialisation 59
social landscape 154–8
social life 49, 119
social order 52
  sexually ordered 67
social position 72
social positioning 75
social practices 17–18
social relations 16–17, 72
social science 51
social status 123
social systems 70, 71–2
social theory 18, 51
  epistemological orientations 48
social world 29
society formation 48
sociology and ideology 51
socio-political context 17–18
specificity of context 22
statement 38
  embedded 39
  features 39
status and teachers 213–14
Stephens 29
  see life history research 29
stigmatisation 135, 137
structuralists 53
structural properties 194
structural resources 75
structuration, theory of 18, 48, 49, 69–75, 194
  limitations of 75–8
structure 69
  duality of 69, 233
  as embodied 76–7
structure and agency 21, 48, 49, 51, 55, 69
  dialectic relationship 50
structuring properties 69
subaltern positions 79
subject 39
  disassociation from 70
  formation 47, 48–9, 55–65, 83–4
  positioning 79, 93, 106, 110, 145–6
subjection 19, 77
subjective experiences 18, 37, 191–4, *193*
  levels of influence *267*
subjectivity 47, 48, 69–75, 81
subject positioning 47, 79, 193, 241
  and classroom discourse 21
subordination 80
surveilance and teachers
  living in glass houses 215–16
  role modelling 217–218
symbolic capital 60
symbolic interaction 104–5
symbolic power 61–3
symbolic violence 62–3
teacher 17, 18
  engagement 106
  gender and choice 212
  identity and classroom practice 91
  identity in South Africa 113–14
  as individuals 143
  perspectives in South Africa 114–16
  and politics 199–201
  and poverty 201–4
  power to act 109–10
  purpose and role of education 205–10
  responsive rather than active 100
  and teaching 211
'teacherliness', patterns of 261, 304
teaching
  as art 102–11
  as performance 106
  as performative 110–14
  perspectives in South Africa 114–16
  as science 99–102
technological advancement 127
teenage mothers 247–8
theoretical framework of study 20
tradition 251
traditional culture 259

traditionalist positivist positions 101
traditional moment 97
training, impact of 140
transformation 107–8
transmission of HIV/AIDS
misconceptions about 257–8
prevention 265–6
trust 127
unconscious 73–4
understanding 29
unintended consequences 75, 305
universal or general good 62
urban environments 169
values 48, 251
white teachers 114–15, 259, 287–8
women
roles of 120
subordinate role to men 259
vulnerable to infection 160–1
youth
knowledge 140–1
sexually active 14